The Fight for Life
The Medical Services in the Gallipoli Campaign, 1915-16

John Dixon & Ritchie Wood

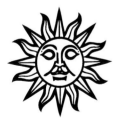

Helion & Company

Helion & Company Limited
Unit 8 Amherst Business Centre
Budbrooke Road
Warwick
CV34 5WE
England
Tel. 01926 499 619
Email: info@helion.co.uk
Website: www.helion.co.uk
Twitter: @helionbooks
Visit our blog at blog.helion.co.uk

Published by Helion & Company 2024
Designed and typeset by Mach 3 Solutions (www.mach3solutions.co.uk)
Cover designed by Paul Hewitt, Battlefield Design (www.battlefield-design.co.uk)

Text © John Dixon and Ritchie Wood 2024
Images © as individually credited
Maps, diagrams and sketches drawn by Terrence Powell

Cover: HS *Assaye* and unidentified field ambulance at Anzac Cove. (SRG 435/1/282 and
PRG 280/1/12/231 respectively)

Every reasonable effort has been made to trace copyright holders and to obtain their permission for the
use of copyright material. The author and publisher apologize for any errors or omissions in this work
and would be grateful if notified of any corrections that should be incorporated in future reprints or
editions of this book.

ISBN 978-1-804513-25-5

British Library Cataloguing-in-Publication Data.
A catalogue record for this book is available from the British Library.

All rights reserved. No part of this publication may be reproduced, stored in a retrieval system,
or transmitted, in any form, or by any means, electronic, mechanical, photocopying, recording or
otherwise, without the express written consent of Helion & Company Limited.

For details of other military history titles published by Helion & Company Limited contact the above
address or visit our website: http://www.helion.co.uk.

We always welcome receipt of book proposals from prospective authors.

Dedicated to the men and women
of the medical services past and present
in honour of the work they do for all service personnel

Contents

List of Photographs	vi
List of Sketches & Diagrams	viii
List of Maps	ix
List of Abbreviations	x
Acknowledgements	xiii
Preface	xiv
Introduction: Nothing Can Be More Visionary	xvi
1 Military Medical Services: Royal Army Medical Corps (RAMC)	27
2 Based on the Assumption: Medical Services and Planning for the Campaign	50
3 Helles: A Solid Mass of Dead and Wounded	71
4 Anzac: Landing Up Over Our Knees in Water	90
5 The Landings: Effectiveness and Criticisms	108
6 Myriads of Flies: Helles May–July	115
7 Man with the Donkey: Anzac May–July	142
8 We Had Nothing for Them: Hospitals on Lemnos	166
9 A Night of Bloodshed and Pain	178
10 An Inferno of Shrapnel: The Suvla Landings	200
11 Only the Dead Remained in the Trenches	210
12 The Physical Condition of the Troops is Very Serious	217
13 The Australians and New Zealanders Are Suffering	224
14 Men Who Had Suffered So Much	244
15 The MO Died in His Sleep: The Storm	259
16 Some Were Dying, Some Found Dead	270
17 Evacuation: Tents Left Standing and Flags Flying	281
18 Not Equal to the Task	303
Conclusions	309
Appendices	
I A Note on the Turkish Medical Services during the Çanakkale Wars	312
II List of Hospital Ships Serving during the Gallipoli Campaign	320
Bibliography	323
Index	335

List of Photographs

Former naval hospital at Bighi on the southern side of Valletta Grand Harbour, Malta.   56
C ward on the HS *Sicilia*.   79
Matron K. F. Fawcett, QAIMNS.   80
HS *Gascon*.   97
Grave of Private John Simpson, 3rd AFA, at Beach Cemetery.   146
ANZAC Commemorative Medallion, issued by the Australian Government in 1967.   147
Bronze statue commemorating the ANZACs near the Melbourne War Memorial.   148
Officers' ward of the HS *Grantully Castle*.   154
Some of the first casualties to reach Mena House (No. 2 AGH) in Egypt, taken
    during May 1915.   164
Australian nurses at No. 2 AGH at Gezireh Palace Hotel, Cairo, in mid-1915.   164
Patient's record card from No. 2 AGH.   165
Matron Jean Miles Walker, AANS, in 1918.   165
ADS of the 4th AFA at Anzac.   184
Suvla Bay as seen from Plugge's Plateau to illustrate the main areas of the landing
    in August.   203
Members of the 1/1st WFA, taken during the last annual camp before the Great War
    started.   206
Private William 'Bill' Watkins, 1602, 1/1st WFA.   209
Private Samuel Powell, 1/1st WFA.   209
Private Walter Harris, 1700, 1/1st WFA.   209
Embarking stretcher cases by winch onto the HS *Sicilia*.   213
Nurses and MOs on the HS *Gascon*.   225
1st ALHFA, near Walker's Ridge.   229
Grave of Private D. J. White at Pieta Military Cemetery, Malta.   230
Unidentified field ambulance at Anzac Cove.   236
Grave of Lyle Everard Hodges, a 22-year-old blacksmith from Fairfield, New South
    Wales.   237
HS *Assaye*.   252
Nursing staff and MO on board the HS *Assaye*, probably taken in early autumn 1915.   252
Grave of Private Daniel John of C Company 2nd SWB, wounded in action at Gallipoli
    and died of wounds at Gibraltar, aged 28.   258
Snow at the 4th AFA (B Section) in Hotchkiss Gully, Anzac, following the blizzard.   266
A routine death.   299

Turkish field medical unit during the Çanakkale Wars (Gallipoli Campaign).	313
Embarking wounded on a hospital ship for transfer to Istanbul.	315
An operating theatre in one of the larger, more permanent hospitals during the Çanakkale Wars (Gallipoli Campaign).	315
A temporary hospital nearer the front.	317
Field disinfector or steriliser.	319

List of Sketches & Diagrams

Sketches

Layout of the 11th CCS at Helles in May 1915.	119
Layout of No. 1 CSH at West Mudros.	175
Sanitary arrangements at Suvla in September 1915.	246
Layout of the 35th Field Ambulance at Suvla.	255
Final layout of the 108th IFA as it was left after evacuation.	290

Diagrams

General schematic for the chain of command in the medical services at Gallipoli.	43
Schematic for the evacuation of wounded.	46

List of Maps

The Gallipoli Peninsula and the nearby Aegean Islands that became important during the campaign.   59

The landings on the Gallipoli Peninsula.   73

The medical services at Cape Helles – final situation   85

Anzac Cove   91

Suvla Bay   201

Lines of evacuation at Helles   298

List of Abbreviations

AAH – Australian Auxiliary Hospital
AAMC – Australian Army Medical Corps
AANS – Australian Army Nursing Service
ABC – Army Bearer Corps
AC – Ambulance Carrier
ACCS – Australian Casualty Clearing Station
ADMS – assistant director of medical services
ADS – advanced dressing station
AFA – Australian Field Ambulance
AGH – Australian General Hospital
AIF – Australian Imperial Force
ALHFA – Australian Light Horse Field Ambulance
AMS – Australian Medical Service
ANS – Army Nursing Sisters
ANZAC – Australian and New Zealand Army Corps
AOC – Army Ordnance Corps
AOD – Army Ordnance Department
ASC – Army Service Corps
ASH – Australian Stationary Hospital
AWM – Australian War Memorial
BCCS – British Casualty Clearing Station
BGH – British General Hospital
BHQ – brigade headquarters
BPGH – Bombay Presidency General Hospital
BSH – British Stationary Hospital
CAMC – Canadian Army Medical Corps
CCS – casualty clearing station
CGH – Canadian General Hospital
CGS – Chief of the General Staff
CO – commanding officer
CRE – Commander Royal Engineers
CSH – Canadian Stationary Hospital
CWGC – Commonwealth War Graves Commission
DADMS – deputy assistant director of medical services

DAG – deputy adjutant general
DAQMG – deputy assistant quartermaster general
DCM – Distinguished Conduct Medal
DDMS – deputy director of medical services
DGAMS – Director General of Australian Medical Services
DGMS – director general of medical services
DMS – director of medical services
DSO – Distinguished Service Order
EAFA – East Anglian Field Ambulance
ELFA – East Lancashire Field Ambulance
EMBFA – Eastern Mounted Brigade Field Ambulance
EPIP – Eight Person Indian Pattern
FFNC – French Flag Nursing Corps
GHQ – general headquarters
GOC – general officer commanding
GSO1 – General Staff Officer (1st Grade)
HE – high explosive
HMAT – His Majesty's Australian Transport
HMBFA – Highland Mounted Brigade Field Ambulance
HMS – His Majesty's Ship
HQ – headquarters
HS – Hospital Ship
IFA – Indian Field Ambulance
IGC – Inspector General Communications
IMS – Indian Medical Service
ISMD – Indian Subordinate Medical Department
KOSB – King's Own Scottish Borderers
MC – Military Cross
MEF – Mediterranean Expeditionary Force
MiD – mentioned in despatches
MO – medical officer
NAA – National Archives of Australia
NCO – non-commissioned officer
NZANS – New Zealand Army Nursing Service
NZEF – New Zealand Expeditionary Force
NZFA – New Zealand Field Ambulance
NZMBFA – New Zealand Mounted Brigade Field Ambulance
NZMC – New Zealand Medical Corps
NZMCNR – New Zealand Medical Corps Nursing Reserve
NZMFA – New Zealand Mounted Field Ambulance
NZMRB – New Zealand Mounted Rifles Brigade
NZSH – New Zealand Stationary Hospital
OC – officer commanding
PCANS – Princess Christian's Army Nursing Service
PCANSR – Princess Christian's Army Nursing Service Reserve

PDMS – principal director of medical services
PMO – principal medical officer
POW – prisoner of war
QAIMNS – Queen Alexandra's Imperial Military Nursing Service
QAIMNSR – Queen Alexandra's Imperial Military Nursing Service Reserve
QARNNS – Queen Alexandra's Royal Navy Nursing Service
QARNNSR – Queen Alexandra's Royal Navy Nursing Service Reserve
QMG – quartermaster general
RAMC – Royal Army Medical Corps
RAP – regimental aid post
RMO – regimental medical officer
RMS – Royal Mail Ship
RND – Royal Naval Division
RRC – Royal Red Cross
SAS – sub-assistant surgeon
SEMBFA – South Eastern Mounted Brigade Field Ambulance
SLSA – State Library of South Australia
SMO – senior medical officer
SMS – *Seine Majistäts Schiffe* (His Majesty's Ship)
SS – Steam Ship
SWB – South Wales Borderers
SWMBFA – South Western Mounted Brigade Field Ambulance
TAHO – Tasmanian Archive and Heritage Office
TF – Territorial Force
TFNS – Territorial Force Nursing Service
TFNSR – Territorial Force Nursing Service Reserve
TNA – The National Archives
VC – Victoria Cross
WFA – Welsh Field Ambulance

Acknowledgements

The work for this volume commenced following a series of discussions over cups of coffee (and muffins) as we thrashed out some ideas with which we could both be happy working and were satisfied to put forwards as a proposal to Helion & Company. Thereafter, there has been a lot of hours spent researching and reading everything we could find to do with medical services and the Gallipoli Campaign. So the first people to whom we have to offer heartfelt thanks are our wives, Francesca and Marilyn, who have suffered hours of abandonment as we have buried ourselves in the research.

We have not written the book in isolation, in spite of the Covid-19 crisis, and there have been many people who have offered encouragement and help throughout the course of the research. Dr Anita Jordan read the early drafts of the text and made helpful suggestions, and, to her, we are grateful. Some sources have been tricky to track down, and we have been helped in the search by friends like Pat Evans in the United Kingdom and Robert Johnston in Australia, and we thank them for helping to make the work easier for us.

Thanks to Dr Anusha Sivasuriam, who helped us understand the means of the spread of infectious diseases that occurred during the Gallipoli Campaign and how these diseases affected those men infected. The expertise of Terry Powell has been indispensable for the preparation of the maps and sketches we required to illustrate the text, and we thank him for his suggestions on ways to improve the overall presentation.

Thanks to Kristi Snodgrass for her work editing the manuscript.

Writing a book such as this during the Covid-19 crisis has presented challenges that neither of us had faced before, especially in the context of making spur-of-the-moment decisions to visit a place of interest or an archival source. It was possible to visit the Museum of Military Medicine at Aldershot. The staff there assisted with the booking process and walked us through the archive they hold on the campaign, and we are grateful to them for allowing us to spend as long as we needed at the museum to complete the research in one visit.

Special thanks must go to Ahmet Senol Ozbek, our friend in Turkey who has not only supported and taken interest in the research we carried out but has also completed some of his own research on the medical services of the Turkish Army that we include it in this work as an appendix. We are grateful to him and are only sorry that we have been unable to travel to Turkey during the research as a result of the pandemic. We hope that we can remedy this.

Thanks also to the manager of the Military Book Shop at the Garrison Church Crypt in Valletta, who provided information on an interesting web page relating to Malta that included an excellent account of the part played by Malta during the campaign. Whilst there have been many people involved, we are responsible for the content of this work throughout.

Preface

There have been many books written about the Gallipoli Campaign over the years since its failed attempt to defeat the Ottoman Empire. There has been much discussion, much finger pointing and much blame apportioned ever since the publication of the Dardanelles Commission's *Final Report* in 1919. The medical services have not escaped entirely from this process of blame and recrimination, and there are a number of books that deal with certain aspects of the medical services in some detail, such as that those of Michael Tyquin. However, as pointed out by Professor Maury Klein, '... history is at bottom the story of people, and that the stuff of people's lives is no less important than their public record'.[1] It is for this reason that we have sought to tell the story of the medical services at Gallipoli not only through the official documents such as war diaries and official histories but also through the personal accounts of those who served. Sometimes, the boundaries are blurred, as some accounts in the war diaries of medical officers (MOs) are clearly of a personal nature and not only relate to the official requirement to keep a record of events but also record their frustration, hopes and fears as the campaign progressed and ultimately failed. Of course, the people who took part were not only MOs. Some accounts of the medical services come from those who were tended by them, and these, too, form part of the overall picture of the services provided by doctors, nurses and orderlies of the various medical units.

The experience of the medical services at Gallipoli differed from that of the Western Front, in that, for instance, the medical services largely and heavily relied upon sea-based transport to supply it, maintain its effectiveness and remove the wounded and sick from the beaches. This, in itself, produced significant issues that were not addressed fully at any time during the campaign and that are reflected in both official and personal accounts. The level at which the account was written will often reflect the level of understanding of the events as seen from the viewpoint of the writer. A wounded soldier clearly had a different view of the medical services than did a senior officer of the same service. We have written this book in attempt to bring together some of these views from the wounded soldier to the nurse and orderly who cared for him to the senior medical officer (SMO) who may have operated upon him and recorded some of his treatment. We have attempted to address the neglect that the medical services have suffered as an integral part of the whole campaign and, indeed, the Gallipoli story. In so doing, we hope that we have highlighted the work of a dedicated group of men and women who cared for the fighting troops.

---

1   Maury Klein, *Days of Defiance: Sumter, Secession, and the Coming of the Civil War* (New York: Vintage Books, 1999), p.xi.

It should be noted that all the quotations used in the text are, with the exception of the addition of minor punctuation to allow easier reading, reproduced as in the original, including the spelling and word usage that may be less familiar with modern readers.

To avoid confusion with the names of medical units, we have adopted a certain nomenclature. All field medical units, such as field ambulances or casualty clearing stations (CCSs), have been written using ordinals – thus, the 1st Australian Field Ambulance (1st AFA), the 11th British Casualty Clearing Station (11th BCCS) and so on. All lines of communication units, such as stationary and general hospitals, have been written as 'No. 1 Australian Stationary Hospital' (No. 1 ASH), 'No. 27 British General Hospital' (No. 27 BGH) and so on. It is hoped that this helps to keep the units separate in the minds of the readers. We have also specified the nationality of the units, as seen above, although they were not necessarily addressed this way at the time of the campaign.

Introduction: Nothing Can Be More Visionary

The work of the medical services in any theatre of the First World War is generally underrepresented in studies of the conflict. This is particularly true of the Gallipoli Campaign, where even the *Official History of the Medical Services* dismisses the work in 60 pages of a five-volume history. This is not because of the shortage of data, for the records of the campaign appear to be as good as they can be under the circumstances of the war. Perhaps the dismissal of the campaign by the British official historian has more to do with the fact that the campaign ended in defeat and that the medical services came in for some considerable criticism in the Dardanelles Commission report of 1919. These factors seem to have affected the Australian historian much less, for their official account, covering almost 500 pages, is longer by some margin and deals thoroughly with the Australian medical services input to the campaign. It also does not hesitate to be critical of the British medical leadership and organisation. Perhaps this is to be expected in any Australian history of the campaign. Nevertheless, the history has been rather neglected, and, for whatever the reason, the stories of the men and women who served have been, to a considerable extent, ignored.

The relatively short campaign saw a number of stages of development and adaptation of the medical services as the military campaign developed and, ultimately, failed. Much of the planning and organisation of the medical services could, undoubtedly, have been better, but much of the work carried out by them was reactive, as the expectations of the military campaign were never realised. It is perhaps the failure of the military part of the campaign that has been overlooked when criticism has been levelled at the medical services.

Much of this criticism, particularly in Australian accounts, is levelled at the provision of transport for the wounded along the lines of communication to base hospitals some distance from the fighting. Generally, this takes the form of criticism over the lack of provision of suitably equipped hospital ships that could be used in evacuation of wounded. This complaint arose at the time of the campaign, and MOs recorded in war diaries and personal accounts their frustration at their inability to get wounded men off the beaches around the peninsula. Whilst these frustrations are not unique to any one officer, medical unit or nationality, it seems that this shortage had a greater impact on the Australian's interpretation of the events that took place during the campaign. There seems to have been more post-war argument and recrimination over this issue than the failure of the campaign as a whole. This, in turn, seems to have weighted many accounts over the years since the campaign.

The lack of an understanding of the work of the medical services is, perhaps, not surprising since, for those interested in the progress of battles and the strategy and tactics relating to them, it is usually enough to quote casualty figures with little thought to what may lie behind.

There is little effort, generally, to understand the impact of casualties on the support networks lying behind the front line. In battles of the First World War, the number of men killed was a relatively small proportion of those who became casualties. Those who were killed, perhaps as high as 30 percent, were generally beyond help, but the larger proportion needed aid of one sort or another. There was, in the first instance, the stretcher-bearers who removed them to a place of safety and subsequently doctors and nurses to administer the care required for recovery. In a battle where thousands of casualties resulted, it is worth remembering that most of these would have passed through the medical services at some point. Thus, when there was large-scale engagement, it was possible for the medical services to become more or less overwhelmed as large numbers of wounded arrived from the battlefield over a very short period of time. The Gallipoli Campaign was no different to anywhere else in this respect.

The Gallipoli Campaign differed considerably from, for instance, the Western Front since, by the end of the campaign, approximately two-thirds of the casualties had been caused by sickness such as dysentery and enteric fever, not by enemy action. This high sickness rate, particularly in the second half of the campaign, produced large strains on the medical services, which still had to cope with, and accommodate, battle casualties. This factor has to be kept in mind when examining the work, and indeed the effectiveness, of the medical services throughout the campaign.

The medical services were not confined to the peninsula, but those on the peninsula were integrated into a large international network of hospitals in Egypt, across the Mediterranean and Great Britain. Whilst Britain was a seafaring power, the supply and maintenance of a major campaign distant from the main base placed considerable logistical issues on the navy and military commanders. The medical services were part of this and did not operate in isolation outside the overall logistical effort of the country. This, too, is sometimes forgotten when the shortage of hospital ships, or indeed medical equipment, is considered. It is perhaps too easy to think of things in today's terms, setting out modern parameters to deal with problems that occurred over 100 years ago. Whilst the First World War saw considerable technical innovation, there were difficulties in, for instance, communication that could affect the conduct of the war in distant theatres. In the case of communication affecting seaborne transport, it was not impossible for a ship to become effectively lost for a few days with consequential issues arising. There are instances during the Gallipoli Campaign when the loss of communication directly affected the medical services.

To understand the work of the medical services during the Gallipoli Campaign, it is necessary to have a measure of understanding of both the origins of the campaign as a whole and the motives that drove Great Britain and her Empire to embark upon what was ultimately an ill-fated misadventure.

The invasion of the Gallipoli Peninsula in April 1915 had come about as a result of the Allies, mainly Britain, looking for a different approach to fighting the Germans on the Western Front. It had been preceded by months of discussion at the very highest level in London, where the British Government struggled to balance the needs of the developing war with the limited resources at its disposal. The origin and development of the campaign was closely related to the overall foreign policy of the British Empire and how that had developed in the late Victorian period and in the years leading up to the outbreak of the First World War. Consideration of the campaign and its outcome suggests that it was a hastily developed operation. Whilst this may be true at the time of the First World War, the concept of fighting in the Dardanelles, against a defended coastline, had been developed over many years with political and both naval and military assessments made to consider different scenarios for an attack against the Ottoman Empire. All these previous assessments needed to be considered in the context of what would prove to offer the best outcome for the great power that was the British Empire in 1914.

The Dardanelles separated Europe from Asia. The narrow inlet of the Mediterranean Sea connects it to the Sea of Marmora and hence the Black Sea and, in so doing, allows access to the countries bordering the River Danube and to Russia. For Russia, this route was of considerable importance since it offered the only ice-free route by which the Russian Empire could maintain its winter trade with the rest of the world. The British Empire could not consider the possibility of any sea route that could be closed to its navy, and this perhaps made the passage through the Dardanelles every bit as important as it was to the Russians. Of course, the Ottoman Empire recognised the importance of the route and the power it could wield by controlling it. To that end, the Ottomans spent many years constructing and arming a series of forts along the narrow waterway to ensure that it could control both the waterway and the ships that passed along it. It is in the control of the narrow waterway that the origins of the Gallipoli Campaign can be found.

For over 100 years before the First World War, the Royal Navy had been concerned with the issue of ensuring that the waterway remained open. In 1807, Admiral Sir John Duckworth took a fleet through the Dardanelles to bring pressure to bear upon Constantinople (present-day Istanbul). The surprise had been complete, and the firepower of the forts had been completely outmanoeuvred by the sudden approach adopted by Duckworth. However, the admiral soon realised that there was little he could do within the Sea of Marmora without military support, and, after three weeks doing little more than worry the Turks, he was forced to return through the Dardanelles, where his passage out was less comfortable than it had been on the way in.[1]

Even at this time, it was recognised that the Dardanelles were largely controlled by the Gallipoli Peninsula. This had been ignored by Duckworth, and, although he made a successful passage, it had been rather fortunate. It was clear that, to control the Dardanelles, the peninsula also needed to be subdued, and this was beyond the power of the Royal Navy. Thus, in the early nineteenth century, it was recognised that, for success, any mission against the Dardanelles would need substantial military input to support the navy.

The question of the use of naval power in the Dardanelles was examined again in 1877, when Admiral Sir Geoffrey Phipps Hornby was placed in command of a fleet to support the Turks in their second war with Russia in a little over 20 years.[2] The problem faced by Phipps Hornby was rather different, in so far as it was considered there was a possibility that Russia could take control of the forts and hence the waterway. Phipps Hornby wrote to then Foreign Secretary Lord Derby, 'There seems to be an idea that this fleet can keep the Dardanelles and the Bosphorous open. Nothing can be more visionary. Not all the fleets in the world can keep them open for unarmoured shipping.'[3] Phipps Hornby was in no doubt of the difficulties involved in such an operation and was making it clear to the home government that controlling the Dardanelles required more than naval power. Thus, in the 70 years since Duckworth's mission, little had changed in the thinking about the Dardanelles. On this occasion, a treaty was signed between Russia and Turkey, and the British were not called upon to act. However,

---

1   Geoffrey Penn, *Fisher, Churchill and the Dardanelles* (Barnsley: Leo Cooper, 1999), p.21ff.
2   Penn, *Fisher, Churchill and the Dardanelles*, pp.118–19.
3   Penn, *Fisher, Churchill and the Dardanelles*, pp.118–19.

the Turks looked at their forts along the Dardanelles and set about modernising and rearming them in preparation for such a future threat.

By the time the next crisis arose in the area in 1904, Admiral Sir John Fisher had been appointed First Sea Lord. He was acquainted with the area since he had commanded a battleship in Phipps Hornby's fleet and had been commander-in-chief of the Mediterranean Fleet from 1899. Fisher considered any naval action against the forts of the Dardanelles to be 'mightily hazardous', even with military cooperation.[4] Fisher's attitude in 1904 had not substantially changed by the start of the First World War.

Nevertheless, a review in 1906 did suggest that the Dardanelles could be rushed using 'His Majesty's least valuable ships', but, without significant military support, these ships would be left in much the same, and rather useless, position as Duckworth's fleet was some 100 years earlier. Thus, such an undertaking based solely on naval power was 'much to be deprecated'.[5] By this time, it had become almost conventional thinking that the Royal Navy could do nothing against the Dardanelles on its own. Whilst it may have been accepted that a large military operation would be required for any operation against the Turks, it was not thought that a sufficiently large force could be gathered without giving them some indication of the intentions. Without the navy giving a guarantee of covering such a force and subduing the forts, it was considered that 'However brilliant as a combination of war, and however fruitful in its consequences such an operation would be if crowned with success, the General Staff, in view of the risks involved, are not prepared to recommend its being attempted.'[6] Although this question was revisited in 1908 and 1911, there was little to change the overall informed opinion concerning an attack on the Dardanelles. This was the situation up to the start of the First World War.

Whilst it is sometimes considered that the invasion of the peninsula was the result of the poor situation on the Western Front in 1915, this is only part of the story. It is true that, with no sign of a quick victory on the Western Front, some politicians were looking for alternatives to attack the Central Powers. However, the reasons behind this run deeper, for, as early as 31 August 1914, there were some preliminary discussions concerning the capture of the Dardanelles and 'forcing the Narrows'. This was perhaps premature since, at that time, Turkey (or, more precisely, the Ottoman Empire) was neutral and it was hoped that it would stay that way. The relationship between British and Turkish governments had not been improved when Winston Churchill, then First Lord of the Admiralty, detained two warships that were being built in Britain for delivery to Turkey.[7] The first of these ships had been completed before war started, and a Turkish crew had arrived in Britain on 3 August ready for the handover, which did not happen. Although Churchill considered his actions as 'perfectly legal', it strained the relationship and assisted in pushing neutral Turkey towards an alliance with Germany. It had been hoped that a neutral bloc could be formed in southern Europe, where Greece, Turkey, Bulgaria and others did not take either side. As time progressed, this became increasingly unlikely and was not helped by action such as those taken by Churchill, no matter how well they could have been justified.

---

4   Penn, *Fisher, Churchill and the Dardanelles*, p.118.
5   Brigadier General C. F. Aspinall-Oglander, *Official History of the Great War, Military Operations: Gallipoli* (London: William Heinemann, 1932), vol. 1, p.28.
6   Aspinall-Oglander, *Military Operations*, vol. 1, p.29.
7   The two ships were to be named the *Sultan Osman I* and the *Resadiye*; they were renamed HMS *Agincourt* and HMS *Erin*.

xx   The Fight for Life

At this point, Germany offered an inducement to Turkey in the form of two warships, the SMS *Goeben* and the SMS *Breslau*, as more or less direct replacement for the ships detained by Churchill. Turkey accepted these ships, and, after successfully eluding the Royal Navy in the Mediterranean, they passed through the Dardanelles at the end of October 1914. On 29 October, the Turkish government declared war on the Triple Entente of France, Russia and Great Britain. Britain reciprocated by declaring war on Turkey on 3 November.

It was at this point that, perhaps, the first mistake of the war against Turkey was made by the British. As the British Ambassador left Constantinople, the Royal Navy bombarded forts on the Dardanelles for about 10 minutes. This did some damage – some emplacements were destroyed – but it also seems to have given warning to Turkey, and its German advisors, sufficient for a reorganisation of the Dardanelles defences to begin immediately. It was with this reorganised and strengthened defensive system that the invasion force was to contend in April 1915.

Turkey's entry into the war created another front, which was probably more than needed for the already rather stretched resources of the British fighting on the Western Front. It had been a very difficult autumn for the British Empire, with a continued lack of success on the Western Front. It has also suffered its first naval defeat in 100 years when Rear Admiral Sir Christopher Cradock's squadron was destroyed at Cape Coronel by the more modern German Pacific Squadron on 1 November 1914.[8] It was with these matters in mind that thoughts of politicians and, perhaps to a lesser extent, some military commanders began to look for alternatives to the stalemate of the Western Front. It is to be expected that views on the prosecution of the war were divided. There were those who thought Germany could be weakened, and ultimately defeated, by knocking out its allies. This, of course, included defeating the Turks. On the other hand, there were those who believed that Germany could only be defeated on the Western Front. These two camps were essentially mutually exclusive. Nevertheless, at the end of November 1914, the capture and control of the Dardanelles was discussed at a meeting of the newly formed War Council. This was the first time that the topic had been discussed at such a high level, but nothing could be agreed upon at that time, although, a month later, serious questions were being asked about the validity of sending all available troops to France. Clearly, there was a movement to consider alternatives. Thus, by the end of 1914, the capture of the Dardanelles was on the table for discussion along with other ideas to break the deadlock that had deepened on the Western Front during the first winter of the war.

On 1 January, a paper, prepared by Lieutenant Colonel Maurice Hankey, secretary to the War Council, was presented to examine alternative proposals for continuing the war. This included the possibility of attacking Turkey and opening the Black Sea, which, at this time, would have assisted Russia. Whilst this implied an attack on the Dardanelles, it was not stated explicitly.[9] David Lloyd George, Chancellor of the Exchequer, presented a similar assessment to that of Hankey on the very same day, spelling out four criteria that he considered necessary to be met before any operations against Turkey could be undertaken:

1.   That it should not involve the absorption of such a large force as to weaken our offensive in the main field of operations;

8   Sir Julian S. Corbett, *Naval Operations* (London: Longmans, Green and Co., 1920), vol. 1, p.341ff.
9   Aspinall-Oglander, *Military Operations*, vol. 1, p.51.

2. That we should operate at a distance which would not be far from the sea, so as not to waste too many of our troops in maintaining long lines of communication and so as also to have the support of the Fleet in any eventualities;
3. That it should have the effect of forcing Turkey to fight at a long distance from her base of supplies and in country which would be disadvantageous to her;
4. That it should give us the chance of winning a dramatic victory, which would encourage our people at home, whilst it would be a corresponding discouragement to our enemies.[10]

Although Lloyd George's assessment was concerned with a landing in Syria to meet the Turks in the Middle East, the general approach of the politician was similar to that of the soldier in seeking to a way to end the unsatisfactory situation on the Western Front by knocking out what was perceived to be a weak ally of Germany.

It is perhaps a coincidence that, the day after these papers had been presented, a telegram was received from St Petersburg in which the Russians asked for help from its ally to fight against the Turks in the Caucasus Mountains. Whilst there is no doubt that the Russians were being pressed, it is difficult to understand what they expected Britain to do since any response, even a diversionary attack elsewhere, could only have been too late to bring any relief to the Russians. However, the Turks, led by Enver Pasha, pushed themselves too hard. There is no doubt that the Turkish Army was unprepared and ill-equipped for a winter campaign in the mountains, which ultimately ended in disaster. The Turkish assault halted in snow and freezing conditions, which left most of the force frozen to death on the slopes near Sarikamiş.[11]

The relief of the pressure on the Russians that this Turkish defeat produced was not known in Britain for some time. However, by that time, Britain had already committed to give whatever assistance it could whilst accepting that there was little immediate action it could take. The government recognised that support was more morale than physical. It was into this situation that Admiral Fisher threw his ideas on 3 January. His scheme was a grand mixture of those proposals presented by Hankey and Lloyd George only days before and relied upon forces from Greece, Serbia and Rumania to join in an attack on the common enemy. Within this scheme, Fisher proposed a joint military and naval attack to 'force the Dardanelles'.[12] The scheme was essentially unworkable because it relied on certain elements that were outside the home government's control and included the removal of 100,000 men from the Western Front. The latter would not have been received positively by the French. Nevertheless, Fisher's proposal opened the door to allow Winston Churchill to bring forward a proposal for the Royal Navy to attack the Dardanelles alone.

The assumption made by Churchill that Fisher would back such a proposal was the beginning of the end of the working relationship that the two men had developed before the war. Churchill sought to adapt his plan further, and, as the War Council began marginalising both its military and naval advisors, this task became easier. Fisher never supported Churchill's plan, but his silence in subsequent War Council meetings was taken as tacit approval.[13]

---

10 David Lloyd George, *War Memoirs* (London: Odhams Press, 1938), vol. 1, p.224.
11 Roger Ford, *Eden to Armageddon: World War 1 in the Middle East* (London: Phoenix, 2010), p.126ff.
12 Penn, *Fisher, Churchill and the Dardanelles*, p.128.
13 Penn, *Fisher, Churchill and the Dardanelles*, p.128ff.

In an effort to strengthen his plan, Churchill approached the commander-in-chief of the East Mediterranean Squadron, Admiral Sir Sackville Carden, for his opinion on the proposal for a naval attack on the Dardanelles. Carden replied, 'They may be forced by extended operations with a large number of ships.'[14] Churchill seized upon this response from Carden, and, with enhanced belief in and enthusiasm for his idea, he responded to the admiral, 'Your view is agreed with by high authorities here. Please telegraph in detail what you think could be done by extended operation, what force would be needed for, how you consider it should be used, and what results could be obtained.'[15] Whilst Carden may have been surprised by the First Lord's response, it left him little alternative but to look at the matter more closely. Churchill, on the other hand, still had little support, and no 'high authority' had actually agreed to the plan. However, Sir Henry Jackson and the chief of staff appear to have given the matter a favourable hearing, and that was enough for Churchill. Admiral Jackson had no official appointment at the Admiralty, but that did not prevent Churchill from seizing upon his apparent support.

Churchill argued that Fisher had not offered a negative opinion, although it was clear that Fisher did not support any such operation, deeming it impossible to bring to a successful conclusion. Fisher's silence in War Council meetings was not tacit approval, for he was there essentially as the navy's senior advisor and would only advise if he were asked. Churchill was not about to do that and throw doubt on a scheme in which he believed. Whilst Churchill would probably have preferred the admiral's support, he made it absolutely clear that he did not need it and was happy to proceed without Fisher to push the proposal along. On 11 January, Churchill received a response from Carden that gave a four-stage approach to a naval operation against the Dardanelles:

> Possibility of operations:
> (A) Total reduction of defences at the entrance.
> (B) Clear defences inside of Straits up to an including Kephez Point Battery No. 8.
> (C) Reduction of defences at Narrows, Chanak.
> (D) Clear passage through minefield, advancing through Narrows, reducing Forts above Narrows, and final advance to Marmora.[16]

Carden not only suggested that a fleet of no less than 60 ships would be needed but also stressed that any operation required good weather if it were to succeed.

Fisher's position was clear, in so far as he considered that a naval operation could not succeed without considerable military support. Lord Kitchener, the Secretary of State for War, had made it clear that there were no troops to spare to support any such naval operation. Whilst that should have been the end of it, Churchill took this to mean that the naval operation could proceed without military assistance. With Churchill pushing the government and directing policy towards a naval assault against the Dardanelles, it is hardly surprising that, on 13 January, the navy was informed that a decision had been made to bombard the forts of the Dardanelles. This was relayed to Carden on 15 January, and, at the same time, he was told that his fleet would include the recently completed HMS *Queen Elizabeth*. It was considered that the huge 15-inch

---

14   Penn, *Fisher, Churchill and the Dardanelles*, p.123ff.
15   Winston S. Churchill, *The World Crisis: 1915* (London: Thomas Butterworth, 1923), vol. 2, p.68.
16   Churchill, *World Crisis*, vol. 2, pp.69–70.

guns of this warship, which were still undergoing trials and calibration, could be useful against the targets in the Dardanelles.

At a meeting of the War Council on 28 January, it was decided that the attack would commence during February, and the navy was told to make the necessary arrangements. At this time, something of an olive branch was offered to Fisher, in so far that, if the attempt looked like it was failing, the ships would be withdrawn and the operation would be considered no more than a demonstration. Whilst this did not fully satisfy Fisher, the admiral took full responsibility for the operation then being planned.[17] The decision of 28 January is seen by the *Official History* as 'the first great landmark in the history of the Dardanelles Campaign'.[18] There could be no going back as the navy prepared for the work. Nevertheless, the Admiralty was, by mid-February, having some misgivings. Even Churchill recognised the value of military support, as he sent two battalions of the Royal Naval Division (RND) to assist in the action by providing landing parties. The belief in the need for military support at the Admiralty led one of Churchill's supposed supporters, Sir Henry Jackson, to write on 15 January that there was a need for 'strong military landing parties'.[19] The following day, a decision was made to send the only regular division remaining, the 29th Division, to support the naval attack. However, this decision was cancelled, as the government vacillated and continued to discuss options. It was 10 March before the 29th Division was finally ordered into the Dardanelles area of operation.

Although there had been much discussion and indecision at the War Council, Churchill finally got his way, and naval operations against the Dardanelles commenced on 19 February. There was a measure of success during the first day of bombardment, but then the weather changed, and, for five days, the operations were suspended. It was, by this time, becoming clear that military input was going to be necessary. The War Council now considered that the operation could not be stopped, as had been intimated to Fisher, without loss of face and that military action was becoming inevitable. Lloyd George was unhappy with this situation, particularly objecting that the army was being used 'to pull the navy's chestnuts out of the fire'.[20]

The naval assault continued in March, and the outer forts were reduced by a combination of shell fire and landing parties. No progress was made against the inner defences, and Carden could do no more until the minefield protecting the approach to these defences could be swept. He reported this to the home government on 9 March, and, although some effort was made to clear the mines, it was some days before shelling recommenced. By this time, Carden was ill and was replaced by Vice Admiral J. M. de Robeck on 17 March. Although the attack was continued, by 22 March, it was seen that the operation was not making progress, and de Robeck informed the War Council that a force needed to be landed on the peninsula to assist the attack.

To some extent, this had been anticipated in London, and, on 12 March, Kitchener had appointed General Sir Ian Hamilton as commander-in-chief of the force being prepared to assist the navy. The following day, Hamilton left for the Dardanelles with 13 officers of his operational staff. Significantly, he did not take any of his administrative or medical staff with

---

17   Lord Fisher before the Dardanelles Commission. See Aspinall-Oglander, *Military Operations*, vol. 1, p.61fn.

18   Aspinall-Oglander, *Military Operations*, vol. 1, p.61.

19   Lord Fisher before the Dardanelles Commission. See Aspinall-Oglander, *Military Operations*, vol. 1, p.61fn.

20   Aspinall-Oglander, *Military Operations*, vol. 1, p.75.

him, although these could have proved to be useful in planning for the military assault on the Gallipoli Peninsula. Hamilton arrived at the island of Tenedos on 17 March, where he had immediate discussions with de Robeck to grasp the situation as quickly as possible. The admiral pointed out that he believed the navy had the firepower to subdue the forts but could not handle the enemy's mobile artillery because he simply could not locate it from the sea. This was the point where the military support was needed. Kitchener had resisted all attempts to include the 29th Division in the military force, but, in the end, his options were limited, and the division was sent to the Dardanelles in preparation for the invasion. Meanwhile, in Egypt, General Birdwood's Australians and New Zealanders were being prepared ready for action. This force, together with the RND, was considered to be sufficient military presence to bring the entire operation to a rapid and successful conclusion.

With the final acceptance that there was to be a military component to the assault on the Dardanelles came the need for a forward base within range of the Dardanelles and from which both the navy and the army could be supplied. Of necessity, this pointed towards one of the islands near to the Dardanelles. For the navy, it also meant that there was a need for a suitable harbour to which it could return to be supplied with ammunition and food, as well as fuel to run the large warships. For the military, a forward base was necessary, if only temporarily, to allow it to supply its needs as the land campaign progressed. The need for a large base to be established on an island depended largely upon the success of the operation. If the assault was a complete success and the military advanced quickly, then the forward base would need to move with it to keep the supply lines open and available. That is, if the campaign was relatively short, the need to utilise the islands in the Aegean diminished correspondingly.

Of the nearby islands of the Aegean, most were mountainous and offered little in the way of suitable harbour facilities to allow the development of a forward base. Imbros, close to the Dardanelles, could offer only a small harbour at Kephalos. Lemnos, on the other hand, had a fine harbour in the form of Mudros Bay but was 60 miles west of the Dardanelles. It was, nevertheless, to become the most important harbour for the duration of the campaign.

Following the naval action at the Dardanelles during February, the 3rd Australian Infantry Brigade began arriving in Mudros Harbour on 6 March. Lieutenant Colonel Alfred Sutton of the 3rd Australian Field Ambulance (AFA) was to record, 'This harbour is very, very beautiful … the soil is a poor sandy loam, the men are very fine, big built and sturdy and the children are dark eyed, handsome, well-nourished kiddies and the women are really beautiful … The inhabitants are very polite'.[21] This was the unit to which 'the man with the donkey', John Simpson, was attached, and it was amongst the first Australian units to disembark at Mudros. More will be said of this unit and soldier later.

The 3rd Australian Brigade was to remain at Mudros since General Birdwood had received orders from Lord Kitchener that one of his brigades should be specially trained in landing and re-embarking; Colonel E. G. Sinclair-MacLagan was ordered to conduct this training with the 3rd Brigade. This unit was to spearhead the Australian landings, acting as the covering force when the landings on the peninsula eventually took place on 25 April.

---

21 Tom Curran, *Across the Bar: The Story of 'Simpson', The Man with the Donkey: Australia and Tyneside's Great Military Hero* (Brisbane: Ogmios Publications, 1994), p.186.

In addition to the use of the island's harbour, Mudros also became the location of the major Allied hospitals supporting the Gallipoli campaign. These hospitals were staffed by British, Canadian, New Zealand and Australian Army medical staff. By the end of the campaign, Mudros was the site of two general hospitals, four stationary hospitals and two convalescent depots, with a total capacity of slightly more than 13,000 beds. Wounded soldiers and sailors were treated initially on the peninsula at field ambulances and casualty clearing stations (CCSs) and evacuated by hospital ships to a number of destinations depending on their wounds. Amongst these destinations were West Mudros and East Mudros, where more advanced medical and surgical care was possible.

The island of Imbros also played its part in the attempt to wrest the peninsula from the Turks. Imbros is the closest of the Aegean islands to the Gallipoli Peninsula, lying as it does about 16 miles from Anzac Cove. Shortly after the landings on the peninsula, it was decided that Imbros would be the site for the general headquarters (GHQ) camp. However, the disadvantage of Imbros was that, at times, transport could be difficult across the narrow stretch of water separating it from the peninsula. The small harbour there could not provide shelter for ships from all directions of the wind, and hence there were some difficulties in landing stores, and later wounded, at the island. This also created problems for staff officers needing to visit the peninsula: not only could ships not approach during a gale, but it was also difficult for them to leave if the wind was in the wrong direction. At the start of the campaign, the General Staff was based on the liner RMS *Arcadian*. It was not long before Hamilton realised that perhaps it was better for the staff to be on land, and, on 14 May, the *Arcadian* sailed for Imbros and remained there with the staff on board. GHQ was established on Imbros from 31 May 1915.

From May 1915 until well into 1916, Imbros was used by the British forces in the area. It saw the development of a GHQ and an infantry camp to hold a division at rest, and, indeed, it was from Imbros that the 11th Division embarked for the landings at Suvla Bay. By the time the forces were evacuated from the peninsula, there was a significant military presence on Imbros that went far beyond the GHQ camp there and was more like a temporary town that accommodated men, stores, equipment and munitions – all requiring such things as water supply and roads. It is difficult to estimate the number of men stationed there at any one time since the garrison was essentially mobile, with men coming and going within a matter of days. However, it should be considered that there was a camp there capable of billeting one division, plus the GHQ camp and all the logistical staff that kept everything running, plus the work force that kept all the sites functioning as a military base. It would not be too unrealistic to expect that the population of the small town that resulted could have been upwards of 20,000 men.

To summarise, the ideas for the Gallipoli Campaign, or an attack on the Dardanelles, had a long history and had gone through many iterations before it came to the stage where both naval and military forces were despatched to the area to fight. Despite all assessments that had gone before, suggesting that any attack would be difficult, the final decision was made largely at the continual prodding and pushing by Churchill. The planning was ultimately very rushed, and Hamilton was given little time from his appointment in March to the invasion in April. Hamilton was forced to prepare what can only be seen as a hasty scheme, and it was within this scheme that his medical services were forced to operate, though not until it was a full-fledged scheme in which the medical services had no input. The following chapters look at the work of the medical services.

1

Military Medical Services
Royal Army Medical Corps (RAMC)

Medical services in the British Army date from the formation of the standing Regular Army in 1660 after the Restoration of Charles II. This was the first time when there was opportunity for a medical man to make a career within the military. At this stage, the medical services were provided on a regimental basis, with each battalion providing its own MO and, when necessary, finding its own medical supplies and hospital as required. In 1793, a more centralised approach was adopted, and general military hospitals were established throughout England during the following decade. Nevertheless, it was not until 1873 that the regimental appointments of MOs were abandoned when a more coordinated approach, requiring MOs to pass further examinations, was set up. At this stage, the MOs did not hold a military rank, though they were allowed some of the privileges of officers, such as living quarters and fodder for a horse. This lack of military status became a bone of contention, as the medical services failed to have the recognition of the other professional arms of the services, such as the Royal Engineers or Army Service Corps. The British Medical Association and the Royal College of Physicians lobbied for a change, and, in 1898, this resulted in the formation of the Royal Army Medical Corps (RAMC), with the first colonel-in-chief being Prince Arthur, the Duke of Connaught.

At this time, the structure of the RAMC was based on bearer companies and field hospitals, which was soon shown to be inadequate in times of war as the newly formed force took its place in the South African War of 1899–1902. During this war, there were bearer companies and field hospitals for two army corps. This amounted to one bearer company and one field hospital for each brigade, with each division being provided with an additional field hospital for 100 sick and wounded patients. These were accompanied by seven stationary hospitals and three general hospitals. Additional personnel were found from the civilian medical practitioners and by using an increased number of nursing sisters. Combined, these facilities were insufficient, as they provided capacity for less than three percent of the total force involved.[1]

The weaknesses in the RAMC exposed by the South African War, together with information coming out of the Russo–Japanese War in Manchuria in respect of large numbers of casualties,

---

1   Major General Sir W. G. MacPherson, *History of the Great War Based on Official Documents: Medical Services* (Facsimile edition, Uckfield: Naval & Military Press, n.d.), vol. 1, p.1.

indicated to the British Army that there needed to be considerable reorganisation of its medical services. During the South African War, it was recognised that the use of the title of 'principal medical officer' (PMO) had created confusion since this was often applied to the commander of the field force, the officer in charge of medical services in the lines of communication and the SMOs of divisions. This resulted in misdirected orders and communications, leading to delay and confusion within the medical services.[2] In 1907, the following reclassification of officers was introduced, which was to be largely used during the First World War:

Classification of MOs

South African War	From 1907
Principal medical officer (PMO) of field force	Director of medical services (DMS)
Assistant to PMO of field force	Assistant director of medical services (ADMS)
PMO of lines of communication	Deputy director of medical services (DDMS)
Assistant to PMO of lines of communication	Deputy assistant director of medical services (DADMS)
PMO of division	Administrative medical officer (MO) – in 1912, this became 'deputy director of medical services' (DDMS).
PMO of hospital	Officer commanding (OC)
PMO of base	Senior medical officer (SMO)

Immediately following the South African War, the director general of medical services (DGMS) was a member of the War Office, but, when that office was replaced by the Army Council in 1904, that ceased to be the case, and medical services were placed under the adjutant general's remit. In 1907, an inspector general of forces was appointed, and an inspector of medical services was placed on his staff. This, too, was placed under the control of the adjutant general's office in 1909. This arrangement, where the medical services were subservient within the administrative arm of the forces, was to have a particular impact during the Gallipoli Campaign.

During the South African War, the inadequacies of the medical services had been recognised, and, in 1901, it had been proposed that the bearer companies and field hospitals be combined to form what was then called a 'field ambulance'. This was not acted upon until 1905. At this point, the field ambulance ceased to be brigade troops and became divisional troops, with two field ambulances per division and a further one provided as corps troops.[3] The field ambulance was the basic unit of the medical services of the field force during the First World War. At this time, field ambulances were also organised for each cavalry or mounted brigade.

The field ambulance was the fundamental unit of the medical services and was divided into the bearer division and tent division. Each of these divisions was further subdivided into three sections, except in the cavalry, where only two sections of each division were employed. There was also a provision for 10 ambulance wagons for each ambulance, and the capacity of each ambulance was the care of 50 sick or wounded in each section, a total of 150 cases. In association

2   Macpherson, *History of the Great War: Medical Services*, vol. 1, p.3.
3   Macpherson, *History of the Great War: Medical Services*, vol. 1, p.8.

with the field ambulances were the regimental medical officers (RMOs), and together these 'represented the whole medical organization in front of the lines of communication for an army in the field'.[4] The establishment resulting from these changes in 1905 was given as:

- One field ambulance for each of three cavalry brigades
- Two field ambulances for each division
- 14 stationary hospitals
- 10 general hospitals
- Two advanced medical depots
- Two base medical depots
- Two ambulance trains
- Two hospital ships.

This was a considerable improvement upon that supplied for the South African War but, in light of the casualty rates seen in the Russo–Japanese War, was still considered to be inadequate for the casualties likely to occur in fighting a European war. It will also be noted that there was no allowance for clearing hospitals as part of the lines of communication. It was thought highly likely that, in the event of large casualty numbers, there would be congestion in the field ambulances, and this brought about the concept of the clearing hospital, which was designed to form a link between the field ambulance and the lines of communication in the evacuation of the wounded from the forward areas.[5] With the addition of the clearing hospital, the treatment and evacuation of sick and wounded was seen as:

- RMOs and field ambulances – the collection of wounded from the battle zone
- Clearing hospitals and ambulance trains – the evacuation of wounded to rear areas
- Stationary and general hospitals – the long-term or permanent treatment of the casualties.

In its original form, the clearing hospital was formed by the conversion of stationary hospitals; that is, a 200-bed stationary hospital became a 200-bed clearing hospital but used only field equipment and, notably, did not have beds or nursing sisters. This was not thought to be suitable for use in war since it was considered that these hospitals would become responsible for the clearing of casualties from the entire division to which it was attached, making the capacity of 200 beds far too low. This was all reviewed in 1907, and, along with increased capacity, it was recognised that the clearing hospital should be essentially mobile and hence provided with its own transport.

With this review, it was also recognised that much of the problem encountered in South Africa had been the result of disease, some of which could have been prevented by better control of hygiene and sanitation. As a result, it was recommended that each unit in the field was to form a sanitary detachment of a non-commissioned officer (NCO) and eight men. On the lines of communication, sanitary arrangements were looked after by 'special technical units of the RAMC'.[6]

---

4   Macpherson, *History of the Great War: Medical Services*, vol. 1, p.9.
5   Macpherson, *History of the Great War: Medical Services*, vol. 1, p.10.
6   Macpherson, *History of the Great War: Medical Services*, vol. 1, p.15.

30   The Fight for Life

Slowly, the organisation of the medical services was evolving during the years immediately before the First World War. Part of this evolution was the recognition that there was a lack of suitable hospitals in the United Kingdom that could be used in the event of a large-scale war. In 1911, a scheme was approved by which a further 4,750 beds were made available at a number of barracks throughout the country that could be used for convalescent purposes. In the event of war, it seemed likely that the barracks may not be available, and so provision for hutted and tented accommodation was made.[7]

Under the 1907 arrangements, the organisation of the RAMC was given as:

- Four cavalry field ambulances to the cavalry division
- One cavalry field ambulance to each of two mounted brigades (army troops)
- Three field ambulances to each division (six divisions allowed for)
- Two field ambulances as army troops
- Six clearing hospitals
- 12 stationary hospitals
- 12 general hospitals
- Three advanced depots
- Three base depots
- Six ambulance trains
- Six hospital ships
- Two sanitary sections
- 11 sanitary squads.

This was essentially the organisation that applied in 1914, with the exception that the allowance for the mounted brigades was removed and replaced by those of a 5th Cavalry Brigade. It was recognised, even in 1907, that there was a likely to be problem with the number of hospital ships because of the likely shortage of such vessels, but this was to some extent countered by the consideration that a European war would make sea transport short and hospital ships perhaps less important. This assumption was to prove to be an oversimplification when fighting in more distant theatres such as the Gallipoli Peninsula.

Whilst this organisation looked better on paper, there was still a problem with manpower since the units mentioned did not all exist in peacetime. Thus, if war resulted in mobilisation of an expeditionary force of 140,000 men, the RAMC was hundreds of officers and thousands of other ranks short of the establishment to take to the field. In the first decade of the twentieth century, there were a number of schemes brought forwards to assist with the recruitment of personnel to increase the manpower of the RAMC. In the case of officers, one such approach was to allow civil surgeons to be taken as part of the medical services, but a restriction was placed so that these surgeons did not form more than 45 percent of the establishment. This was partly because such men would not be able to serve entirely under military conditions, as they lacked the necessary training. In the case of other ranks, there were initiatives such as offering men approaching the end of their service the opportunity to

---

7   Macpherson, *History of the Great War: Medical Services*, vol. 1, p.19.

finish it in the RAMC. These approaches went some way to allowing the RAMC to reach the required establishment.[8]

While this was coming into existence, the Territorial Force (TF) was also coming into being, and with it the territorial arm of the RAMC. Haldane's reforms of the volunteers in 1908 allowed for the formation of 14 territorial divisions, and these were to be provided for with the requisite number of RAMC units, which, by 1914, resulted in the formation of:

- 14 mounted field ambulances (TF)
- 42 field ambulances (TF)
- 23 general hospitals (TF)
- Two sanitary companies (TF)
- 14 casualty clearing hospitals (TF).[9]

Whilst these TF units were designed for service in home defence, it was not long before that concept was abandoned, and many territorial units were serving overseas before the end of 1914. Indeed, some of the territorial field ambulance units were destined to serve during the Gallipoli Campaign.

In parallel with the development of the medical services in the RAMC, there was also considerable development and expansion of the nursing services. In 1896, Princess Christian had initiated the army nursing service (PCANS) of 88 trained nurses, who were further supplemented by a reserve (PCANSR) of nurses. Some of these ladies served during the South African War alongside the RAMC. In 1902, Queen Alexandra's Imperial Military Nursing Service (QAIMNS) was initiated by Royal Warrant.[10] At this time, the establishment was set at one matron and eight trained sisters for every 100 beds, which gave an allowance for 230 nurses. This figure was gradually increased to 382, and, in 1910, a reserve (QAIMNSR) was formed, providing further trained nurses and into which Princess Christian's nurses were eventually absorbed. In a similar manner to the RAMC, the nurses were also involved in the TF with the formation of the Territorial Force Nursing Service (TFNS), which was to be used for the staffing of the 23 TF general hospitals. This organisation also formed a reserve (TFNSR), and, by the outbreak of war in 1914, the TF nurses numbered 713 exclusive of the 2,576 in the 23 general hospitals.[11] Similarly, the Royal Navy also formed a nursing service in 1884, which became known as 'Queen Alexandra's Royal Navy Nursing Service' (QARNNS), with a reserve (QARNNSR) formed in 1910. During the First World War, the service was greatly expanded, and many of the service saw duty on the Royal Navy hospital ships during the Gallipoli Campaign.

Thus, by the onset of the First World War, there was a reasonably well-organised medical service that had grown in size since the South African War in an effort to meet the exigencies of a European war. However, in a matter of months, there was a need to increase the size of not only the medical services but also the entire British Army to meet the increased fighting on the Western Front. Nevertheless, the structure of the RAMC was essentially to remain the same as

---

8   Macpherson, *History of the Great War: Medical Services*, vol. 1, p.21ff.
9   Ray Westlake, *The Territorial Force, 1914* (Newport: Ray Westlake, Military Books, 1988), pp.76–83.
10   Yvonne McEwen, *In the Company of Nurses: The History of the British Army Nursing Service in the Great War* (Edinburgh: Edinburgh University Press, 2014), p.9.
11   Macpherson, *History of the Great War: Medical Services*, vol. 1, p.34.

32   The Fight for Life

that envisaged before the war, and, although it was to become involved most deeply in the war in western Europe, the RAMC was to see service in all theatres where the British Army served. One of these was, of course, Gallipoli.

Australian Army Medical Corps (AAMC)

The establishment of the Australian Army Medical Corps (AAMC) can be traced to two basic sources. The first is the medical provisions made for the small permanent force, and the second is for the provisions made in the unpaid volunteers or partially paid militia forces of the colonies that later became federated as the Commonwealth of Australia. Up to 1870, the medical services were largely dependent upon the medical staff attached to the small garrison of British troops in the country. This was not a universal service since it mostly served only the officials of the country and had a supervisory role in the public hospitals.[12]

Following the withdrawal of the British troops in 1870, no provision was made for MOs within the permanent force until 1891. At this time, New South Wales formed the 'Medical Staff Corps'. Alongside the permanent forces, the volunteers, which had existed since 1801, also provided medical staff, though in this case it was not well organised and relied on doctors giving up time from their civil practices as and when needed. This was similar in the militia, and each colony had its own militia and medical staff throughout the nineteenth century.

New South Wales was the first colony to form an official Voluntary Medical Staff Corps in 1888, and, from this, the first permanent Medical Staff Corps was recruited. In the years immediately before federation (1901), all of the colonies had an army medical service, but, except for New South Wales, they were little more than rudimentary. For instance, the service comprised only 20 all ranks in Western Australia and 23 all ranks in Tasmania, whereas, in New South Wales, it was 158 all ranks. In 1900, New South Wales sent a bearer company and a field hospital of 62 all ranks to South Africa.[13] This was not the first time that New South Wales had sent MOs overseas to support its army. In 1885, it had sent a small contingent under PMO Colonel W. D. C. Williams to take part in the Suakin Campaign during the Sudan War.

During the South African War, the involvement of the Australian medical services was considerably more developed, with a number of contingents being sent overseas in 1899 and 1900 at the expense of the colonies while the contingent of 1901, known as the 'Imperial Draft', was sent overseas at the expense of the British Government. Once again, Colonel Williams was responsible for the organisation of these contingents and for completing the formation of the Australian Medical Service (AMS). In 1901, he was able to send both a bearer company and a field hospital to South Africa. By the end of the war, a total of 30 officers and 338 other ranks had served overseas, and a number of nursing sisters had seen service.

Colonel Williams had also taken responsibility for adapting field equipment to suit Australian conditions. This did not go unnoticed in South Africa. When the official report was compiled, Surgeon General Sir W. D. Wilson, PMO of the British forces, was to comment:

---

12   A. G. Butler, *The Official History of the Australian Army Medical Services in the War of 1914–1918: Volume I: Gallipoli, Palestine and New Guinea* (Facsimile edition of 1938 edition, Uckfield: Naval & Military Press, 2019), p.2.
13   Butler, *Official History of the Australian Medical Services*, vol. I, p.3.

The Colonial medical units were more mobile than the regulation field hospital or bearer company. This was partly due to the difference in the equipment and in the waggons … The equipment was exceedingly good and practical … (the NSW unit) had its own draft animals and was thus quite independent and self-contained. Its success is an example of what may be done by a field unit which is not dependent on local conditions for its mobility …[14]

Captain N. R. Howse was awarded the Victoria Cross (VC) for gallantry in South Africa and became the first member of the AMS to receive the award. Howse became an important figure in the AMS during the First World War and was assistant director of medical services (ADMS) for the 1st Australian Division at the beginning of the Gallipoli Campaign.

Federation saw the formation of one Australian Military Force and brought about the formation of an AAMC by the general order of 30 July 1902:

The whole of the existing Army Medical Services of each State will be dealt with as one Corps and will be styled the Australian Army Medical Corps. The Corps shall comprise:
a. Permanent Army Medical Corps (nucleus only)
b. Militia Army Medical Corps.
c. Volunteer Army Medical Corps.
d. Reserve of officers.
e. Army Nursing Service Reserve.[15]

The Permanent Army Medical Corps provided only a small instructional cadre, whilst the Militia and Volunteer Medical Corps provided:

- Regimental medical establishments
- Mounted bearer companies
- Infantry bearer companies
- Field hospitals.

This was certainly progress towards a unified force, but there were still no provisions for either lines of communication medical services or for base hospitals or provision for dental care, and pharmaceutical services were very poorly organised at this stage. Nevertheless, it was organised in much the same manner as the British medical services and, in that context, suffered from the same omissions. Surgeon General Williams was determined to give the AAMC its own character and continued with the move towards their own design of medical vehicles and tentage for their specific needs.

During the years prior to the First World War, there were issues in maintaining the required level of personnel, and there was a need, for instance, to train regimental stretcher-bearers from the men in those regiments. Moves were made to make all regimental bandsmen train as stretcher-bearers so that, in wartime, their role was determined.

---

14 Butler, *Official History of the Australian Medical Services*, vol. I pp.4–5.
15 Butler, *Official History of the Australian Medical Services*, vol. I, p.5.

When the medical services in the Great Britain were reorganised in 1907, the AAMC followed similar lines, with the bearer companies and field hospitals combining to form the field ambulance. Each field ambulance had personnel of 10 officers and 224 other ranks divided into tent (nursing and administrative) divisions and bearer divisions. There was still no inclusion of lines of communication units and, in a similar manner to the British formation, no immediate allowance for casualty clearing hospitals. However, a reserve of MOs was formed at this time. This was followed in 1909 by the inclusion of pharmaceutical officers with the honorary rank of lieutenant and a number of command sanitary officers to advise the PMO, though sanitary work was still carried out by regimental fatigues. This was to form the nucleus for expansion during wartime.

By 1914, there had been further reorganisation, and the inclusion of the lines of communication troops had occurred so that the need for CCSs and base hospitals had been recognised and were established in line with that adopted by the RAMC in Great Britain. In 1914, the permanent force medical service comprised only four officers and 29 other ranks, but the militia and the newly named 'Citizen Force' had a total of 183 officers and 1,649 other ranks. This allowed the formation of:

- 16 field ambulances
- Five light horse field ambulances
- Three-and-a-half sanitary companies
- 121 regimental establishments.

There was also an unattached list of 33 officers and a reserve of 231 officers, and the Australian Army Nursing Service (AANS) had 108 nursing sisters in its ranks. This did not allow for any formation larger than a brigade.

In September 1914, the AAMC had developed its lines of communication medical units to comprise:

- No. 1 CCS (raised and equipped in Tasmania)
- No. 1 Stationary Hospital (raised in South Australia)
- No. 2 Stationary Hospital (raised in Western Australia)
- No. 2 General Hospital (raised in New South Wales)
- No. 1 General Hospital (Commanding Officer (CO) Colonel Ramsay Smith from South Australia, while officers were from Victoria and other staff from Queensland).[16]

It was with this general establishment and organisation that the AAMC went overseas at the end of 1914.

The history of the AANS cannot be discussed without mention of Principal Matron Ellen Julia Gould, who was born in 1860 in Wales, where her father was a mining agent. At the age of 19, Ellen became a governess and moved to Germany, where she lived until a visit to relatives in Australia in 1884. Ellen decided to stay in Australia and began her training as a nurse in the

---

16   James W. Barrett and P. E. Deane, *The Australian Army Medical Corps in Egypt During the First World War* (London: H. K. Lewis and Son, 1918), pp.15–16.

Prince Alfred Hospital (Royal Prince Alfred) in Sydney in the same year. She completed her training and worked in several hospitals, where she gained a broad knowledge and experience of nursing before being promoted to matron in 1891.[17]

In 1899, Matron Ellen ('Nellie' as she was known) Gould was approached by Colonel William Williams and asked for help to form an army nursing service reserve that would be attached to the New South Wales Army Medical Corps. In May 1899, 26 nurses were sworn in, and Ellen Gould was appointed lady superintendent of the newly formed New South Wales Army Nursing Service. Early in 1900, Ellen left Australia in charge of 13 nursing sisters for service in South Africa during the South African War, where she served for two years. The Australian service was modelled on the PCANSR, which was operating at that time in the United Kingdom. Other Australian colonies also sent nurses to South Africa, such as the South Australia Transvaal Nurses, who left for service in February of 1900.[18]

At first, the Australian nurses met with some entrenched opinions and prejudice from British MOs who were not entirely sure of the value or, indeed, the role of a nurse in war. There was also a belief at the time that Australian nurses would not work with their counterpart in the Imperial service in the same hospitals: 'On handing in my Papers to the PMO he groaned, "My God, Australian Sisters, what shall we do?" On my asking the reason he said that they did require help but he understood we could not work with the RAMC [sic] sisters.'[19] Lady Superintendent Nellie Gould soon corrected this attitude, and it was not too long before most MOs began to recognise the value of the work and dedication of the trained nurses in their hospitals.[20] According to Miss Gould, the way in which the Australians were accepted by the British nurses was, to a large extent, due to their lady superintendent, Miss Oram, who treated the Australian nurses as professionals at all times, accepting that they were there to do the same job and were equally capable of that job.[21]

The women who served as nurses during the South African War provided Australia's first real experience of military nursing. However, at this stage, the nurses were mostly employed in looking after the sick whilst the wounded were still cared for mainly by doctors and male orderlies. During the South African War, sickness caused more deaths than the fighting, and all nurses were kept busy carrying out the essential caring for thousands of men who fell ill with diseases such as enteric fever or malaria. The nurses worked for 14 hours a day, and 'no one complained'.[22] Although there was little first-hand experience with battle casualties, there were many lessons learned that were taken back with the nurses and used to improve the base of military nursing in the various military districts. Not least of these was, perhaps, the need for good organisation of the medical services and for close cooperation between MOs and nurses to run hospitals efficiently and effectively for patients, whether wounded or sick.

---

17 Perditta M. McCarthy, 'Ellen Julia (Nellie) Gould (1860–1941)', *Australian Dictionary of Biography* (2006), <https://adb.anu.edu.au/biography/gould-ellen-julia-nellie-6437/text11013>, accessed Aug. 2019.

18 Jan Bassett, *Guns and Brooches: Australian Army Nursing from the Boer War to the Gulf War* (Melbourne: Oxford University Press, 1992), pp.11–28.

19 Australian War Memorial (AWM) AWM41/975: [Nurses Narratives] Principal Matron Ellen Julia Gould.

20 Bassett, *Guns and Brooches*, pp.11–28.

21 AWM: AWM41/975: [Nurses Narratives] Principal Matron Ellen Julia Gould.

22 AWM: AWM41/975: [Nurses Narratives] Principal Matron Ellen Julia Gould.

36   The Fight for Life

Whilst military nursing was essentially as a reservist, increased contact with the military through the AAMC was encouraged, indeed was required, if a nurse was to remain efficient for the military. This was achieved by establishing a requirement that all nurses wishing to remain efficient should attend a minimum of three out of four lectures a year given by an MO in the relevant military district. The purpose of this approach was for each, that is, nurses and MOs, to understand the work of the other and to develop ways in which they could combine to produce something workable for the soldiers in their charge in time of war. However, by the start of the First World War, although there was a framework in place, it was not very well organised, and it took a lot of work by both the medical men and the senior nurses to arrive at the point where the service could be described as 'efficient'.

Upon federation, Matron Gould became responsible for the organisation of the army nursing service reserve in New South Wales, becoming the principal matron of the state. Ellen Gould remained a driving force behind the army nursing service and served throughout the First World War.

Although the groundwork started by Matron Gould, and her contemporaries, had made significant advances, the problems associated with a nursing reserve attached to the AAMC remained. Perhaps the most significant problem, and one that affected nurses up to the first year of the First World War, was that they had little understanding of the military and its processes. Whereas, in Great Britain, there was the professional QAIMNS with trained nurses belonging to the army, in Australia, the nurses were simply attached reservists who had little contact with the realities of military service. Nevertheless, by the end of 1914, there were sufficient trained nurses in the AANS to be mobilised with the AAMC to provide the nursing care in both the general hospitals and stationary hospitals that soon appeared in Egypt in the early months of 1915.

New Zealand Medical Corps (NZMC)

The history of the New Zealand Medical Corps (NZMC) can be traced back to 1845, when surgeons were first attached to each of the three militia regiments then in existence. By 1862, the involvement of the medical services in the military life of the islands had grown to match the increasing number of militia regiments in the county. This was to be known as the 'Colonial Medical Services' to separate it from those services provided for the Imperial forces then in New Zealand. The development was slow and tended to depend upon the enthusiasm for the militia movement as a whole and to the crises faced by the country. However, by 1897, there had been some reorganisation of the medical services available, and, in each of the four military districts in the country, a bearer company was organised, each comprising two officers and 25 other ranks and answerable to the PMO of the district concerned.[23]

At the beginning of the South African War, there was an increase in the number of volunteers coming forwards for overseas service, and, during this war, a total of 26 MOs were sent to support the 6,500 volunteers who served in South Africa. Some of these men served as RMOs, while some served in hospitals. Following the war, there was a sharp decline in the interest in

---

23   A. D. Carberry, *The New Zealand Medical Service in the Great War 1914–1918* (Facsimile edition, Uckfield: Naval & Military Press, n.d.), p.4.

the volunteer movement in New Zealand, and, by the time Surgeon General Skerman introduced reforms to the medical services in 1905, it was considered to be in a poor condition and in need of change. However, Skerman's reforms brought about the formation of the NZMC, which, in 1908, was reorganised along the lines of the RAMC. At this time, the bearer companies were formed into field ambulances, and an army nursing reserve was established. Each field ambulance comprised four officers, one quartermaster and 46 other ranks. Four such units were formed at this time.

Obligatory training for all young males was introduced in 1909, and this helped to keep the numbers up to establishment so that, by 1913, each of the four military districts in the country had a field ambulance and a mounted field ambulance to support the other military arms in the district. However, although there was a framework in place, there was no permanent medical staff, and, on that basis, the NZMC could not have been considered as ready for the war of 1914.[24]

On 7 August 1914, the New Zealand Government cabled the British Government, offering the services of a New Zealand Expeditionary Force (NZEF). This was accepted on 12 August and brought about the mobilisation and embarkation of the New Zealand first contingent during the months from August to November. A total of 48 officers and 328 other ranks were mobilised by the NZMC and were organised into one mounted field ambulance and one field ambulance. This was essentially the organisation that served as part of the New Zealand and Australian Division, which landed on Gallipoli in April 1915.

The military nursing services in New Zealand were much less well developed at the start of the war than in other countries that served during the Gallipoli Campaign. At the start of the First World War, there was no official army nursing service in the country, though there was a matron-in-chief of what was little more than an idea. According to Lieutenant Colonel Carberry, 'The New Zealand Branch of Queen Alexandra's Imperial Nursing Service [sic], founded in 1913, with Miss H McLean [sic] as Matron-in-Chief, had as yet no names on its roll.'[25] This brief statement hides the work that the New Zealand nursing service had required to get to the point where there was even recognition in the military for a need for such a service. There was no organised military nursing at the time of the South African War. Nevertheless, New Zealand nurses were approved to travel overseas. In the course of the war, a total of 27 nurses served in South Africa, though all of them served with the PCANSR and not with New Zealand medical units.

In 1907, Princess Christian wrote to the New Zealand Government to suggest that a committee should be formed to enrol nurses in an affiliated branch of the QAIMNS. This led to the formation of the New Zealand Medical Corps Nursing Reserve (NZMCNR) in 1908, and the first matron-in-chief, Janet Gillies, was appointed to set up the nursing service and enrol suitable nurses. This was the first time that nursing had been considered as part of the defence forces of New Zealand.[26] There was immediate interest from nurses, but, for a variety of reasons, mostly administrative, none were enrolled. This remained the situation until 1910, when Matron Gillies was forced to resign and replaced by Matron-in-Chief Hester Maclean, who took up the post of the renamed 'New Zealand Army Nursing Service' (NZANS) in 1910 and remained in position until 1923. Matron Maclean's job was a very difficult one, in so far

---

24 Carberry, *New Zealand Medical Service in the Great War*, p.12.
25 Carberry, *New Zealand Medical Service in the Great War*, p.13.
26 'New Zealand Military Nursing', *NZANS*, <nzans.org>, accessed 9 Feb. 2021.

38   The Fight for Life

that, although there was support in some quarters for the military nursing service, there was considerable inertia in actually getting it organised to a useful service. One of the first steps was to appoint district matrons throughout New Zealand, but it was impossible to enrol nurses since the necessary rules and regulations of their service had not been agreed with the military or the government.[27] This was unfortunate since, upon the outbreak of the war, as Carberry intimated, the nursing service simply did not exist.

However, by the end of August 1914, Matron Maclean had managed to win a concession: she was allowed to appoint six nurses to accompany New Zealand troops sent to occupy German Samoa, where they served for seven months before returning to New Zealand. However, the army nursing service still did not exist, and Minister of Defence James Allen refused to agree to the attachment of nurses to the first New Zealand soldiers to sail for Europe in October 1914. Allen appears to have considered that this was to presume on the needs of the Imperial Government.[28] Pressure was brought on the minister from a number of sources, and, on 25 January 1915, he finally agreed to offer 50 nurses to the British Government, which gratefully accepted. The 50 nurses were chosen from as wide a range of hospitals throughout New Zealand to give a range of knowledge and experience to the service, and they were embarked on the SS *Rotorua* in Wellington on 8 April 1915. This group of nurses travelled via England to Egypt, where they disembarked at Alexandria on 3 June 1915. They were destined to serve in British hospitals in Egypt for the rest of the Gallipoli Campaign. While these nurses were being selected, a request came from the Australian Government for 12 nurses to join a contingent of Australians being prepared. These were provided and embarked on the *Kyarra* at Melbourne on 13 April.[29] New Zealand also sent a stationary hospital (No. 1) to Egypt, but, on 23 October 1915, the HT *Marquette*, carrying the hospital, including its nurses, was torpedoed in the Mediterranean on the way to Salonika, and 10 nurses were drowned.[30]

In addition to these nurses, a further 11 nurses were sent from New Zealand, together with a fully equipped hospital ship, the *Maheno*, in July 1915, and this ship served during the latter half of the Gallipoli Campaign.

Although the NZANS had been rather slow to get involved, before the end of 1915, a total of 278 nurses had embarked for overseas service.[31] By the end of the war, 550 nurses of the NZANS had served overseas.

Canadian Army Medical Corps (CAMC)

The Canadian involvement in the Gallipoli campaign was limited, in so far as it did not send any fighting troops to the peninsula.[32] Nevertheless, the Canadian Army Medical Corps (CAMC)

---

27   'New Zealand Military Nursing', *NZANS*, <nzans.org>, accessed 9 Feb. 2021.
28   'New Zealand History', *NZHistory*, <nzhistory.govt.nz>, accessed 9 Feb. 2021.
29   Peter Rees, *The Other Anzacs: Nurses at War, 1914–1918* (Crows Nest: Allen and Unwin, 2008), p.71.
30   Rees, *Other Anzacs*, p.115ff.
31   Carberry, *New Zealand Medical Service in the Great War*, p.536, Appendix A. Eleven of these nurses were embarked for service in Samoa.
32   Note that the Newfoundland Regiment was attached to the 29th Division from September 1915 but that Newfoundland was not a part of Canada at this time, being the tenth province to join the confederation in 1949. At the time of the campaign, Newfoundland was a sovereign state.

was involved in providing three stationary hospitals during the course of the campaign and in the evacuation of sick and wounded by hospital ship on one occasion.

In 1867, the British forces were removed from Canada, and, similar to Australia, the military medical services were removed with them. In that year, the first four provinces formed the Confederation, with a further five provinces joining by 1905. The Dominion of Canada was left with no provision for its military at this time, and the void was filled by the formation of militia regiments in the various provinces as the need arose. Development of its military was slow, as was the medical services within it. At this time, each militia regiment had its own surgeon attached, though, as to be expected, these men mostly maintained their civilian practices whilst being involve in the militia. There was no specific training in military matters for the MOs thus involved, and the military relied on the local practitioners to meet their need.

A small permanent medical force developed as the permanent military force began to develop around garrisoned towns throughout the country, but the development was slow such that, by 1885, at the time of the Riel Rebellion, the 'medical services were crude'.[33] Nevertheless, in such a small campaign involving no more than 4,000 men, the medical services were adequate if not properly organised.

It was not until 1896 that the medical sub-department of the militia was created, and it is from this point that the Canadian Army Medical Service developed. At this time, there was the Permanent Active Medical Corps, of the permanent force, and the Army Medical Corps of the Militia. The combination of these two aspects was an important feature of the development, and, for the first time, a DGMS was appointed in the form of Colonel Hubert Nelson. Nelson had trained at Netley in Great Britain and had been attached to the RAMC for a number of years, and so it was, perhaps, inevitable that he urged the Canadian Army to adopt the medical provisions similar to those of the RAMC. There had been a bearer company, along the lines of those in Great Britain, prior to this, but, under the leadership of Nelson, six bearer companies and six field hospitals were formed by 1899. This was thus the formation of the Army Medical Corps. Alongside this, the Regimental Medical Service was also formed, drawing its officers from those RMOs of the existing regiments.

During the South African War, the Canadians sent fighting troops to assist with the campaign, and the Regimental Medical Service was thus represented. In January 1902, the 10th Canadian Field Hospital was also sent to support the troops already there. The Canadian unit took its own specially adapted equipment and wagons with it. Most notably, perhaps, was the 'Hubert tent', named for the first DGMS.

Following the South Africa War, the development continued much as that of the RAMC, and the field ambulance was formed. In Canada, this was not done by combining the existing bearer companies and field hospitals but rather by enlarging each section to provide the staff each was lacking.[34] However, the biggest difference in the formation of the field ambulance was that Canada only looked to provide one section of each unit. That is, instead of a wartime establishment of 10 officers and 241 other ranks, each Canadian field ambulance was to have a peace-time establishment of 10 officers and only 75 other ranks. In this manner, a framework was formed of experienced and trained officers and men in each ambulance whose ranks could be filled in

---

33   John G. Adami, *War Story of the Canadian Army Medical Corps: The First Contingent, to the Autumn of 1915* (London: The Rolls House Publishing Co., 1918), vol. 1, p.12.

34   Adami, *War Story of the Canadian Army Medical Corps*, vol. 1, p.20.

wartime. In 1904, the medical services officially became the CAMC. Throughout the years to the start of the First World War, the MOs worked hard at training their units so that, by 1914, the Canadian medical services were probably better prepared for warfare than most of the other combatant nations, and there had been a particular drive in training men in the importance of sanitation, especially by making it more or less part of everyone's responsibility, and the understanding of how bacteriological influence affected armies in the field. As part of this growth in the medical services, the need for hospitals was also recognised, and, immediately upon the outbreak of war, the Canadian Medical Corps began to mobilise a number of stationary and general hospitals, again along the lines of those adopted in the RAMC. No. 1, No. 3 and No. 5 Canadian Stationary Hospitals (CSHs) played a role in the Gallipoli Campaign.

In Canada, the military nursing services were well organised and, in at least one aspect, different to those nursing services in other countries. This was because, when the service was created as the Army Nursing Sisters (ANS), it was done so as part of the army medical services. That is, the nurses had the same chain of command as the other medical personnel in the army, and they were not, as in other countries, an auxiliary service to the military. At the same time as the service was created, rules and regulations were set down as to qualifications and training required and that all fully trained nursing sisters would enter the armed forces as lieutenants. This gave the members of the army nursing service immediate military status.[35] This avoided some of the administrative problems that arose in other nursing services. Their first matron was Miss G. Pope, who had been awarded the Royal Red Cross (RRC) for her service in the South African War.

As the Canadian nurses were within the armed forces, it meant that they were more familiar with the methods of their army, and so, before the war, there was a body of well-trained nurses experienced in the ways of the military and ready to take to the field. Although the Canadian Medical Service played a relatively minor part in the Gallipoli Campaign, the army nursing service was represented in all three of the stationary hospitals provided by Canada.

Indian Medical Service (IMS)

The Indian Medical Service (IMS) was essentially a military medical service, although the serving officers usually had some commitment to civil practice during their stay on the subcontinent. The IMS traced its origin to the surgeons on the first ships of the East India Company to trade there in the early 1600s. However, it was not until the second half of the eighteenth century that the service began to be organised, with the formation of the Bengal Medical Service. This was the first of the Presidencies of British India to set out the fixed grades for MOs and the necessary rules for promotion of those officers. This was soon followed by the Presidencies of Madras and Bombay, which developed their medical services along similar lines. During the nineteenth century, the medical services associated with the presidencies grew, and, in 1855, the first Indians entered the service. They were thereafter to form an integral part of the service.[36]

---

35   Adami, *War Story of the Canadian Army Medical Corps*, vol. 1, p.33.
36   'Indian Medical Service', *Wikipedia*, <https://en.wikipedia.org/wiki/Indian_Medical_Service>, accessed 2 Feb. 2021.

During the nineteenth century, the IMS became an effective reserve of MOs for the military in India, and its members took part in almost all the conflicts on both the sub-continent and overseas where the Indian Army was involved.[37] In 1891, IMS officers were first given military rank and afforded the privileges of those ranks. In 1895, the three Presidency Armies amalgamated, and the medical services of those armies likewise amalgamated on 1 April 1896.[38] At this stage, there was some reorganisation of the service, and as the profession as a whole grew in India so did the military medical service. There was a tendency for the service to follow the approach that was being adopted at this time in Britain, but there were significant differences that continued to the First World War.

The MOs of the service had made significant steps in the control of disease by instructing the Indian Army in hygiene and sanitation so that, by the beginning of the First World War, the Indian soldier was considered to be well disciplined in sanitation and conservancy, that is, the disposal of waste.[39] This was to prove to be of considerable importance in the context of the Gallipoli Campaign.

At the beginning of the war, the establishment of medical services for the Indian Army was such that five field ambulances were allotted to each division. This was two more than allotted to a division in the British Army at the time. Each division of the Indian Army comprised both British and Indian battalions, and this was reflected in the arrangements for field ambulances since each division had two that served only the British battalions while there were three that served the Indian battalions. The former units were known, confusingly, as 'British field ambulances' and the latter as 'Indian field ambulances'. Each field ambulance comprised four sections, with a capacity to treat 25 sick or wounded at any one time. This meant that a field ambulance in the IMS had accommodation for 100 patients whilst, in the British Army, the total accommodation was 150 patients. However, since there were five field ambulances in a division, this gave a total accommodation for 500 patients in the division to which it was attached. This was slightly lower in the British equivalent, with accommodation for 450.[40]

Each field ambulance had a staff of five MOs supplemented by eight assistant or sub-assistant surgeons (SASs) of the Indian Subordinate Medical Department (ISMD). In the British field ambulances, the officers were of the RAMC, with the required number of assistant surgeons. In the Indian field ambulances, the officers were all from the IMS, with the required number of SASs. In the Indian divisions, the staffing of British field ambulances was:

- Four pack store sergeants
- One supply and transport sergeant
- Eight nursing orderlies selected for the British infantry battalions of the division
- 50 men of the Army Hospital Corps (Indian staff) who served as ward servants, cooks, water carriers and sweepers
- 133 men of the Army Bearer Corps to act as stretcher-bearers.[41]

---

37 Donald MacDonald, 'The Indian Medical Service. A Short Account of Its Achievements 1600 – 1947', *Proceedings of the Royal Society of Medicine*, 49:1 (1955), pp.13–17.

38 Lieutenant Colonel D. G. Crawford, *A History of the Indian Medical Service, 1600–1913* (London: W. Thacker & Co., 1914), vol. 2, p.328.

39 Lieutenant Colonel J. W. B. Merewether and Lieutenant Colonel Sir Frederick Smith, *The Indian Corps in France* (London: John Murray, 1918), p.494.

40 Macpherson, *History of the Great War: Medical Services*, vol. 2, p.117.

41 Macpherson, *History of the Great War: Medical Services*, vol. 2, p.118.

In Indian field ambulances, the staffing was similar except that the 50 men of the Army Hospital Corps were replaced by eight ward orderlies and a total 14 cooks, water carriers and sweepers found from the Indian battalions of the division. A similar arrangement was adopted for cavalry divisions in India, but, in France in 1914, this was modified to form a combined ambulance where one section was of a British field ambulance and two sections were of an Indian field ambulance.

At the regimental level, the IMS provided an establishment of one RAMC officer, one assistant surgeon, 12 men of the Army Bearer Corps and one man of the Army Hospital Corps for each British battalion. In an Indian battalion, one MO of the IMS was provided, together with one SAS and 12 men of the Army Bearer Corps. These regimental units were allotted only four field stretchers or half that of equivalent units in the British Army.

It should be noted that, at Gallipoli, the Indian Army provided only the 29th Indian Brigade, which comprised four Indian battalions. As such, it is to be expected that the total number of the IMS personnel was reduced to one field ambulance (108th Indian Field Ambulance (IFA)) to serve on the peninsula and one (110th IFA) to serve on Mudros. The 137th Combined IFA also served on the peninsula, serving the 7th Indian Mountain Artillery Brigade.[42]

In keeping with the other armed forces of the day, the IMS also provided for casualty clearing hospitals, though these were usually small units not designed for prolonged stay. Although three went to France, none were provided specifically for the Gallipoli Campaign. However, one CCS, the Indian Clearing Hospital, was established at Ismailia in Egypt on 27 January 1915.[43] In the autumn of 1915, the 108th IFA, then serving at Anzac, established a casualty clearing hospital, by utilizing one of its sections, for the evacuation of Indian troops.

Indian troops had been sent to Egypt early in the war to provide security to the Suez Canal, and a number of medical units also served in Egypt from this time. There were nine field ambulances serving there by the end of 1914, while No. 5 and No. 8 Indian General Hospitals were in Egypt from December 1914. At the same time, the Indian Bombay Presidency General Hospital (BPGH) was also established there, and, since it served there until early 1916, it is reasonable to assume that it acted as a general hospital for those Indian troops serving at Gallipoli as well as those who remained in Egypt defending the Canal.[44]

French Army Medical Service (*Service de Santé des Armées*)

The French Army Medical Service (*Service de Santé des Armées*) was started by Louis XIV when he appointed surgeons to his army in 1708. The service expanded during the Napoleonic Wars but remained relatively unsophisticated until the 1890s, when a number of military hospitals and two medical schools were set up in France. Nevertheless, by the start of the First World War, the *Service de Santé des Armées* was seen to be rather backward by the other Allies, and, indeed, it was commented that it was where the British had been at the time of the Crimean War almost 60 years earlier.[45]

---

42   This brigade was classed as 'Corps Troops' and comprised the 21st (Kohat) Battery and the 26th (Jacob's) Battery.
43   Macpherson, *History of the Great War: Medical Services*, vol. 3, p.514.
44   Macpherson, *History of the Great War: Medical Services*, vol. 3, p.516.
45   Anon., 'The French Medical Services during the War of 1914-1918', *BMJ Military Health*, 52 (1929), p.38.

Royal Army Medical Corps (RAMC)

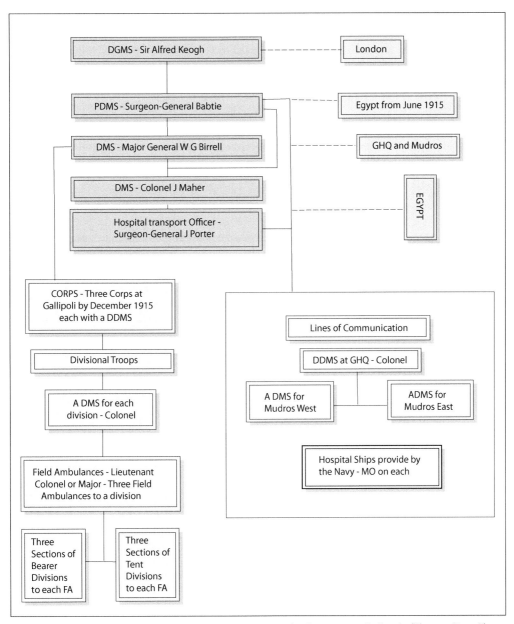

General schematic for the chain of command in the medical services at Gallipoli. (Terence Powell)

44   The Fight for Life

The role of the doctor in the armed forces of France was purely technical, and he served no executive function beyond the command of his own unit. That is, there was no position in the French Army equivalent to the director of medical services (DMS) in the British and Empire Armies of the time. There was, however, provision made prior to the war such that each corps of the army was assigned eight ambulances to serve the two divisions within the corps, and this was the case for the two French divisions serving at Gallipoli.[46] There was some difference between the ambulance of the French service compared with the British model. A French ambulance was, perhaps, rather nearer to that of the bearer division of a British field ambulance, in so far as it was required to give treatment at the equivalent of an advanced dressing station (ADS), or divisional collecting post, before moving the casualty farther down the line to a field hospital, roughly the equivalent of the tent division in the British model. At the outset of the First World War, the philosophy of the French medical services was to get wounded men as far away from the front as possible. This often entailed long journeys to, for instance, Bordeaux. The results of such a policy were considered 'disastrous' since the long journeys had terrible effects upon the badly wounded. However, by 1915, the French had established the principle of a first aid station directly behind the front line, with surgical (mobile or stationary) ambulances a few miles farther back. This was the first point where a wounded man could receive surgical care.[47] It is with this sort of arrangement that the French medical services were engaged in Gallipoli.

As an example of how the French *Service de Santé des Armées* was organised at Gallipoli, it is useful to consider the position of Major Joseph Vassal. Vassal was the SMO for the 6th Mixed Colonial Regiment, which comprised three battalions. This gave him command over no less than 21 MOs distributed throughout the regiment and within the field ambulances serving his brigade.[48] He was ultimately answerable to the divisional surgeon and hence to the director of the *Service de Santé des Armées*. The units worked similarly to the British medical units, but, because of the different organisation of the battalions within a regiment, the role of an RMO was different and required a relatively senior officer, in this case Vassal, to coordinate the work of the battalion MOs with that of the field ambulance and clearing stations. The senior RMO was also responsible for the setting up and running of the dressing stations and was heavily involved in the work of the initial treatment of wounded passing through. The model for the Gallipoli Campaign also provided for the use of a hospital ship, the *Duguay-Trouin*, and a number of transports to evacuate the wounded. Initially, these transports acted much as clearing stations, as wounded were successively evacuated to the hospital ship.[49]

General hospitals were also provided for in the general lines of communication for the French forces. During the Gallipoli Campaign, the Bombay Presidency Hospital, in Alexandria, and its staff of the IMS, was handed over to the French as a 500-bed general hospital for wounded French soldiers from the peninsula.[50] In a similar manner, the French also had hospitals, under

---

46   Anon., 'French Medical Services', p.40.
47   Daniel P. Rignault, *The History of the French Military Medical Corps* (Paris: Ministère de la défense, Service de Santé des Armées, 2004), pp.37–40.
48   Anon. [Joseph Vassal], *Uncensored Letters from the Dardanelles* (London: William Heinemann, 1916), p.59.
49   Anon., *Uncensored Letters*, p.66.
50   Butler, *Official History of the Australian Medical Services*, vol. I, p.186 fn. This hospital had arrived in Egypt in December 1914.

the control of the French naval medical director, roughly equivalent to the principal hospital transport officer, at East Mudros during the campaign. This also required the use of at least one French hospital ship to transfer patients to either Alexandria or Mudros throughout the eight months of the campaign. Furthermore, the French Army was to supply a bacteriological laboratory at Helles, and this was of considerable importance until others were established at Mudros, Anzac and Helles by the British.[51] Thus, overall, the approach to the removal of the wounded, and sick, from the battlefields was generally similar to that of the other Allies on Gallipoli but differed somewhat in detail.

At the outbreak of the war, there was a complete lack of organised system of trained nurses in the French military machine. This is partly because nursing had traditionally been carried out by nuns. Whilst this had largely disappeared by the time of the war, there had been little move to improve the situation in the military. Schools for nursing, such as that of Dr Anna Hamilton at Bordeaux, had been established, but few women had passed through them by the outbreak of war. After the Battle of the Marne in 1914, the lack of preparedness of the French medical services became very clear, and senior staff of the French Army recognised the need for good nursing. Miss Grace Ellison presented a scheme to General Troussaint by which trained British nurses could be employed by the French, and he accepted. These nurses became known as the 'French Flag Nursing Corps' (FFNC) and started their service in October 1914.[52] During the course of the war, between 250–300 British nurses served with it. It is not known how many, if indeed any, such nurses served with the French services during the Gallipoli Campaign, but it is to be expected that the French provided some nurses to assist on their hospital ships and in the hospitals based on Mudros at this time.

Medical Services and Evacuation of Wounded

At this stage, it is necessary to consider the basic outline of the medical services that were to operate during the campaign. The medical services of the Allied nations were broadly similar in their approach to delivering care. The general approach to the evacuation of the wounded from the front line can be summarised briefly:

- Regimental aid post (RAP) – usually the first point of contact for a wounded man with the medical profession
- ADS – set up by a field ambulance to care for wounded coming from the line
- Field ambulance – essentially a field hospital serving the wounded of a brigade
- CCS – used to clear the wounded from the field ambulances, the first stage of the lines of communication
- Stationary hospital – the next stage in the lines of communication, often a large hospital that would accommodate wounded from more than one CCS
- General hospital – a large base hospital with capacity for around 1,000 sick and wounded.

---

51 Macpherson, *History of the Great War: Medical Services*, vol. 4, p.43.
52 Captain G. R. Bruce, 'Military Hospitals in Malta during the War: A Short Account of Their Inception and Development', *ScarletFinders*, <http://www.scarletfinders.co.uk/190.html>, accessed 13 Feb. 2021.

46 The Fight for Life

MOVEMENT OF A CASUALTY

The general movement of a casualty from the front to hospital during the Gallipoli Campaign can be summarised as shown below:

		Place	Medical Stage	Staff	
BATTLE ZONE			Regimental Aid Post	Regimental MO (RAMC etc)	**Divisional Troops**
		Peninsula under Field Ambulance control	Advanced Dressing Station and Dressing Station	Medical Officers and Orderlies Bearers of RAMC, etc	
LINES OF COMMUNICATION		Peninsula	Casualty Clearing Station	Medical Officers and Orderlies RAMC, etc	
		At Sea - Navy control	Tows from shore	Orderlies and on occasion MO's	**Transport Ships provided by Navy Staffed by RAMC**
			Hospital Ships	MO's Nurses and MO's	
			Hospital Carriers	MO's and Orderlies not permanent	
			Fleet Sweepers	MO's not permanent	
		Mudros and Imbros	Casualty Clearing Stations	Medical Officers and Orderlies RAMC, etc	
		Mudros, Imbros (Peninsular late in Campaign)	Stationary Hospital	MO's Nurses and Orderlies. (nurses did not serve on peninsular)	
		Mudros	General Hospital	MO's Nurses and Orderlies	
	BASE	Egypt, Malta and UK	General Hospitals	MO's Nurses and Orderlies	

This is simplified in so far as not all casualties would have experienced each of the stages and some of the stages such as collection posts, etc., have been omitted

Schematic for the evacuation of wounded. (Terence Powell after Butler 1938)

The RAP was essentially an MO, the RMO, attached to a battalion to offer immediate care in or very near the firing line. This MO was given the service of regimental stretcher-bearers, who moved any casualties needing further treatment to the ADS.

The ADS was in an advanced position, was staffed by members of a field ambulance and followed the advancing infantry closely so as to offer medical assistance close to the firing line. There was little capacity for holding patients, and there was a reliance on the availability of stretcher-bearers to move the casualties rapidly to the main field ambulance.

The field ambulance was the main medical care facility for the units in the line. That is, they were part of an infantry division usually assigned to a brigade and usually took casualties from that brigade. The ambulance was, in reality, a field hospital offering basic medical care, sometimes including surgery, that was necessary to save a life before the casualty was moved down the line. The field ambulance had a capacity for about 100 casualties depending on the situation, but, during the Gallipoli Campaign, this was often exceeded since casualties tended to accumulate quickly during offensives.

Close to the front, the larger hospitals geared more towards emergency medicine were known as CCSs. In the early days of the war, these hospitals were staffed only by MOs and orderlies, and, although on the Western Front these were later to have nurses on their staff, this was never the case at Gallipoli. These essentially mobile hospitals brought a high standard of medical care as close as possible to the fighting. Here, the care was primary, cleaning and dressing wounds, preventing bleeding, administering basic surgery and moving the casualty along the lines of communication as quickly as possible. There was no intention for long-term care at the CCS – the patient was moved as soon as his condition was stabilised. Here, the patients spent as short a time as possible, and the turnover was very high, as they were evacuated, often within hours, for more intensive care farther down the line. CCSs eventually worked in pairs on the Western Front, with wounded being directed to one at a time until it was full and the other came online. This helped to prevent overcrowding and chaotic treatment occurring; it also helped with the evacuation of wounded since convoys were better able to cope with a more controlled flow of wounded. This level of organisation was never reached on the Gallipoli Peninsula. The lack of success of the overall campaign, including the lack of space on the beachheads, did not allow for this approach.

The stationary hospital was the next type of hospital in the hierarchy of the medical services. It was a hospital that was similar to a general hospital, in that it offered a wide range of facilities for treatment of sick and wounded but was not really set up for long-term care. Frequently, these hospitals were closer to the front than the general hospitals, and, during the Gallipoli Campaign, a number were set up on Lemnos, where they ultimately offered support to the general hospital. Later in the campaign, two such hospitals were set up on the peninsula. In the normal situation, evacuation of patients from the stationary hospitals would take place by motor ambulance or rail, but, at Gallipoli, the transport was by sea in the first instance, using fleet sweepers or hospital ships. The principle was that the hospital referred to the staff and equipment, and the hospital could be moved easily when required.

The final point of the evacuation on the lines of communication was the general hospital. General hospitals, as the name suggests, were large hospitals equipped to give long-term care, if necessary, to a wide variety of cases, both wounded and sick. They were the base hospitals and were, of necessity, situated at a distance from the front line. The general hospital should not be considered as a building since it was really the staff and equipment that constituted the hospital so that, when it was necessary to move as a result of the exigencies of war, the whole hospital could be re-sited elsewhere with minimum disruption. Thus, No. 3 Australian General Hospital (AGH) was first set up at Lemnos during the Gallipoli Campaign, moved to Egypt after the evacuation of the peninsula and successively served in Brighton in the United Kingdom and thence in Abbeville in France. The organisation of the hospital remained essentially the same. Staff changed slowly, but the hospital remained No. 3 AGH.

Related to the general hospital but separate from it was the auxiliary hospital. These were set up to offer long-term, often specialist care for soldiers who were recovering from severe trauma. They were not convalescents but were recovering and, in many cases, were on their way to being declared fit for front-line duty. No. 1 Australian Auxiliary Hospital (AAH) was set up in Egypt during the campaign and essentially acted to support No. 1 AGH at Heliopolis in Egypt.

Another important aspect of the medical services, which is sometimes overlooked, was that of the hospital ships. These ships provided the transport for the wounded from rear areas of battlefields to general hospitals and provided care for the wounded in many areas of the conflict. They were also particularly well developed during the Gallipoli Campaign since their sea journeys were generally longer than those associated with, for instance, the Western Front. Here, the hospital ship acted very much like a CCS, in that they were stationed very close to the peninsula and the beaches from which they frequently received the wounded more or less directly. During the campaign, the hospital ships began by carrying most of the wounded back to Alexandria, where they were distributed amongst the general hospitals in both Alexandria and Cairo. All hospital ships carried nursing sisters, except those serving the Indian forces for instance, and, for nurses, the hospital ship was an immediate contact with the fighting and the treatment of the wounded. It was also the closest that nursing staff came to the fighting on the peninsula. For many nurses, service on such ships was considered vital to the survival of the patient. At first, the use of hospital ships did not progress well, but, as the organisation improved, the hospital ships provided the early care that helped to save lives. As the campaign progressed and hospitals in Egypt became full, it was necessary to take wounded to other places such as Malta, and the hospital ships traversed the Mediterranean over many months, carrying their patients to relative safety. For the nurses, the hospital ships were seen as important because of the immediate care they were able to offer, but there was a price to pay since nurses often found the conditions difficult as they fought overcrowding and lack of supplies in the heat of the summer in the Mediterranean, and, for some, a few months on board such a ship was more than enough. The work was hard, and there was no relief from the problems in the closed environment of the ship. Nevertheless, there were always nurses ready to step forwards and take their place on the ships.

During the evacuation from the battlefield, the soldier was likely to have experienced many of the types of hospitals discussed above, though not necessarily all of them. Soldiers arriving, for instance, at an ADS would probably have received little attention other than perhaps the application of a field dressing, more than likely applied directly upon a dirty wound as the soldier was carried away from the battlefield. At the field ambulance or CCS, the first response was to begin cleaning both the soldier and, more crucially, his wound. In many cases, the extent of the wound would not necessarily have been clear until layers of dirty uniform had been cut away and the surrounding tissue cleaned. However, this was sometimes not possible because of the rapid influx of wounded, which resulted in men being transferred to a hospital ship more or less untreated where the wound was then attended to, in the first instance most likely by a nursing sister.

The proximity to the firing line impacted the work that was possible, both from the point of view of the need to evacuate the men quickly and because of the danger in which the medical staff worked. This, too, can be said of the hospital ships, which were considered by some the most hazardous work in which a nurse could be engaged during the war.[53] In the case of hospital ships serving to evacuate the wounded from Gallipoli, they were little more than floating CCSs and were frequently within range of the Turkish guns whilst nurses carried out the washing, cleaning and dressing of wounds and prepared the more seriously wounded for surgery. It was common for the hospital ships in such places to receive the wounded directly from the battlefield in much the same way as a CCS on land.

Of course, not all hospital casualties were the result of traumatic injuries on the battlefield. From the outset of the war, military hospitals found it necessary to accommodate a variety of infectious diseases amongst their medical cases. Some diseases such as measles and mumps would be considered little more than a childhood inconvenience today, but, 100 years ago, an outbreak of such a disease in a military camp could cause many hospital admissions. For trained medical staff, these would have been more familiar complaints to handle since they would have come across them frequently and knew that, with care and appropriate management, there was every chance of recovery. For staff serving in Egypt during the time of the Gallipoli Campaign, there was a first rush of wounded men caused by the heavy fighting. As the months passed, the casualties arriving from the peninsula were increasingly suffering from enteric fever, diarrhoea and dysentery. The care for such patients was often intensive to ensure recovery, which did not always occur. There was strict attention to diets and, above all, to sanitation and cleanliness. In wards full of patients with gastrointestinal conditions, the need to keep the patient, ward and medical staff thoroughly clean was essential, and, as ever, the protocols in place were adhered to and enforced by the nurses. In some places, such as at Choubra in Egypt, special hospitals for infectious diseases were established. Choubra caused a certain amount of trepidation amongst the nurses sent there for duty, but the practices set in place to care for the sick prevented medical staff from succumbing to the diseases they treated.[54]

The level to which the medical services were able to work during the campaign was largely dependent upon the situation on the peninsula. At times of great stress during the main offensives, the medical services struggled to cope with the influx of cases, and this was not only in the immediate battle zone but also all along the lines of communication to the base hospitals around the Mediterranean theatre of operation. The following chapters will examine the work of the medical services throughout the campaign.

---

53 Christine E. Hallett, *Containing Trauma: Nursing Work in the First World War* (Manchester: Manchester University Press, 2009), p.134.
54 Australian War Memorial (AWM) PR85/374: Samsing, Hilda Theresa Redderwold (Sister, b.1871–d.1957), 'Diary of Samsing (1914-1918)'.

2

Based on the Assumption
Medical Services and Planning for the Campaign

The naval bombardment of the forts in the Dardanelles commenced on 19 February 1915, and it is from this action that the remainder of the campaign flowed. It was initially intended to be a naval assault on Turkey, without the need of support from ground troops, to force the Narrows and thereby attack Constantinople and bring about a Turkish surrender. It soon became clear that this would not be the case, and troops of the British Empire were soon involved. However, there was much procrastination before a decision was finally made to use a military force to secure the fortresses that had been reduced by the firepower of the Royal Navy. On this same day, 19 February, it is interesting to note that the DGMS, Sir W. Keogh, at Whitehall appointed Colonel J. Maher as DMS for the Mediterranean. This post, at this time, included supervision of the medical establishments from Gibraltar to Egypt. It is probably the only time during the entire 1915 campaign in the Mediterranean of which it can be said that the medical services took the initiative without awaiting the direction of the War Council in London. However, as there were no military forces in the planning for an assault against Turkey, Keogh's appointment of Maher must be seen as fortuitous rather than prescient.

General Sir Ian Hamilton was appointed commander-in-chief of the yet-to-be-formed Mediterranean Expeditionary Force (MEF) on 12 March 1915 and started planning for what became the Gallipoli Campaign. This was a week after the first Australian troops, the 3rd Australian Brigade, had arrived in Mudros Harbour and had signalled the ultimate intentions of the Allies in their approach towards Turkey. It was clear to the Turks a month before the landings on the peninsula were finally made that the intention was to land upon their shores. Turkey only needed to know exactly when and where, but that did not stop them from making some preparations.

To his credit, Hamilton did what he could to get things moving, arriving on Mudros on 17 March, just days after his appointment as commander-in-chief. He completed a 'sail by' reconnaissance of the coastline of the Gallipoli Peninsula the following day. Whilst he was, at that time, beginning to make plans for the military assault on the peninsula, he did not have a complete staff and no medical input to the plans he was making. The medical issues were not uppermost in his thinking at this time as he considered the strategic aim, of knocking Turkey out of the war, of his campaign.

Before looking at the medical services planning for the Campaign, it is significant to consider the overall medical provisions in the Mediterranean theatre that were available to Hamilton or that could be called upon and expanded as and when needed.

Egypt was to prove to be crucial to the initial planning of the medical services for the campaign and became increasingly important as the months wore on and casualties mounted. The pre-war garrison of Egypt, all regulars, had a small medical establishment comprising 20 officers and 116 other ranks of No. 33 Company RAMC. This unit was, in early 1914, distributed amongst hospitals in Cairo, Alexandria, Khartoum and Cyprus.[1] The main hospital was the Citadel in Cairo, which had an accommodation of 200 beds but was capable of being expanded from stores already in Egypt to over 540 beds. Ras-el-Tin in Alexandria accommodated 100 beds, and Khartoum only 70. The two small hospitals on Cyprus, used mainly for convalescents from Egypt, accommodated only 16. There was also a small hospital at Abbassia under a SAS of the ISMD to care for the Indian establishment of the pre-war garrison. Added to the RAMC and ISMD establishment were 17 members of the QAIMNS distributed between the hospitals in Cairo, Alexandria and Khartoum. There were also two modern Egyptian Army hospitals under PMO Lieutenant Colonel H. A. Bray, which were generally reserved for the Egyptian Army garrison.

When war began, most of the British garrison of regulars was withdrawn to assist in completing the formation of the 28th and 29th Divisions in the United Kingdom. The regular troops were replaced by units of the TF from the 42nd Division. At this time, of course, there was little thought of an assault on Turkey. The main purpose of the forces in Egypt was to secure the Suez Canal, on which so much depended for the British cause. To this end, further Indian units arrived during November 1914 and were formed into the 10th and 11th Indian Divisions.[2]

During this general reorganisation of the garrison in Egypt, most of the RAMC was also withdrawn, leaving Colonel N. Manders as deputy director of medical services (DDMS) and Major H. V. Bagshawe as deputy assistant director of medical services (DADMS) sanitation. Lieutenant Colonel H. T. Knaggs was then the SMO in Cairo, and Lieutenant Colonel T. B. Beach held a similar post in Alexandria. The 42nd Division had its own ADMS in Colonel J. B. Mann and its associated field ambulance units. Colonel W. H. B. Robinson of the IMS was DDMS for Indian forces in Egypt, whilst Surgeon General William Williams, AAMC, was the SMO for the Australian forces that began arriving in Egypt at the beginning of December 1914. This organisation tended to produce duplication in the medical administration, which was, at least to some extent, solved by the appointment of Surgeon General R. Ford to DMS to Sir John Maxwell's staff in Egypt, making him the senior officer in Egypt, from mid-December onwards. The senior medical staff in Egypt at that time was:

- Surgeon General R. Ford, DMS, Egypt
- Colonel N. Manders, ADMS, Cairo
- Colonel T. B. Beach, ADMS, Alexandria
- Colonel W. H. B. Robinson, IMS, DDMS Indian forces and Canal Defences (ADsMS appointed to each of the new divisions)

---

1   Macpherson, *History of the Great War: Medical Services*, vol. 4, p.363. Khartoum is in Sudan but was, at this time, under British administration.
2   Macpherson, *History of the Great War: Medical Services*, vol. 4, p.364.

- Surgeon General William Williams, SMO Australian and New Zealand forces, Egypt
- Colonel N. H. Howse, ADMS 1st Australian Division
- Colonel W. T. Will, NZAMC, ADMS New Zealand and Australian Division.

The 42nd (East Lancashire) Division TF was accompanied by its field ambulances, but, initially, hospital accommodation was that provided mainly by the Citadel in Cairo and Ras-el-tin in Alexandria. With the arrival of the Australians and New Zealanders in December 1914, things began to change. The first convoy from Australia also included 25 nurses, nominally under Matron Nellie Gould, who were, for the most part, sent to set up a hospital in the Mena House Hotel near the pyramids at Gizeh.[3] This hospital was first staffed by the RAMC, with Sister M. E. M. Grierson of the QAIMNS as acting matron. This changed in early 1915, by which time the hospital was serving the Australians then in training at the nearby Mena Camp. At this time, the Australian Army Medical Service took over, Matron Gould was placed in charge of the nursing staff, and Major R. J. Millard, 1st AFA, AAMC, was placed in temporary command of the hospital.[4] The Australians had recognised the need to provide both general and stationary hospitals, and these arrived in Egypt in early 1915 when:

- No. 1 AGH was set up in the Heliopolis Palace Hotel from 25 January.
- No. 1 Australian Stationary Hospital (ASH) was set up at Mena Camp but soon moved to Suez Canal following Turkish attacks there.

Both these hospitals were initially set up to serve the New Zealand and Australian Division.[5] At the same time:

- No. 2 AGH was set up at Mena House from 25 January 1915.
- No. 2 ASH was set up on an adjacent site at Gizeh.

These hospitals served the 1st Australian Division and came under the overall control of ADMS Colonel Neville Howse VC.[6]

No. 1 and No. 2 ASHs both later served during the Gallipoli Campaign: No. 1 ASH was based at Lemnos until November when it landed on the peninsula, while No. 2 assisted in staffing hospital ships and hospital carriers until it set up a hospital at Mudros West. The development of these hospitals in Egypt became an important part of the medical services in Egypt during the Gallipoli Campaign. No. 2 AGH moved to the larger Gezireh Palace Hotel, using Mena House as an overflow building to allow a total accommodation of 1,000 beds. No. 1 AGH expanded into buildings near the Heliopolis Palace Hotel, including the Luna Park fun fair, the so-called 'Atelier' and other buildings, which eventually gave the hospital a total accommodation of 8,000 beds. The general hospitals had some problems in coping with buildings that were not designed as hospitals. No. 1 AGH was in a very smart hotel, but that did not make it

---

3 John Dixon, *Army Nurse: The Matron Who Went to War* (Llangan: Cwm Press, 2019), p.72.
4 AWM: AWM 1DRL/0499, RCDIG0000181: Typescript Extracts from Diary of Sir Reginald Jeffery Millard.
5 Butler, *Official History of the Australian Medical Services*, vol. I, p.62.
6 Butler, *Official History of the Australian Medical Services*, vol. I, p.61.

a building at all suited as a hospital, and it was described as '… an immense place and has not proper wards'.[7] Sister Annie Kidd-Hart was detailed for duty at No. 1 AGH and was placed in charge of an officers' ward but found it very difficult to manage because of the number of small rooms she was required to supervise. However, Sister Kidd-Hart also pointed out that the hospital was very well equipped.[8] As this hospital expanded, first to Luna Park, similar problems were met:

> I was sent to No. 1 AAH, Luna Park, Heliopolis, which was in its early stages of organization and very chaotic. The conditions were very bad indeed. Food, clean linen and clothing were all most difficult to obtain and the heat and the flies and the dust made life a misery. Later, as the place became more organized, things were adjusted. We had the overflow patients from No. 1 AGH and they were all very badly wounded. There were men who arrived from Gallipoli still having their field dressings on after five or six days.[9]

There were also practical problems involved in adapting buildings to use as military hospitals. Luna Park, for instance, had problems getting water to all the various parts of the hospital, and it relied on a lot of local labour to ensure that patients could be washed and wounds cleansed.[10] Also, in most of the commandeered buildings, there were no adequate sanitary facilities, and, in most cases, one of the earliest jobs was to provide sufficient latrines and sluice facilities. Nevertheless, Luna Park, as No. 1 AAH, eventually had accommodation for approximately 1,600 cases.

By June 1915, the accommodation available in Egypt was becoming overcrowded, and more buildings were adapted: 'The Atelier was a large shed which had previously been a furniture depository and held about 800 beds. We took in all kinds of patients, surgical and medical. The flies, dust and heat proved a great nuisance and we suffered much discomfort from them.'[11] To accommodate 800 patients, it was necessary for the Atelier to expand into tented wards in the grounds, but, in the early days, 'It was very badly equipped and, therefore, everything was muddled'.[12] Whilst it had been anticipated that there would be a need for general hospitals in Egypt, the scale of the need had been greatly underestimated, and the adaptation of the medical services to the pressures of the time showed much skill and determination to achieve the final accommodation that was made available in Egypt. The Australians also provided the only CCS in Egypt at this time, No. 1 Australian Casualty Clearing Station (ACCS), and this unit moved to the Gallipoli Peninsula with the opening of the campaign.

Whilst the need for hospitals in Egypt may have been recognised in Britain at the end of 1914, the immediacy was not realised until the planning for operations in the area had been started.

---

7   AWM: AWM41/1072: [Official History, 1914-18 War: Records of Arthur G Butler:] Interviews Containing Accounts of Nursing Experiences in the AANS [Australian Army Nursing Service]. These Nurses Were Interviewed by Matron Kellett [Index to Interviews of Members of AANS Included in File], Miss L. Comber.
8   AWM: AWM41/1072: Kellett Interviews, Miss A. Kidd-Hart.
9   AWM: AWM41/1072: Kellett Interviews, Miss C. P. Hodsgson.
10   AWM: AWM41/1072: Kellett Interviews, Miss E. J. Smeaton-White.
11   AWM: AWM41/1072: Kellett Interviews, Miss V. E. Drewett.
12   AWM: AWM41/1072: Kellett Interviews, Miss E. J. Smeaton-White.

54   The Fight for Life

Nevertheless, No. 15 and No. 17 General Hospitals arrived in Alexandria in March 1915, with the former hospital going in the Abbassia Schools buildings and the latter in the Victoria College. These were followed in June by No. 19 and No. 21 General Hospitals, which also moved into buildings in Alexandria. All hospitals were nominally under the newly appointed Surgeon General Birrell, DMS of the MEF, who arrived in Egypt on 1 April.[13]

No. 15 and No. 17 British General Hospitals (BGHs) arrived in Egypt without any nursing staff, and one of their first tasks was to try and find such staff locally. Some were found from the local civilian nursing staff, and some were loaned by the Australians, who, by the time that the British hospitals arrived, had about 200 nurses in Egypt. Miss J. Buchan was one of the Australians who had been sent to No. 15 BGH in Alexandria and pointed out that the '... conditions were very good and the hospital was well equipped'.[14] But, as the Australians had found in Cairo, it was no easy matter to adapt buildings for use as hospitals, and sanitary and cooking facilities were always lacking. It has been recorded that, when No. 21 BGH arrived, Sir Victor Horsley, a surgeon of considerable fame, got down on his hands and knees and helped scrub floors at Ras-el-Tin Barracks in readiness for the hospital to open.[15] With the first rush of wounded from the Gallipoli Campaign, both No. 15 and No. 17 BGHs expanded rapidly to accommodate over 1,000 cases.

The main medical units in Egypt in the months preceding the commencement of the Gallipoli Campaign can be summarised as:

- Field ambulances – arrived with the 42nd Division in September 1914 and were the only medical units immediately available to the British. Field ambulances arrived with the Australians and New Zealanders at the beginning of December 1914.
- CCSs – No. 1 ACCS was the only such unit in Egypt and was removed to Lemnos in March 1915 and thence to Gallipoli.
- Ambulance trains – were constructed in Egypt when the Indian Expeditionary Force arrived in December 1914. Three Indian units (known as X, Y and Z sections) were mobilised in Poona and sent to Egypt to man these trains. Two more trains were formed in June 1915 and staffed from Indian hospitals (see below).
- Hospitals – No. 5 and No. 8 Indian General Hospitals set up with the formation of the 10th and 11th Indian Divisions in December 1914. BPGH arrived in January 1915. No. 1 and No. 2 ASHs and No. 1 and No. 2 AGHs arrived in January 1915. A New Zealand general hospital (later No. 2 New Zealand Stationary Hospital (NZSH)) was formed at Abbassia with the formation of the MEF. No. 15 and No. 17 BGHs arrived in Egypt in March 1915. There was also a French hospital in Alexandria, and, during the campaign, the BPGH was also handed over for the use of French casualties.

By the start of April 1915, the total hospital accommodation in Egypt was 5,000 beds. During the month, there was rapid expansion of some of the hospitals, notably No. 1 AGH, so that, by the end of the month, as casualties began to arrive from the peninsula, the total accommodation

---

13   Macpherson, *History of the Great War: Medical Services*, vol. 4, p.365.
14   AWM: AWM41/1072: Kellett Interviews, Sister J. Buchan.
15   Anon. [a sergeant major], *With the RAMC in Egypt* (London: Cassell & Company, 1918), p.31.

was approximately 15,000 beds. Nevertheless, this was to prove to be inadequate since, by the end of May 1915, more than 17,000 casualties had landed in Egypt.

While all of this had been going on, there had been discussions about the provision of hospital ships for Australian casualties as early as February 1915. These were primarily to be used for the repatriation of Australians and were to work out of Egypt. There seems to have been little done about this issue prior to the actual landings. This was, in part at least, down to the indecisiveness of Australian High Commissioner Sir George Reid and his communications with the Australian Government. Of course, at this stage, there was little thought of the Gallipoli Campaign or the likely needs that it was to throw upon the medical services. This matter of hospital ships for repatriation remained unresolved and, by 26 March, was considered to be a 'very remote' possibility.[16] In a similar manner, the request of the Director General of Australian Medical Services (DGAMS) to Surgeon General Williams for a 1,000-bed general hospital to be provided for Egypt went unheeded, and, as late as 27 March, this was 'still under consideration' by the High Commissioner.[17]

It was not only in Egypt that preparations were being made to receive wounded from the actions on the peninsula. The British garrison in Malta was also to become involved in the provision of medical services for the campaign against the Turks. Malta was similar to Egypt, in so far as it had a peacetime garrison of regular soldiers, and the peacetime RAMC establishment was 23 MOs and 150 other ranks serving with 12 nurses of the QAIMNS. At the outbreak of war, the British regular battalions were recalled and replaced by two battalions of the Malta Militia and TF units, initially of the 1st London Infantry Brigade of the 56th (London) Division.[18] These territorial units were accompanied by TF MOs and by a further four officers and 193 other ranks of the 1st London Field Ambulance, which had arrived on Malta on 14 September 1914. Although the infantry battalions of the division were removed in January 1915, the field ambulance remained and was to form the bulk of the capacity for the medical care on Malta until it, too, was replaced in March 1916 and left to join the division in France. With the recall of the regular forces from the island, Colonel M. W. Russell, the DDMS on Malta, was also transferred, and Lieutenant Colonel R. R. Sleman, RAMC(TF), of the 1st London Field Ambulance took over the position on a temporary basis. In March 1915, Sleman was replaced by Colonel Maher, who was then appointed DDMS for the island, giving up his post as DMS for the Mediterranean with the appointment of Surgeon General Birrell.

The peacetime garrison on Malta was provided with four hospitals. The main hospital and headquarters (HQ) of the RAMC on the island was the Cottonera Military Hospital, close to the southern side of Valletta's Grand Harbour. This hospital had accommodation for 167 patients. There was a comparatively modern hospital at Imtarfa (Mtarfa) in the centre of the island, with accommodation for 55 patients, while at Forrest, near Sliema, there was a 20-bed hospital mainly for venereal cases. In Valletta, there was an old hospital that, although large, had been reduced in capacity in the years before the war so that, by 1914, it had only 36 beds. Added to these four hospitals on Malta, there was also a small military convalescent hospital on Gozo at Fort Chambray and a large naval hospital at Bighi, near to Cottonera.

---

16   Butler, *Official History of the Australian Medical Services*, vol. I, p.101.
17   Butler, *Official History of the Australian Medical Services*, vol. I, p.89.
18   Macpherson, *History of the Great War: Medical Services*, vol. 1, p.235. The four battalions of the London Regiment arrived in Malta with their field ambulance on 14 September 1914.

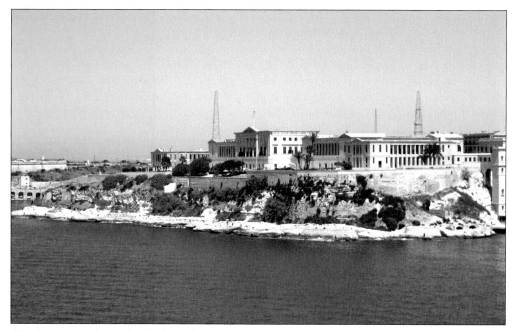

The former naval hospital at Bighi on the southern side of Valletta Grand Harbour, Malta, was one of the many hospitals on the island used during the campaign. (Author)

At first, it was considered unlikely that Malta would become involved in the Mediterranean theatre of operations, but, on 24 February 1915, a telegram was received from Egypt asking what capacity the island could offer for handling sick and wounded. This was responded to immediately, offering 500 beds. At this stage, with the planning for the Gallipoli Campaign still some weeks in the future, it is not surprising that the response from Egypt on 3 March was that the 500 offered beds were not needed. Of course, within weeks, all of that had changed, and the preparations in Malta took on more significance.

Although Malta's offer had been rejected, Governor of Malta Lord Methuen decided to put preparations in place to ensure a measure of readiness on the island should it be called upon. Methuen had taken note of the actions of the Royal Navy against the forts on the Dardanelles to that date and clearly considered that preparation was appropriate. On 14 March, two days after Hamilton had been appointed commander-in-chief of the MEF, Methuen forwarded a plan to the War Office in London for approval. Five days later, he was contacted again by Egypt to ask if Malta could take 500, mostly venereal, patients. The response was positive, and the first patients from Egypt arrived two weeks later. Subsequent to this, on 12 April, the War Office sanctioned the authorities in Malta to look to expand the hospital capacity there to 1,200 beds.

At the beginning of April 1915, the medical personnel of the island were nine MOs, 220 other ranks of the RAMC and 14 nurses of the QAIMNS. To assist with the expansion of the facilities, 25 civilian medical practitioners, 11 nurses and 65 men of the local St John Ambulance Brigade stepped forwards to volunteer to serve until reinforcements arrived from the Great Britain. This helped the expansion to proceed without delay. In addition to these volunteers, on 4 May, the Scottish Women's Hospital, en route for Serbia, disembarked in

Malta and remained for two weeks, giving whatever service it could to help with the expansion. Following its departure, the reinforcements arrived in the form of 82 MOs, 219 nurses and 798 other ranks providing the personnel to complete the work in readiness to receive sick wounded up to the 1,200-bed capacity indicated by the War Office.[19]

The immediate expansion of medical services in Malta affected three of the hospitals of the peacetime establishment. The Cottonera Hospital was expanded from 167 beds to 432 beds by converting the verandas of the existing hospital and taking over the RAMC barracks of the RAMC HQ. The Forrest Hospital was expanded to 186 beds.[20] Finally, the largely disused old hospital in Valletta was reopened and provided accommodation for 524 beds. Elsewhere, the hospital at Imtarfa grew to take 300 venereal cases from Egypt whilst hospitals associated with barracks at St George's and St Andrew's were set up following the commencement of the campaign. These hospitals were to eventually provide 1,685 beds from May 1915, and others were added as the need grew, such as at Tigne and St David's, with a large hospital for 1,184 cases set up at Manoel and opened in November 1915. During the campaign, a total of 28 hospitals on Malta were used by forces involved in the Gallipoli fighting, and a total of 57,991 sick and wounded passed through Malta between the arrival of the first convoy of wounded on 4 May and the end of the campaign.[21] It is not without reason that Malta was known as the 'Nurse of the Mediterranean'.[22]

Situated at the western end of the Mediterranean, Gibraltar was, perhaps, too far from the peninsula to be considered as a location for the provision of major hospital facilities. However, during the campaign, the medical facilities there were expanded and used for a significant number of casualties. The medical facilities at Gibraltar were small but sufficient for its peacetime garrison. At the outbreak of war, the medical personnel comprised 13 MOs, 86 other ranks and nine nurses, providing medical care for a maximum of 160 cases.[23] During the campaign, the hospital facilities were first expanded to 300 beds, and the first wounded were received during May, when seven Australians with badly septic wounds were disembarked from the HS *Letitia*. Thereafter, hospital ships disembarked sick and wounded regularly, and the hospital was expanded to 638 beds. To assist in keeping beds free, a convalescent depot was opened on Windmill Hill to accommodate 579 convalescing soldiers. This, too, was added to later in the campaign. The total capacity at Gibraltar for wounded eventually reached 987 in October 1915.[24] After the evacuation of the peninsula, the hospital accommodation at Gibraltar was reduced rapidly as the need subsided, and, early in 1916, the medical work at Gibraltar fell to what was more or less the same as that of the peacetime garrison. Gibraltar had, nevertheless, provided a valuable medical facility throughout of the campaign.

Two days after Hamilton had completed his reconnaissance of the peninsula from the sea, on 20 March, Surgeon General W. G. Birrell set sail from Great Britain with the rest of the General Staff.[25] Birrell was to take up the position of DMS for the MEF, which was rapidly being

---

19 Macpherson, *History of the Great War: Medical Services*, vol. 1, p.243.
20 Macpherson, *History of the Great War: Medical Services*, vol. 1, p.239.
21 Macpherson, *History of the Great War: Medical Services*, vol. 1, p.247.
22 C. Savona-Ventura, 'Military Hospitals in Malta', *Vassallo History*, <https://vassallohistory.wordpress.com/military-hospitals-in-malta/>, accessed May 2022.
23 Macpherson, *History of the Great War: Medical Services*, vol. 1, p.249.
24 Macpherson, *History of the Great War: Medical Services*, vol. 1, p.250.
25 Colonel W. G. Birrell was appointed surgeon general on 1 March 1915 in order to take up his appointment as DMS of the MEF. He was 55 years of age.

58   The Fight for Life

assembled. As Birrell sailed across the Mediterranean, his commander-in-chief, Hamilton, had cabled Kitchener from Alexandria on 23 March to say that the main features of the landing on the peninsula had been worked out. He had not considered any medical arrangements at that time, concentrating on the higher-level military needs of assembling his force and how he was to deploy it. However, it should have been expected by Birrell that his chief would have allowed some thought to the evacuation and disposal of casualties.

Although Hamilton had made no special consideration of the medical arrangements, they had not been entirely neglected. At an early stage of the planning, the island of Lemnos had been considered as an advanced base for the operations on the peninsula. Colonel Maher visited the island on 15 March to assess its usefulness. Maher's conclusion, which in turn had considerable impact upon the planning for the campaign, was that the island was unsuitable to establish significant medical facilities because of the lack of potable water.[26] This had the result that Lemnos was, at first, only considered as a place for the assembly of troops and not as an advanced base that could provide care for casualties only a matter of hours away from the fighting. Nevertheless, on the same day that Colonel Maher made his assessment, No. 1 ASH was established on the island, complete with 200 tons of equipment, to act as a hospital only for the sick of the units being assembled there.[27] On the other hand, and directly related to Maher's assessment, General Hamilton moved his advanced base from Lemnos to Alexandria and was back in Egypt from 26 March. Alexandria is approximately 750 miles and two-days' sailing from the peninsula. This move was perhaps against Hamilton's better judgement, for, whilst at Lemnos, he recorded:

> Here am I still minus my Adjutant-General; my Quartermaster and my Medical Chief, charged with setting the basic question of whether the Army should push off from Lemnos or from Alexandria. Nothing in the world to guide me beyond my own experience and that of my Chief of the General Staff [CGS] ... I can see that Lemnos is practically impossible; I fix on Alexandria in the light of Braithwaite's advice and my own hasty study of the map. Almost incredible really, we should have to decide so tremendous an administrative problem off the reel and without any Administrative Staff ...[28]

The distance was just one of the challenges for those organising the medical arrangements for the campaign. It was also to be a large-scale seaborne invasion against unknown defences and, possibly, poorly understood topographic and geographic conditions. Although, in theory, the campaign was planned using the *Manual of Combined Naval and Military Operations*, published in 1913, nothing of this type had been attempted before. Thus, the logistical issues were considerable, and everything, including the medical arrangements, had to be completely reconsidered within the framework of the manual to take into account the difficulties that were at least visible to the planners of the campaign.

---

26   Michael B. Tyquin, *Gallipoli: An Australian Medical Perspective* (Newport: Big Sky Publishing, 2012), p.32; Macpherson, *History of the Great War: Medical Services*, vol. 4, p.1. This was presumably based on the report of Colonel Joly de Lotbiniere, Royal Engineers, of some three days earlier.
27   Butler, *Official History of the Australian Medical Services*, vol. I, p.113.
28   General Sir Ian Hamilton, *Gallipoli Diary* (Woking: Unwin Brothers, 1920), vol. 1, p.28.

Medical Services and Planning for the Campaign 59

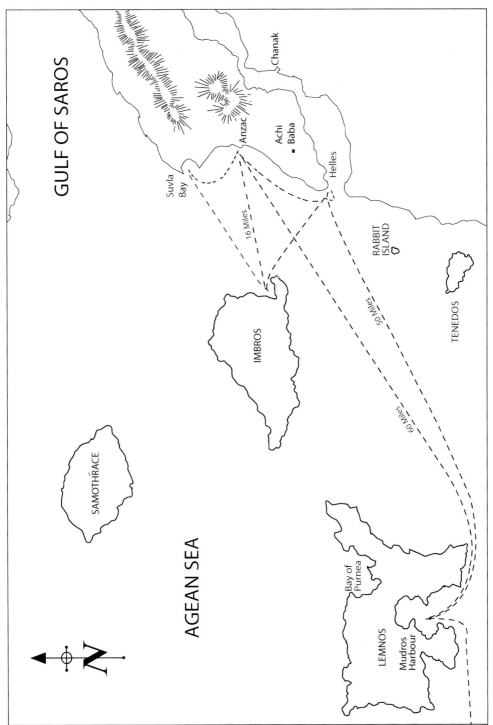

The Gallipoli Peninsula and the nearby Aegean Islands that became important during the campaign. (Terence Powell)

60   The Fight for Life

The medical arrangements that arose were, in their simplest form, considered at this stage by the Staff as follows:

1. Field ambulance units were to land with assaulting troops, with an emphasis on bearer divisions moving first, and then, when appropriate and as necessary, tent divisions or sections of them were to land.
2. CCSs were to land as soon as possible and establish themselves on the beaches as near as possible to the field ambulance unit they were intended to clear.
3. Hospital ships were to stand off ready to receive seriously wounded from the CCSs.
4. The Royal Navy were to provide 'hospital boats' to ferry wounded to hospital ships and temporary hospital ships but not until (i) all infantry had been disembarked and (ii) fighting had moved from the beaches.
5. Temporary hospital ships were to be provided from transports (troopships) to be staffed by members of the field ambulances, CCSs and stationary hospitals depending on availability.
6. All movements of hospital ships and temporary hospital ships were to be controlled by the Royal Navy and not to leave the area until so directed or until they became full.
7. Stationary hospitals were to be landed as soon as it was safe to do so.

According to W. G. Macpherson, 'The whole of the medical arrangements was based on the assumption that a considerable advance inland would immediately follow the landing of the Covering Force'.[29]

This assumption was detrimental not only to the planning for the military campaign and its medical services but also to the care of the wounded as the fighting progressed. Nevertheless, on 4 April, Surgeon General Birrell submitted a proposal to Brigadier General Woodward, Hamilton's deputy adjutant general (DAG), for a ferry service between the Dardanelles and Egypt (or Malta), which would require five hospital ships. Whilst this was acknowledged, the War Office was to inform Egypt three days later that there were only two such ships available, the HS *Sicilia* and the HS *Gascon*.[30] Whilst Birrell was largely excluded from the planning for the campaign, he was making an effort to get his medical service recognised. He was also pointing out to the Staff that there was a need for the lines of communication units to be used in their 'proper sphere' and insisting that a number of stationary hospitals then in Egypt were placed in readiness for their part in the campaign. At first, this was rejected, but the decision was reversed on 17 April, and three hospitals were prepared for departure along with the two advanced medical depots.[31] Even so, the proposals forwarded by Birrell were considered, at that time, to be the minimum for a force of two divisions, and, from the outset, there were to be four divisions included in the opening manoeuvres of the Gallipoli Campaign. It has been said that the medical arrangements, and the campaign as a whole, were based on either total success or total failure, and, as we shall see, neither of these scenarios played out when the landing on the peninsula commenced.[32]

Whilst the overall plan for the attack was completed by 13 April, at that time, there was no plan for the organised disposal of wounded from the four divisions that eventually would

---

29   Macpherson, *History of the Great War: Medical Services*, vol. 4, p.23.
30   Butler, *Official History of the Australian Medical Services*, vol. I, p.102.
31   Butler, *Official History of the Australian Medical Services*, vol. I, p.102.
32   Butler, *Official History of the Australian Medical Services*, vol. I, p.115.

be landed.[33] Even the outline of arrangements given above had not been given to all the units engaged, and, to those who had seen it, there were a number of issues mainly involving the removal of wounded from the beaches. This was further complicated for the Australian and New Zealand Army Corps (ANZAC), in so far as they had little in the way of lines of communication in place. This, according to A. G. Butler, was the responsibility of the Imperial Government, which was 'implicitly undertaking the whole of it' from the provision of hospital ships to all the stores required.[34] It is perhaps in this understanding that much of the problem that later arose with the evacuation of the Australians and New Zealanders can be found. Furthermore, Birrell had been left in Egypt, along with Surgeon General Williams of the AAMC, to arrange the medical facilities there.[35] The only medical representative with the General Staff was Lieutenant Colonel A. E. C. Keble, who was the ADMS for the MEF. Birrell's involvement at an earlier stage probably would have helped both the campaign as a whole and his own understanding of the thinking of the General Staff.

As far as the General Staff was concerned, their concept of how wounded should be dealt with was made on their estimate of no more than 3,000 casualties occurring during the landing. Colonel Keble, acting in the absence of Birrell, disagreed with the figure and set about reviewing and revising the ideas under consideration by the General Staff. A day later, Colonel Keble informed Colonel Howse of the 1st Australian Division, '... that I would probably have to provide a ship for slightly wounded cases and supply 3 MO's and 30 men from FA's [field ambulances]'.[36] By 15 April, Colonel Keble was in the process of consolidating his proposals and issued instruction to the 29th Division, copied to the Australians, to inform both the need for additional transport for wounded. At this stage, he also instructed one tent division to land 'with what they could carry' to act as a dressing station.[37] Keble's intention was that the additional transports would carry both medical staff and the necessary equipment for a 48-hour voyage to Alexandria. There was, at this late stage, some confusion over the transports to be used and how they were to be staffed. Howse was not happy about depleting field ambulances of their staff, and both he and Colonel Yarr, ADMS of the 29th Division, pointed out inadequacies in the overall medical arrangements as late as 15 April. Yarr was told, '... they were the best that could be made under the circumstances'.[38] Colonel Howse was so concerned that he saw the general officer commanding (GOC) of the 1st Australian Division, Major General W. T. Bridges, that day and asked specifically about the arrangements for:

1. Transports for less serious cases
   a. officers and personnel for these,
   b. equipment to be supplied.
2. Hospital ship for seriously wounded cases.[39]

---

33 That is, the 29th Division, the RND, the 1st Australian Division and the New Zealand and Australian Division.
34 Butler, *Official History of the Australian Medical Services*, vol. I, p.86.
35 It is sometimes suggested that Birrell had remained in Egypt because he was sick. There appears to be no clear evidence for this.
36 AWM: AWM4/26/18/5: War Diary, 1st Australian Division ADMS, 14 April.
37 Butler, *Official History of the Australian Medical Services*, vol. I, p.117.
38 The National Archives (TNA) WO 95/4307: War Diary, 29th Division ADMS, 15 April.
39 AWM: AWM4/26/18/5: War Diary, 1st Australian Division ADMS, 15 April.

He was asked by the GOC what arrangements he would support, but, although he was assured that a hospital ship would be provided and a CCS would land, he was not given details of how the transports for less serious cases would operate. Colonel Howse provided recommendations to his corps commander, General Birdwood, through the capable administrator General R. A. Carruthers, detailing that he would select necessary transports and personnel. However, he remained critical of using personnel of the field ambulances and the equipment of the CCSs.[40] This was based on the grounds that he considered that field units should be maintained as such and that lines of communication units should be employed for most of the work away from the fighting zone. He pointed out that No. 2 ASH, a lines of communication unit, was available in Egypt and ready to move at short notice and should be used for staffing transports. This plan was accepted, and both No. 2 ASH and No. 15 British Stationary Hospital (BSH) were sent for to serve this purpose. No doubt as a result of Howse's intervention, the order for men of the field ambulances to work as personnel on transports was cancelled on 16 April. The objections Howse made concerning the use of equipment from the CCSs also prompted an order to No. 5 Advanced Depot Medical Stores to embark for Lemnos along with the two stationary hospitals.

At the same time as Colonel Howse was making his recommendations, Colonel Yarr of the 29th Division was ordered to '… inspect three transports as hospital ships'.[41] He was forced to reply, '… it is physically impossible, not a case of "I will not" but "I cannot"'. He had plenty to do, working to organise the 29th Division's medical units and the 11th CCS allotted to it, which also came under his control, but his main reason for his response was that transport was not available to get to the transports in the harbour. The Royal Navy had no boats available to take the hard-pressed ADMS around Mudros Harbour in search of suitable transports to act as temporary hospital ships. Colonel Keble, who had issued the order, responded that he, too, was in the same position and agreed that there was nothing that could be done while the navy was unable to provide the necessary boats. However, this meant that more time was lost in sorting out the problems associated with selecting suitable transport for the work. The longer the delay in the selection of the transports the less likely it became that they could be suitably cleaned, equipped and staffed in readiness to take casualties.

On 18 April, operation orders were issued, and they were inadequate in the details for the medical services. On this date, Surgeon General Birrell arrived in Mudros Harbour and joined the General Staff on the *Arcadian*. To this date, Birrell, DMS of the MEF, had made little input to the medical planning. He was then informed of the general arrangements that Hamilton's staff had made for handling casualties. This was based upon an estimated 3,000 casualties, which had been considered to be inadequate by Keble some days before.[42] Keble had prepared a plan but had not presented it to the General Staff, presumably awaiting the arrival of Birrell as senior officer before that was done. It has been suggested that the difficulty of communication within the Mudros Harbour also hampered Keble in presenting his proposals to the General Staff. Nevertheless, the General Staff had gone ahead with their planning without reference to medical

---

40   AWM: AWM4/26/18/5: War Diary, 1st Australian Division ADMS, 15 April. Also see Butler, *Official History of the Australian Medical Services*, vol. I, p.118.
41   TNA: WO 95/4307: War Diary, 29th Division ADMS, 16 April.
42   Part of the General Staff plan drawn up on 13 April. Colonel Keble was later to claim that the plan was drawn up by Major Cuthbert Graham Fuller, Royal Engineers. See also Mark Harrison, *The Medical War: British Military Medicine in the First World War* (Oxford: Oxford University Press, 2010), p.175.

personnel until the arrival of Surgeon General Birrell, who, upon his arrival, saw the plan and also considered it inadequate. Birrell was not alone in seeing the inadequacies of the General Staff's plan. Birrell's arrival on Lemnos coincided with that of Major General E. M. Woodward, Hamilton's DAG, who took up the surgeon general's suggestions that allowance should be made to provide facilities for the evacuation and distribution of 10,000 casualties from the landing phase of the operation. Woodward wrote to the CGS the same day. His memo outlined the existing plans as he saw them, and he commented, 'The provision for evacuation of casualties from the force appears to be altogether inadequate and I would strongly urge that the following proposal should be adopted.'[43] He then proceeded to give details of his proposals to handle the numbers of casualties he considered likely. He also wrote a similar memo to the quartermaster general (QMG) and gave further details of the transports that he considered to be necessary:

The position as regards Hospital Ships is as follows:

> *Sicilia*: accommodation 400 serious cases, Mudros
> *Gascon*: accommodation 300 serious cases, due on Tuesday.

> In the event of serious fighting those two ships will not provide sufficient accommodation for evacuating wounded from the shore.

> It is proposed in the case of the 29th Division to utilize the following ships

Troops Accommodated

Officers	Other ranks	
100	2,000	B2 *Caledonia*
230	1,800	B7 *Aragon*
140	1,600	*Southland*

> For the Australian and New Zealand Corps

Troops Accommodated

Officers	Other ranks	
200	1,200	A3 *Devanaha*
135	1,790	A25 *Lutzow*
900	2,000	A1 *Ionian*
220		A10 *Derflinger*
34	1,050	A29 *Sewing Bee* [sic; *Seang Bee*]

It is proposed to provide personnel and medical and surgical equipment for the above ships from Nos 15 and 16 Stationary Hospitals and No 2 Australian Stationary Hospital, and to evacuate direct to Alexandria.

The ships when loaded with wounded could remain off shore for 48 hours so as to be available for re-embarking troops if necessary. But the ships could not be kept waiting for more than 48 hours.

---

43 Macpherson, *History of the Great War: Medical Services*, vol. 4, p.20.

> Have you any objection to the above arrangements being carried out? If not, I propose to take steps at once to ascertain the number of wounded cases that could be accommodated on each of the above-mentioned ships. The matter is one of great urgency as without some such arrangement it will be impossible from a medical point of view, to commence serious operations.[44]

This memo certainly struck the right note with the General Staff, and both the CGS and QMG agreed with proposals as of 18 April. However, it is, perhaps, noticeable that Woodward suggested that transports full of wounded could remain offshore in the event of a re-embarkation becoming necessary, that is, the event of failure of the landing force to secure a beachhead. This would not have seemed like a very good idea to the MOs, and it would not have been the best practice for the wounded on those ships. It is also noticeable that Woodward had selected ships that were capable of carrying large numbers of troops – these may not have been the most suitable for carrying wounded. He had, however, managed to get the go-ahead for a considerably greater number of wounded to be considered within the plan for the campaign. Woodward had also recognised the critical importance of the lines of communication, particularly the stationary hospitals, and these were embarked at Alexandria on 20 April on the *Hindoo*.[45] This was too late for the original planned date of the landings of 21 April. However, as this date slipped, the *Hindoo* arrived in Mudros on 23 April as the task force was making its final preparations for the landings on 25 April.

Also on 20 April, Birrell informed Colonel Manders, SMO of ANZAC, and Colonel Howse, ADMS of the 1st Australian Division, that No. 2 ASH would be placed under Manders' control when it arrived and that he was to use it to staff and equip the transports supplied for the evacuation of the Australian and New Zealand wounded. This was to become part of the medical arrangement circulated by Birrell on 24 April and included the 29th Division. However, matters were further complicated in ANZAC because there was no administrative MO to oversee their arrangements. The appointment of a DDMS had not been made, and it was with some reluctance that Colonel Manders took on this role only days before the landing commenced.[46] This lack of administrative support was to hamper the medical services' efforts at Anzac.

Although Birrell was better informed by this date than he had been at the time of his arrival in Mudros Harbour, his part in the overall planning was little more than peripheral, and, to some extent, this was reflected in the manner in which evacuation occurred during the opening phase of the operations. On 22 April, he was informed that he would not accompany the General Staff on the HMS *Queen Elizabeth* during the landing operations but would instead have his HQ on the HMT *Arcadian*. These ships were not in regular contact, and hence Birrell became more marginalised as operations began. This was further reinforced by the fact that he was told at the same time that, once operations commenced, the evacuation of wounded would be controlled by a member of the General Staff and, since his input was not needed, that he was not required on the *Queen Elizabeth*. Thus, the most senior MO in the Mediterranean theatre of operations was not to be consulted or have any direct input on the medical arrangement at this critical point of the campaign.

---

44 AWM: AWM4/26/3/1: War Diary, DMS MEF, Appendix 2, April 1915. See also Macpherson, *History of the Great War: Medical Services*, vol. 4, p.21.

45 It is worth noting that the *Hindoo*, although carrying medical staff and equipment, was not a hospital ship and was not equipped, or intended, to be used as one.

46 Colonel Howse refused the appointment at this time, preferring to be with his divisional troops.

Even though the General Staff had accepted Woodward's general proposals, it took Birrell until 24 April, the eve of the landings, to provide the details by which the medical services were to operate. In general, they followed the concepts of Colonel Keble and General Woodward, with the appropriate variations to the ships suitable as temporary hospital ships. Birrell accepted that there would be two hospital ships available but modified the capacity of the *Gascon* so that it took 500 serious cases evacuated from the Australian beachhead. In his statement of the medical arrangements, he went on to say:

> I understand from the Senior Naval Transport Officer that the Navy will commence the transfer of wounded from the shore to the ships about 2 pm.

> The means of evacuation are as follows:

> Three launches each capable of holding twelve cots are available for the 29th Division and the same number for the A & NZ Army Corps.

> These launches are to be towed to the hospital ships and other ships in which the men are to be accommodated.

> The following transports are allotted to the 29th Division for accommodation of casualties:

> | | | |
> |---|---|---|
> | B2 *Caledonia* | 400 serious cases | 1200 – 1550 slight |
> | B7 *Aragon* | 400 serious cases | 1200 – 1550 slight |
> | B9 *Dongola* | 400 serious cases | 1200 – 1550 slight |

> Allotted to the A and NZ Army Corps:

> | | | |
> |---|---|---|
> | A25 *Lutzow* | 200 serious cases | 1000 slight |
> | A1 *Ionian* | 100 serious cases | 1000 slight |
> | A15 *Clan McGillivray* | 100 serious cases | 600 slight |
> | A31 *Seang Chun* | 100 serious cases | 600 slight |

> Medical personnel and surgical equipment for the *Caledonia*, *Aragon* and *Dongola* have been provided by No 15 Stationary Hospital and for the *Clan McGillivray* and *Seang Chun* by the A & NZ Field Ambulance, at present, and later by No 2 Australian Stationary Hospital.

> The *Lutzow* and *Ionian* to be supplied later with medical and surgical equipment by No 2 Australian Stationary Hospital

> The personnel of No 16 Stationary Hospital kept in reserve.[47]

---

47   Macpherson, *History of the Great War: Medical Services*, vol. 4, p.22.

In addition to the ships mentioned here, the Royal Navy provided two hospital ships: the HS *Rewa* and the HS *Soudan*. These ships were provided for casualties arising on the ships involved in the bombardment of the peninsula and to supply hospital transport for the casualties of the RND. However, both were used throughout for any casualties of the fighting at both Helles and Anzac as and when needed. Whilst these arrangements were made available to the Staff, they were not widely distributed amongst the units involved. There was clearly a move forwards in the planning for the evacuation of wounded at this stage, but there were still a number of issues that had not been sorted out at this late stage. Notably, two of the transports had not been allotted any staff in readiness for their service at the ANZAC landing site, although a provision had been made for No. 2 ASH to supply them 'later'. It is difficult to understand that, as late as the evening before the landing, there was no more concrete proposal than that these ships would be supplied later.

As part of the arrangements Birrell made was the fact that No. 4 Advanced Depot on the *Anglo–Egyptian* was placed at the disposal of the ANZACs while No. 5 was placed at the disposal of the 29th Division. There is no clear statement that either were immediately available, though both had arrived in Lemnos on the *Hindoo* on 23 April. It is also noted that it was proposed to evacuate all casualties from the landing direct to Alexandria and Malta in keeping with the arrangements then being made in those destinations. The final point of note in Birrell's arrangements was that No. 1 ASH, then at Mudros, was to remain and act as the hospital to handle the sick from the mass of shipping then using the harbour.

The medical arrangements, as worked out mainly by the General Staff and modified later by a number of MOs, was considered to be sufficient before the landing took place. That it later proved to be inadequate was largely due to the overoptimism of the General Staff in expecting the landing to be successful enough to allow for all medical establishments to land and deal with casualties on shore as they arose. Essentially, all planning, not just that of the medical services, was based on complete success of the landing. Although it has been suggested that the planning was based on either complete success or complete failure, there was little belief in the latter in the General Staff, and, had it failed, the effect on medical services can only be guessed. In the case of failure, it is likely that the problems faced during the landing would have been compounded, as high casualties would have been likely to have been suffered during re-embarkation. The landings, however, may be considered as a partial success, or, indeed, as a partial failure, and the result was that much of the planning provided proved to be ineffective, as different parts of the plan were either forced to be abandoned or only utilised incompletely. The problems that arose on the beaches undoubtedly had a significant impact on hospitals in Egypt, for instance, and hence the need to expand accommodation from 5,000 at the start of April to over 15,000 by the end of the month. The planning arrangements for the medical services can be split into a number of elements:

a.   Onshore after landing (field ambulances and CCSs)
b.   Evacuation (hospital ships and transports)
c.   Onshore at Lemnos (stationary hospitals), which became more important later
d.   Onshore at Egypt and later Malta (general hospitals).

Each of these phases, or parts, needed to be functioning correctly, and as planned, for each of the units in the hierarchy to function properly. The fact that the landing of 25 April did not meet expectations put immediate stress on the first link in the chain for the evacuation of the wounded, that is, the field ambulances and their associated dressing stations. This, in turn, impacted the disposal of the wounded to seaborne transport and subsequently those units farther along the lines of communication. Whilst planning for the medical services had been subordinate to the main organisation of the General Staff and was, perhaps, ill-judged and rather rushed, the problems encountered ultimately resulted from a lack of clear thinking at the highest level of command. In the end, the issues arising from the lack of thorough planning for medical services, which has raised much discussion and criticism in the years since, stem entirely from a lack of understanding and a lack of foresight on the quality, and behaviour, of the enemy as the forces landed on the beaches.

The manner in which the medical services at all levels handled this unforeseen and undesired outcome will be examined further in subsequent chapters as each of the phases of the campaign is examined.

Hospital Ships

In the above discussion on planning for the campaign, it can be seen that there was a significant emphasis placed upon the number of hospital ships available and needed for the opening phase of the campaign. The need for ships for evacuation is clear, but the types of ships both called and used as hospital ships has been misunderstood and, in some cases, misused. It is perhaps appropriate to discuss the meaning for each of the terms that occur in the histories of the campaign, both official and unofficial, that refer to evacuation procedures. Over the years since the campaign, and, indeed, during the campaign itself, there has been confusion over the terminology of the transports used for evacuation. In some cases, even the people serving on the peninsula used terms more or less interchangeably, with 'hospital ship' being used basically for any ship transporting wounded or sick. It should be stressed that this is unusual in the medical services, but it still occurred occasionally.

According to Article 1 of the Hague Adaptation of the Principles of the Geneva Convention to Maritime War, signed on 18 October 1907:

> Military Hospital Ships, that is to say, ships constructed or adapted by States for the particular and sole purpose of aiding the sick, wounded, and shipwrecked, the names of which have been communicated to the belligerent Powers at the commencement or during the course of hostilities and in any case before they are employed, shall be respected, and may not be captured while hostilities last.
>
> Such ships, moreover, are not on the same footing as war ships as regards their stay in a neutral port.[48]

This article sets out the purpose and function of the ships and, significantly, the need for all such ships to be notified to warring nations. It would seem that this was the first step in the protection of hospital ships during the early part of the First World War. The Adaptation goes on to

---

48   Barrett and Deane, *Australian Army Medical Corps in Egypt*, p.199.

68   The Fight for Life

set out the rules for privately owned ships, and again, providing there was notification, they were to be treated in the same manner. Article 5 of the Adaptation states, in part:

> Military hospital ships shall be distinguished by being painted white outside with a horizontal band of green about a metre and a half in breadth.
>
> The boats of the said ships, as also small craft which may be used for hospital work, shall be distinguished by similar painting.
>
> All hospital ships shall make themselves known by hoisting, with their national flag, the white flag with a red cross provided by the Geneva Convention, and further, if they belong to a neutral State by flying at the mainmast the national flag of the belligerent nation under whose orders they are placed.[49]

It is within these two articles that the basic requirements for a hospital ship are set out, and it was these that were followed during the Gallipoli Campaign. The recognition of such ships by their colour was significant since ships in this livery could easily be distinguished at distance by the warring nations. As such, any ship not so liveried and notified through the necessary channels would not be classified as a hospital ship. There is nothing in the convention to state how the ships were to be fitted out except to say that they were fitted for the carrying of sick, wounded and shipwrecked. The standard of the fit does not appear to be the concern of the Adaptation, and, as such, it could be very thorough or, indeed, basic.

The issue of hospital ships at Gallipoli is one that raises many questions and is fraught with difficulties because of the various types of transport that were used to evacuate wounded and the manner in which the ships are referred to in everything from war diaries to histories of the campaign.

The requirements for a ship to be used as a hospital ship is quite clear under the Geneva Convention, but, even when the official histories of the medical services were compiled, there seems to have been confusion over the usage. For instance, Butler suggested that painting a ship white with red crosses (no mention of a green line) and fitting it as a full hospital were required.[50] This was clearly not the case. It may have been desired for a ship to be fully fitted as a hospital, but it was not necessary under the terms of the Convention. However, Butler noted that the fitting out of any merchantman as a hospital ship was both a lengthy and costly process. These points are important since there can be no doubt that there was a shortage of hospital ships from the start of the Gallipoli Campaign, leading to some lengthy, if not acrimonious, discussion at the time and in the years since.

To assist with the evacuation of sick and wounded from the peninsula, a practise was adopted whereby ships known as 'hospital carriers' were utilised. This had been developed by the navy to reduce the pressure on the hospital ships and to aid the medical services in clearing the beaches of the peninsula. A hospital carrier was considered as an 'inferior sort of hospital ship', and they were used as follows:

- Merchantmen fitted out as well as time would allow
- Painted as hospital ships

---

49   Barrett and Deane, *Australian Army Medical Corps in Egypt*, p.200.
50   Butler, *Official History of the Australian Medical Services*, vol. I, p.222.

- Registered as such under the Geneva Convention
- Improved as necessary from time to time
- Either fully fitted as a hospital ship or returned to the merchant service
- Staffed with reserve of MOs and nursing sisters.

This was followed wherever possible, but the fitting out was often delayed, and the painting of the ship did not always rank highly when it was necessary to remove thousands of sick and wounded from the beaches. These ships were in service from quite early on during the campaign, with the *Neuralia* being the first to be fitted out and in service by 12 June 1915.[51] This would seem to be a clear distinction on the types of vessels and how they were used. However, it is clear from the war diaries and similar accounts and histories that, in many cases, any ship set aside for sick and wounded was simply called a 'hospital ship'.

Given that hospital carriers were required to be painted white and notified under the Geneva Convention, it is hardly surprising that there was some delay in their entry to service and confusion over their role in the evacuation process. During the early stages of the campaign, there were far more wounded than could be coped with by the hospital ships, and, since there were few other sources of transport available to the commanders, troop transports were quickly, and often crudely, adapted to be used for getting wounded off the beaches. The hospital carriers, at least until they became suitably liveried, were often classed along with these merchantmen, and, since they were all black-hulled ships as opposed to the white-hulled hospital ships, all became known as 'black ships'. The black ships were emptied troop transports often in very dirty condition from carrying horses and equipment, as well as men, and were totally unsuitable for the transport of wounded. In some cases, medical staff was found from the field ambulances, and these men worked under difficult conditions of limited equipment and medical supplies to maintain some level of medical cover. Some of the ships had little or no medical cover, and, on such ships, the wounded often suffered unacceptably. The black ships are synonymous with the lack of planning for the whole campaign and the lack of readiness of the whole of the medical services for the number of casualties that the landing and early stages of the fighting on the peninsula brought about.

As early as 8 May, there were moves to reduce the number of hospital ships serving the peninsula. The campaign had started with two: the *Sicilia*, serving Helles, and the *Gascon*, serving Anzac. These were shortly joined by four others, but, by May, there had been an acceptance of the fact that, to handle the large number of casualties, it would be necessary to use the black ships. In this case, the HS *Guildford Castle* was removed from the service, and its nursing staff were placed upon the *Neuralia*, described as '… a finer vessel but not fitted for hospital work. A number of bunks were put in and with the Red Cross flag we went to Lemnos'.[52] Thus, the *Neuralia* served as a black ship before her role was redefined as a hospital carrier. Other transports were also nominated as 'temporary hospital ships', and instructions were issued concerning the HT *Caledonia* as early as 15 April that it would equip itself with medical stores from a CCS (possibly the 11th CCS) and that three MOs and 20 other ranks were to be taken from a field ambulance to act as staff. Whilst it was common amongst everyone from the nurses serving on

---

51 Butler, *Official History of the Australian Medical Services*, vol. I, p.223; Macpherson, *History of the Great War: Medical Services*, vol. 1, p.366.
52 Butler, *Official History of the Australian Medical Services*, vol. I, p.219, quoting a member of the AANS.

the ships to the general staff directing them to call these ships 'black ships', they were officially known as 'ambulance carriers'.

Added to these vessels were the fleet sweepers. According to Butler, these should be considered as the equivalent of the motor ambulance convoy.[53] They were generally small vessels of between 500–1,000 tons and were taken from those vessels brought into the area by the navy for mine-sweeping work. There were essentially two main types of vessels:

- Packet boats – larger boats, with about five being used for medical purposes
- North Sea trawlers – smaller and used to ferry between larger ships.

Packet boats were better suited to the evacuation of wounded than were trawlers, although both types carried limited medical equipment and were staffed by MOs of both the army and the navy. Trawlers tended to be used for evacuation only when there were large numbers of casualties caused by large-scale operations on the peninsula and were generally not as well staffed or equipped.[54] The fleet sweeper *Clacton* was a 320-ton packet boat and had a medical staff of two MOs and six other ranks from the 1st AFA. It made its first trip carrying wounded on 21 May, and, thereafter, it was arranged for it to make the trip every 24 hours. The process was that stores were carried to the peninsula from Lemnos on the ship and wounded carried back: '... After discharging, barges in charge of a "middy" would range alongside; stretchers were taken in by hand – very awkward at night or if the sea were rough. Light cases were taken from the hospital ship. First instructions were for 150 lightly wounded, but soon all classes of case were sent and frequently over 300 carried'.[55]

In a similar manner, the *Newmarket* (833 tons) and the *Hythe* (509 tons) were also staffed from time to time by the Australian field ambulances, and, from May to July, they worked the route from Helles and Anzac.[56]

In this manner, the evacuation was supposed to be carried out as follows:

- Light cases by sweepers or carriers to Imbros or Lemnos
- More serious cases by ambulance carriers to Egypt or Malta
- Most serious cases by hospital ships to Egypt and Malta.

All black ships were required to report to Mudros before proceeding to base.

Whilst the foregoing suggests that there was at least some measure of planning in place, under the exigencies of war, it was not always possible to maintain even this imperfect approach.

---

53   Butler, *Official History of the Australian Medical Services*, vol. I, p.215.
54   Butler, *Official History of the Australian Medical Services*, vol. I, p.216.
55   Butler, *Official History of the Australian Medical Services*, vol. I, p.216.
56   The HMS *Hythe*, a converted cross-channel paddle steamer, was sunk in a collision on 28 October 1915 whilst ferrying troops from Lemnos to the peninsula with the loss of 154 lives.

3

Helles: A Solid Mass of Dead and Wounded

The landing at Helles on the south-western tip of the peninsula was allotted to the 29th Division, together with support from two battalions of the RND. The 29th Division was the last division formed from regular battalions of the pre-war British Army. These battalions had returned to Great Britain after the start of the war from postings throughout the Empire, mainly from India and Burma. None had any experience of the war except for the 2nd Battalion of the South Wales Borderers (SWB), which had taken part in the action to wrest Tsingtao, in China, from the hands of the Germans.[1] By January 1915, the 29th Division was mobilising around the HQ in Leamington Spa. When the division was completed, it comprised 11 regular battalions and one TF battalion. The attached units of the RAMC, Royal Engineers, and Army Service Corps were also units from the TF. The landing on the Gallipoli Peninsula was the first operation of the division.[2]

General Sir Ian Hamilton took barely a month to prepare a seaborne invasion, and he had to do this with a limited supply of almost everything: there were limited troops available, a shortage of artillery and shells to go with it and limited intelligence on the ground over which he was to fight. The peninsula has a very rugged coastline. That much would have been obvious to anyone viewing the coastline from a ship cruising towards the narrows in peacetime. There were very few and narrow beaches often backed by steep cliffs sometimes covered with thorny scrub. From the little information available, Hamilton and his staff decided upon a number of beaches around the south-western end of the peninsula where the landing was to be made. The beaches were designated as follows, working around the tip of the peninsula from the north-west to the south-east:

- Y Beach – 1st King's Own Scottish Borderers (KOSB), A Company 2nd SWB, Plymouth Battalion RND and a detachment of Anson Battalion RND
- X Beach – 2nd Royal Fusiliers, 1st Border Regiment, 1st Royal Inniskilling Fusiliers and a detachment of Anson Battalion RND

---

1 John Dixon, *A Clash of Empires: The South Wales Borderers at Tsingtao, 1914* (Wrexham: Bridge Books, 2008).
2 Captain Stair Gillon, *The Story of the 29th Division: A Record of Gallant Deeds* (London: Thomas Nelson and Sons, 1925).

71

- W Beach – 1st Lancashire Fusiliers and a detachment of Anson Battalion RND, later joined by 1st Essex, 2nd Hampshires, 1/5th Royal Scots and 4th Worcesters
- V Beach – 1st Royal Dublin Fusiliers, 1st Royal Munster Fusiliers, a detachment of Anson Battalion RND. A half company of the 1st Royal Dublin Fusiliers landed a little farther east at the Camber.
- S Beach – three companies of the 2nd SWB.

There were three field ambulances attached to the 29th Division. The field ambulances were divided as necessary to provide the medical support required during the landing operations. The 87th Field Ambulance landed its bearer division at X Beach, whilst B Section of the tent division landed at Y Beach. The rest of the unit remained on its transport, the *Southland*, and did not land immediately. The 88th Field Ambulance landed at S Beach along with the bulk of the 2nd SWB and remained there until the sector was handed over to the French when their *Service de Santé des Armées* took responsibility for their troops. The bearer division of the 89th Field Ambulance was on board the *River Clyde* at V Beach, whilst the tent division was on board the *Marquette*. This unit eventually landed to operate at both W and V Beaches.[3]

The three field ambulances supporting the RND were landed where they could best serve their division. The 1st Royal Navy Field Ambulance landed at Anzac on 28 April in support of the two partial brigades landed there to assist the Australians. The 3rd Royal Navy Field Ambulance landed at Helles on 29 April, providing the medical cover for the RND units serving there. The 2nd Royal Navy Field Ambulance did not land in this early phase of the operation, providing staff for the transports carrying wounded to Egypt.[4] Also, the 11th CCS landed on W Beach at 7:00 p.m. on 25 April and was to remain in the same general area throughout much of the campaign.

At S Beach, the 2nd SWB, commanded by Lieutenant Colonel Casson, landed from rowing boats together with their RMO, Lieutenant Joseph Arthur Blake, RAMC.[5] The boats soon came under fire, and a number of casualties occurred before landing. Soon after the landing, the SWB captured the enemy trenches at S Beach, the cliffs to De Tott's battery were scaled rapidly by D Company, and the position also captured. The bearer subdivision of the 88th Field Ambulance landed with the battalion and was soon busy, as the battalion began to take casualties. Following the landing, Casson's three companies were expected to join up with the force landing at V Beach, but this never materialised because of the situation that developed there during the day. The SWB were essentially isolated at S Beach, and, although they had succeeded in their landing, the lack of cohesion and communication with the force to their left meant that Lieutenant Colonel Casson ordered his small force to consolidate their position, which they succeeded in doing and, in the process, beat off a Turkish counterattack before the day was finished. By the time that the SWB had consolidated, the rest of the 88th Field Ambulance had also landed.[6]

---

3   Although the 29th Division was a regular division, the field ambulances attached to it were of the TF: the 87th (1/1st West Lancashire) Field Ambulance TF, the 88th (1/1st East Anglian) Field Ambulance TF and the 89th (1/1st Highland) Field Ambulance TF.
4   Macpherson, *History of the Great War: Medical Services*, vol. 4, p.27.
5   Rodney Ashwood, *Duty Nobly Done: The South Wales Borderers at Gallipoli 1915* (Solihull: Helion & Company, 2017), p.67.
6   TNA: WO 95/4307: War Diary, 29th Division ADMS, 25 April.

Helles: A Solid Mass of Dead and Wounded 73

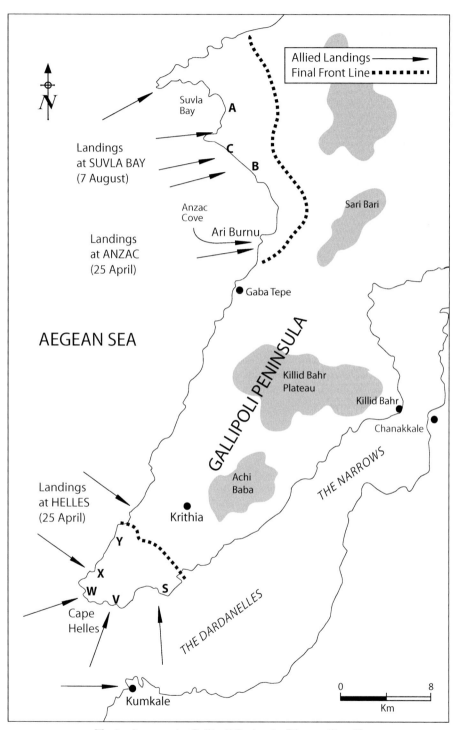

The landings on the Gallipoli Peninsula. (Terence Powell)

74   The Fight for Life

At V Beach, between Sedd-el-Bahr and Cape Helles, tactics for the landing were different to those used elsewhere during the landing. Here, and mainly as a result of the approach championed by Royal Navy Commander Edward Unwin, an old collier, the SS *River Clyde*, filled with soldiers was run aground. This was an attempt to carry the landing force as close to the shore as possible and, in so doing, to prevent its exposure to enemy fire for as long as possible. Once beached, the *River Clyde* was to be used as a breakwater to cover the landing of both men and equipment arriving after the first assault. The collier had been modified by a number of sally ports cut in her sides to allow the troops to disembark quickly. The *River Clyde* could not land troops directly on to the beach, and a system of walkways and floating jetties was required to allow the men to reach the beach. It was perhaps with this detail that things started to go wrong at V Beach.

The SS *River Clyde* was carrying almost two battalions of infantry with supporting troops of the Royal Engineers and the 89th Field Ambulance. The latter two units had been assigned a hold at the stern of the ship for the passage from Lemnos, and disembarkation for them was anticipated to follow that of the main body of infantry. The rest of the landing force at V Beach was carried by Fleet Sweeper No. 1 to attack the Camber a little to the east of the main landing beach.

The landing from the *River Clyde* can only be described as a bloody disaster. The enemy soon brought down withering fire upon the collier, and the disembarking troops suffered heavily, as the improvised gangways failed to provide the anticipated rapid access to the shore and the disembarking men became easy targets for the Turkish machine gunners. In a matter of minutes, the 1st Royal Munster Fusiliers had lost nearly all its officers and a large portion of its men – few made it to the shore uninjured. Similarly, the one company of the 1st Royal Dublin Fusiliers accompanying this attack was almost entirely wiped out before it reached the shore. Meanwhile, conditions on the *River Clyde* were deteriorating, and Lieutenant George Davidson, RAMC, of the 89th Field Ambulance described the conditions in the hold that his unit was sharing with the West Riding Field Company of the Royal Engineers whilst waiting to disembark:

> She was not long aground when the guns on Kum Kale, across the Dardanelles, opened on us, and this fire was kept up the whole day – on us and us only as far as I could make out. It took them some time to get our range and for a considerable time we were not hit all the shells being shorts and overs. At last, they got us, the first shell that hit going through our hold at an angle of 45 degrees, coming through the deck over our heads and going out at the junction of the floor and the side wall. In its course it struck a man on the head, this being splashed all through the hold. Another man squatting on the floor was hit about the middle of both thighs, one leg being completely severed, while the other hung by a thin shred of skin. He fell back with a howl with both stumps in the air.[7]

Heavy rifle and machine-gun fire played on the hull of the ship, and a small number of shells struck the ship, causing casualties, though, as pointed out by Lieutenant Davidson, the shells

---

7   George Davidson, *The Incomparable 29th and the 'River Clyde'* (James Gordon Bisset, 1919, Kindle e-book), location 803.

did not explode since, if they had done so in such an enclosed space, casualties would surely have been high. At one point during the day, things were going so badly on the beach that it was feared that there would be a Turkish counterattack to capture the ship. The men on board began erecting suitable barricades in readiness for such an eventuality, although, as the landings developed and the situation on the beach slowly changed, they became unnecessary.

As the landings continued, wounded were brought back to the *River Clyde*, and the bearer division of the 89th Field Ambulance set up what was really a field hospital in the holds of the former collier. There, they treated as many of the wounded as could be brought on board. The floors in the holds soon filled up with wounded men, and, periodically, a boat came alongside to take the wounded off to the waiting HS *Sicilia* and transports such as the *Caledonia*. This continued throughout the day almost without pause, and the ship was under fire all the time, making the movement of the wounded difficult for the field ambulance. Lieutenant George Davidson had been at work in the hold through much of the day, but it was in the evening that he took the initiative to help those on shore:

> About 8:30 an officer on shore made a dash for our ship, and on describing the terrible condition and suffering of the wounded who had been on the sandbank for about 14 hours, I decided to go to their assistance. We had previously been warned that it would be impossible for any of the ambulance to land before morning, but heedless of this I set off alone over the barges and splashed through the remaining few yards of water. Here most of those still alive were wounded more or less severely, and I set to work on them, removing many useless and harmful tourniquets for one thing and worked my way to my left towards the high rocks where the snipers still were. All the wounded on this side I attended to, an officer accompanying me all the time. I then went to the other side, and after seeing to all in the sand my companion left me, and I next went to a long, low rock which projected into the water for about 20 yards a short way to the right of the *Clyde*. Here the dead and wounded were heaped together two or three deep, and it was among these I had my hardest work. All had to be disentangled single-handed from their uncomfortable positions, some lying with head and shoulder in the tideless water, with broken legs in some cases dangling on a higher level.
>
> At the very point of this rock, which had been a favourite spot for the boats to steer to, there was a solid mass of dead and wounded mixed up together. The whole of these I saw to, although by this time there was little, I could do except lift and pull them into more comfortable positions, but I was able to do something for every one on them. My last piece of work was to look after six men who were groaning in a boat stranded close to the point of the rock. Three lay on each side with their legs inwards; a plank ran the whole length of the middle of the boat, and along this as it rested on their legs, men had been running during the landing. Getting on this plank some of them howled in agony and beseeched me to get off. I then got into the water and as I could do nothing more for them, my dressing being finished some time before, I gave them each a dose of morphia by mouth.[8]

---

8   Davidson, *The Incomparable 29th*, location 729. Davidson was mentioned in despatches (MiD) for his work at Gallipoli.

76   The Fight for Life

Davidson had been working for over three hours on the shore when, at about midnight, the Turks began a counterattack on the beachhead. He had little cover as he stood waist deep in the water near the shore. He made a scramble for the shelter of a boat, where he remained until 4:00 a.m. the following morning (26 April) when, as the clouds crossed the moon, he made a dash for the safety of the *River Clyde*.

The landings at V Beach had been costly: casualties had been heavy in all the infantry units engaged. For instance, the 1st Royal Dublin Fusiliers had suffered all but four officers killed or wounded, together with approximately 550 men killed, wounded or missing.[9] By nightfall of 25 April, the beachhead that had been so expensively won was precariously held, and the tired and shocked men that remained in the battalions that had landed from the *River Clyde* prepared for what may come next.

To the north, the landing at what was known as 'W Beach' was to be affected by the 1st Lancashire Fusiliers, together with one platoon of the Anson Battalion RND, to provide a working party. Three companies of the Lancashire Fusiliers were disembarked from the HMS *Euryalus* to six tows, whilst the remaining company was disembarked to two tows from HMS *Implacable*. W Beach is situated between Cape Helles and Cape Teke in a part of the coastline where steep cliffs give way, for a distance of perhaps 350 yards, to a narrow strip of sandy beach that was W Beach. The area was defended by the Turks with belts of barbed wire, trip wires in the sea and land mines on the beach. The flanks and landward entry to the beach were entrenched by the Turks, and machine guns had been sited to give a good field of fire across the sandy beach. It was the only likely place for a landing along this 1,000 yards stretch of coastline, and the Turks had recognised the possibility when preparing their defences.

The Lancashire Fusiliers were to secure the beachhead and then move inland to link with those troops on either flank. The landing on W Beach was met with severe opposition, and intense fire caused heavy casualties. The belt of barbed wire in front of the Turkish positions provided a difficult obstacle and held up the men trying to move off the beach. Many Fusiliers died in the attempt to clear the wire. Nevertheless, the landing was carried through despite the heavy casualties in the Lancashire Fusiliers. When a roll call was taken later in the day, it was in the absence of 10 officers and 507 men killed, wounded or missing during the hours of the landing. Their landing site was later named 'Lancashire Landing' and is still known as that today.

The work of the 89th Field Ambulance on W Beach is described in the unit war diary:

> B Section Tent Sub-Div landed in second tow from the Mine Sweeper *Whitby Abbey* about 6.30am. Owing to large number of wounded Tent Subdivision was split up into four dressing parties, one under Lt Thomson, one under Lt Whyte, one under Staff-Sergt Gaskin and one under Sgt Gilbert. First aid was rendered and wounded were removed as speedily as possible to the cover afforded by the cliffs west of the Beach. Fires were lit and the cooks prepared Beef Tea for wounded. During the forenoon several boat loads of wounded were got off to the *Implacable* and a Hospital Ship. Later in the day it was possible to evacuate large numbers. Owing to the pressure of work it was impossible to record the names of those men early evacuated but after the Admission and Discharge Book was opened 287 entries were made. During the

9   Aspinall-Oglander, *Military Operations*, vol. 1, p.284.

afternoon the work of identifying the dead was carried out, these had been collected into groups earlier in the day. There were 3 officers and eighty-two men identified. Valuables were secured before burial by the Sgt Clark. The rations carried by the dead and their First Field dressings were used to supplement our stores for the wounded. We were left with about 150 wounded overnight which is testimony to the large number that must have been evacuated.[10]

At about 6:00 p.m. on this day, members of the 11th CCS made their landing, and their equipment followed close behind so that it was not long before they were able to establish the hospital 'on W Beach under a high cliff west of W Beach'. There, they began work immediately, for they found some '250 wounded lying on the beach, all of whom were attended to'.[11] They continued to work throughout the night as more casualties arrived, and the Turkish snipers continued to target anything they could see moving in the area. The hospital had a well-chosen site under the cliff, which prevented any direct fire from the Turkish lines, but it was scarcely what had been anticipated had the landing been a complete success.

The landing at X Beach was largely unopposed until the landing force reached to crest of the steep cliffs and attempted to move inland. Communication with W Beach to the south and Y Beach to the north failed more or less completely, but Hill 114, lying between X Beach and W Beach, was captured. By the end of the first day, the landing force was able to consolidate sufficiently to drive off a concerted Turkish attack. The tent division of the 87th Field Ambulance was immediately at work on this beach, taking in casualties from the fierce fighting.

The story of the landing at Y Beach is, perhaps, one of missed opportunity. The infantry landed without difficulty and, throughout the second half of the day, were able to beat of a number of Turkish counterattacks that penetrated their lines in places. However, lack of good communications with the GOC resulted in the situation developing there being misunderstood when it was necessary to reinforce and resupply the infantry units. It was, perhaps, inevitable that rumours to withdraw began to circulate within this seemingly isolated force. Although there was no truth in any of these, the uncertainly this created inevitably led to a certain number of men making their way to the beach, along with the wounded, to re-embark. Eventually, the lack of communication and inability to resupply meant that there was little option left but to abandon the small gain made at Y Beach, and the force left the area on 26 April – it was to be a month before the ground was captured. The force had not landed at Y Beach without medical support. Each infantry unit had its own RMO, and the bearer division of the 87th Field Ambulance also landed and remained until the beach was abandoned.

During the two days (26–27 April) between the landing and the First Battle of Krithia (28 April), the positions on the beaches were consolidated. At S Beach, the consolidated position was taken over by the French 175th Regiment, and the 2nd SWB moved up to join the main body of the 87th Brigade in the assault on the Turkish positions that was to be known as the 'First Battle of Krithia'. At W Beach, the old fort at Sedd-el-Bahr was captured by 11:30 a.m. on 26 April, and the village an hour-and-a-half later. Further small gains were made during the day, and, at about 4:00 p.m., a Turkish counterattack on the position was repulsed.

---

10   TNA: WO 95/4309: War Diary, 89th Field Ambulance, 25 April.
11   TNA: WO 95/4356: War Diary, 11th Casualty Clearing Station, 25 April.

78   The Fight for Life

Early on 26 April, the units of the 29th Division at V Beach were relieved by the French division, which had evacuated its gains in the diversionary attack at Kum Kale, and the front line adjusted to accommodate the new force. The arrival of the French was, in part, in preparation for the attack upon Krithia and the hoped-for advance across the peninsula during the following days.

The consolidation work at this time involved considerable work by the engineers to ensure that there was as suitable supply of water, that the beaches were clear of obstacles, particularly at W Beach, and that temporary piers were constructed to allow for the more effective landing of stores, including medical equipment.[12] This work was to prove of considerable importance for evacuating the wounded from 11th CCS, which had been established on the beach on the evening of 25 April. The unit war diary records the work on the first day:

> About 4am we were able to embark on ships boats about 80 wounded. About 1pm we embarked 156 including 25 cot cases. About 6pm we embarked 47 wounded including 34 cot cases. During the day 72 were admitted including 4 Officers. Three cases died in Hospital.
>
> The method of embarking was as follows: The cases were carried on stretchers or if able to walk to a pontoon landing stage a distance of about 300 yards. They were put on ships life boats or barges and towed to a Fleet Mine Sweeper where they were easily lifted on to the Main Deck, from there were distributed. The cot cases to the Hospital Ship *Sicilia* and the walking cases to HMT *Caledonia*.
>
> Owing to the great scarcity of water none could be used for dressing purposes; the wounds were well swabbed with iodine and usual dressings applied. Owing to the rocky nature of the ground no tents were pitched. Food supplied was hot Beef Extract, milk, cocoa, 2 field rations.[13]

The wounded were removed from the beaches as quickly as possible, and, as mentioned in the 11th CCS war diary, not all were sent to hospital ships. There seems to have been some effort at triage when the wounded reached the fleet sweepers since the diary mentions that only the seriously wounded, or cot cases, were sent to the hospital ship. It is not clear how effective this process was, but it must have relied upon medical cover in the form of a doctor being available on the sweepers. Initially, only the HS *Sicilia* had been provided for the Helles part of the landings, but this was supplemented by the arrival of a further hospital ship during 26 April. A number of transports, particularly those carrying MOs or medical units, had been earmarked to receive wounded. One such ship was the *Southland*, which had carried the 87th Field Ambulance to the area. This unit had landed its bearer sections at X and Y Beaches, but the tent subdivision had remained on the transport. On 26 April, the CO:

> … was awoke at 5.30am by an officer who came to my berth to report that wounded had been taken aboard.
>
> Arrangements were hastily made for their reception; a room was prepared in which they were re-covered and another fitted up as an operation room – while the necessary

---

12   John Dixon, *A Vital Endeavour: Military Engineering in the Gallipoli Campaign* (Warwick: Helion & Company, 2019), pp.69–92.
13   TNA: WO 95/4356: War Diary, 11th Casualty Clearing Station, 26 April.

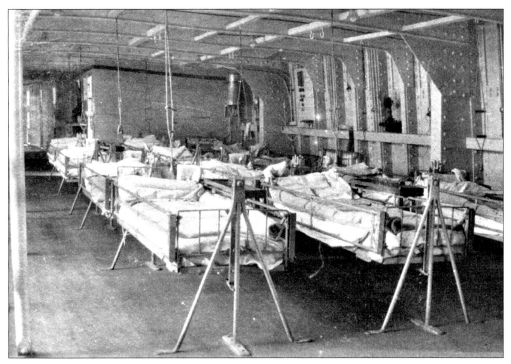

C ward on the HS *Sicilia*. The *Sicilia* was first used at Helles during the landing there but later served the other beachheads. (Tasmanian Archive and Heritage Office (TAHO): NS669/11/1/22)

portion of the equipment was opened up – berths for the wounded were also quickly prepared.

The wounded received numbered 1 officer and 8 men – of these, one (the Officer Lt Rennie SC KSOB) was dangerously wounded in the upper part of right chest and right shoulder and he had evidently bled profusely. Another was a man named Pte A Bagnall RMLI was severely wounded by a gunshot in Right Shoulder – the remainder of the cases were slight.[14]

Lt Rennie was in a very collapsed condition and required the most assiduous care from Major Hope Simpson. The other cases were dealt with by Lt Ryan RAMC. It may be interesting to note that whole of our ship was lying in the position named, shells began to drop about it, eight such shells were counted; the first fire being about 50 yards from us, the sixth and seventh – close to our bow and the eighth whistled thro the rigging – the ship was then moved out one mile further from the shore.

We were again fired at in the afternoon having drifted nearer to the shore, and we soon after saw that the *Andania* was being fired at, and it appeared to us that she was struck by one of the shells.[15]

14 Both Lieutenant Rennie and Private Bagnall appear to have survived the campaign.
15 TNA: WO 95/4309: War Diary, 87th Field Ambulance, 26 April.

In view of the criticism often levelled at the conditions on the transports, it is perhaps as well to remember that they were not universal, and, in many cases, where the medical staff were available, conditions and care were of a reasonable standard, if not up to those in a fully equipped hospital ship. Certainly, over the following days, the 87th Field Ambulance, aboard the *Southland*, although still carrying some troops and stores, maintained a hospital as the numbers of casualties evacuated to it increased as the fighting continued.

For the 88th and 89th Field Ambulances, their work continued. The 88th Field Ambulance had supported the landing at S Beach, but, when the French took over that sector, the unit was moved to W Beach, and all medical care in that sector then transferred to the *Service de Santé des Armées* of the French Army. The 89th Field Ambulance Bearer Subdivision had remained on the *River Clyde* throughout 26 April, where it continued to look after wounded brought into the hospital that it had established in the holds of the old collier. The following day, all its equipment was removed from the ship, and the unit '… got in touch with the 86th Brigade on the heights overlooking the Bay and moved towards the Lighthouse and here an Aid Post was established. All field dressings were collected from the dead and utilized'.[16]

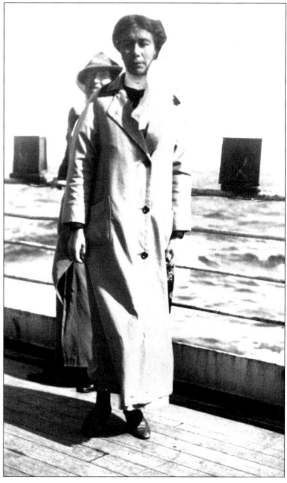

Matron K. F. Fawcett, QAIMNS, was the nurse in charge on both the *Sicilia* and later the HS *Grantully Castle*. Fawcett served for the entire Gallipoli Campaign with nurses of the AANS and was awarded the RRC for her work. (TAHO: NS669/14/1/50A)

However, it was frustrating for those sections of the field ambulances that had been unable to land. Lieutenant Colonel T. Fraser, CO of the 89th Field Ambulance, remained on the troopship *Marquette*, and every effort he made to get A and C Tent Subdivisions landed was blocked either by a lack of communication with the necessary staff or simply by the lack of available small boats to get his unit off the troopship. The frustration felt by Lieutenant Colonel Fraser

---

16 TNA: WO 95/4309: War Diary, 89th Field Ambulance, 27 April.

was echoed by Colonel Yarr, the ADMS, who recorded difficulty in getting ashore and pointed out that '… our tow turn is a long way off'.[17] Nevertheless, when he landed the following day, he seems to have been well satisfied with the progress of the medical units then ashore: 'Large casualties splendidly dealt with, at all beaches and evacuated at night … Have only 3 Bearer Division and 2 Tent Subdivision with only hand carried material and stretchers'.[18]

On 27 April, Yarr was to write that he had been assisting Brigadier General W. R. Marshall (87th Brigade) and the General Staff Officer (1st Grade) (GSO1) in making plans for the attack on Krithia.[19] Although he made it clear that he had not been able to land all his tent divisions, the matter was beyond his control, and, for those days to the end of the month, including the 1st Battle of Krithia, the tent subdivisions were not fully utilised whilst the fighting on the peninsula continued to produce a stream of casualties and increased problems for the stretched medical units that had been able to land.[20]

A joint attack with the French was planned for 28 April with the objective to capture Achi Baba, which was supposed to have been captured on the first day of the campaign. The battle started at 6:00 a.m. on 28 April, and, throughout the day, the men across the Helles sector of the peninsula struggled to gain advantage over the Turks but failed to capture the village of Krithia and Achi Baba at no small cost. The work of the field ambulances was hampered by the lack of transport, but the bearers, both regimental and field ambulance, carried out their work under extremely difficult conditions:

> Bearers were pushed out following the advance along Krithia Road and during the evening they were carrying in wounded on Stretchers from the furthest out tower on that road. This work though very hard on account of the distance (about 2 miles) was continued without break until 5am. Owing to congestion at the CCS, 36 cases had to be retained at the Lighthouse and shelters of stores were built for these. The night was bitterly cold and Bearers gave up their overcoats and ground sheets and even tried to cover the wounded. Hot tea was given to wounded during the evening and night.[21]

At the 11th CCS, their difficulties were different, as they coped with the influx of wounded:

> Still at the same place, very cramped and owing to rocks unable to pitch tents. 204 cases (many other cases not entered in A and D Book owing to the rush) attended to, most of these had a 1st field dressing only and had come straight from the Reg. Aid Posts. Transfers to the ships took place during the afternoon and during the night. Only about 40 remained through the night.[22]

---

17   TNA: WO 95/4307: War Diary, 29th Division ADMS, 26 April.
18   TNA: WO 95/4307: War Diary, 29th Division ADMS, 27 April.
19   At this time, Brigadier Marshall was in command of all troops ashore at Helles. He resumed command of his brigade on 29 April.
20   TNA: WO 95/4309: War Diary, 89th Field Ambulance, 27–30 April.
21   TNA: WO 95/4309: War Diary, 89th Field Ambulance, 28 April.
22   TNA: WO 95/4356: War Diary, 11th Casualty Clearing Station, 28 April.

82   The Fight for Life

Some of those evacuated from the CCS no doubt ended up on the *Southland*, where the tent subdivisions of the 87th Field Ambulance were still working while waiting to disembark:

> Another batch of wounded (50) arrived at about 3pm – began to operate at 7.45pm dealing with urgent cases first – Major McAllister KOSB was among the batch – he was wounded in the right side of abdomen – no wound of exit – and he was very collapsed …
>
> Another batch of wounded (75) arrived about 1.30pm and among them was Lt Col Hulme, Borderers – suffering from a wound in Right hip – bullet passing through pelvis – involving bladder and passing out at an angle corresponding point in left hip.[23] Sent another message to ADMS *Audania* – repeating previous one.[24]

Whilst the medical team on the *Southland* managed the situation in their makeshift hospital ship, the CO was at pains to point out that the casualties from the fighting in front of Krithia had arrived without any notice and added to the difficult situation of handling wounded on the black ship: 'It may be mentioned that no notice was given of wounded being sent to this ship – the wounded were on board before the fact came truly knowledge – nor could I find on whose authority they were sent.'[25]

On shore, the bearer subdivision of this field ambulance was also hard at work:

> In the evening word was brought that Capt. Shubrick RIF was lying badly wounded. Capt. Taylor volunteered to go to him and I volunteered to accompany him, the distance was about 3/4 of a mile but level ground, bullet swept all the way. We got there somehow the bullets ringing and whistling round us. We were unable to do much for the young officer, he have [sic] been shot in the back through the kidneys. We dressed the wound being under fire all the time, placed him in a place of safety, bandaged up a private's leg, RIF, and returned to base.[26]

By 6:00 p.m. on 28 April, the fighting was over. The 29th Division had suffered 2,000 casualties of approximately 8,000 engaged, and the French alongside them had lost 1,000 of their 5,000 men. Colonel Yarr remarked at the end of the day, 'Wounded brought in by regimental and FA bearers who did splendid work. 1500 already evacuated.'[27] Many of the casualties were passed along the evacuation route through the RAP and field ambulances and so to the clearing stations established on the beaches. Many required surgery, and some of those were treated by Lieutenant Colonel J. J. O'Hagan on the *Southland*, where he continued to operate long after the fighting had stopped:

---

23   Lieutenant Colonel R. O. C. Hume, 1st Border Regiment, died of wounds on 1 May 1915 and is commemorated on the Helles Memorial.
24   TNA: WO 95/4309: War Diary, 87th Field Ambulance, 28 April.
25   TNA: WO 95/4309: War Diary, 87th Field Ambulance, 28 April.
26   Museum of Military Medicine (MMM) PE/1/715/Corb.: Diary of Staff Sergeant Corbridge, 87th Field Ambulance.
27   TNA: WO 95/4307: War Diary, 29th Division ADMS, 28 April.

Operated all during the night and left off for a rest and breakfast at 7.45am – began again at 9.30am and continued operating and dressing all day. Another batch of wounded, about 45, arrived at 2am – and another batch arrived about 9.30am (30) – one man (fracture left thigh) was sent from HMS *Implacable*. Lt Shoubrick [sic] RIF and one man died during the night.[28] Communicated with ADMS with regard to the disposal of the dead. Inoculations of anti-tetanus serum given to 14 wounded.[29]

As the fighting faded away, it was clear that the aims of the first day had also faded once again. The Turks were now better prepared, and their losses in the fighting of the days since the landings had bought them sufficient time for their reserves to be mobilised and brought in, or near, the battle zone. For the Allies, there had been significant losses and considerable difficulty in establishing all the elements of the landing. There had been shortfalls at Helles in much of the organisation, as the difficulties of gaining a beachhead had been overcome more slowly than anticipated. However, by 30 April, there was at least some semblance of order to the medical services, in so far as the field ambulances and the CCSs were working together as they were supposed to. There had been difficulties in getting complete field ambulances ashore, but, for the most part, those that were ashore performed as was expected of them. Those on the transports had also worked hard to care for the casualties, as the records for the 87th Field Ambulance show. On 30 April, Lieutenant Colonel T. Fraser of the 89th Field Ambulance wrote:

Seldom if ever can it have happened that a Tent Subdivision of a FA landed with a Covering Force nor occupied with an advanced position in relation to the firing line. The fact that they attained no casualties which prevented men from carrying out their duties is also very noteworthy fact when taken in association with the very large number of wounded dealt with by 19 men and 2 officers during the whole of the 25th.[30]

It is perhaps worth remembering that, whatever the organisation was at the highest level, once battle was entered, it was down to the soldiers on the ground to attempt to achieve what was asked of them. In the case of the medical services, this always came down to the care of the casualties arising from that battle. During the landing on the peninsula, the men of the medical services worked as hard as possible, transporting men on stretchers from the front line to ensure treatment as soon as possible before they were evacuated to waiting hospital ships and transports. Here, their duty was taken over by others, also trying to provide the best care possible, as casualties were moved to the rear:

Continued to operate until 1.30am this morning. Among the cases dealt with was one in which there was 'Ventral' hernia protruding through a bullet wound. Near 'Barneys Spot' right side of abdomen –the bowel – size of an orange – was very tightly gripped and a laparotomy was performed and the bowel returned to the abdomen – this man was very ill and not likely to do well and died suddenly this morning.

---

28   Captain Richard Brian Shubrick, 1st Royal Inniskilling Fusiliers, died of wounds on 28 April and is commemorated on the Helles Memorial.
29   TNA: WO 95/4309: War Diary, 87th Field Ambulance, 29 April.
30   TNA: WO 95/4309: War Diary, 89th Field Ambulance, 30 April.

> A Naval paquet boat came alongside and took off three bodies for burial at sea 10.30 am.
>
> Capt Hare RAMC came aboard and took away with him 55 men who were slightly wounded or convalescing in Hospital.
>
> Went round Hospital and continued to help in dressing all day.[31]

The 87th Field Ambulance, working on the *Southland*, was just one of the units that were used, in part at least, to provide medical cover for the ships that were to be used to transfer the wounded to hospitals in Egypt. At Helles, there was initially only one hospital ship, the *Sicilia*, that was on station of the peninsula as the fighting commenced. This ship, with accommodation for a little over 300 cases, was soon filled to overflowing and left the area for Egypt to be replaced by the RNHS *Soudan*.[32] Thereafter, the distribution of the casualties also involved the use of transports, the so-called 'black ships', such as the *Caledonia* and the *Southland* and others to remove the wounded from the area. Some, such as the *Caledonia*, had been provided with some medical cover in anticipation of this situation, and others, such as the *Southland*, had the good fortune to have been carrying medical units intended for the landing force, which remained on the ships to care for the wounded. In the case of the 87th Field Ambulance, much of its tent subdivision remained on board until early May. Not all the ships were in a fit state, or suitably staffed, for the transport of wounded, and, as a result, there was additional suffering for the wounded on such transports.

The transports from Helles, as from Anzac, carried the wounded to Egypt. In the first instance, the wounded were disembarked to hospitals in Alexandria. Here, a number of general hospitals provided care, but there were shortages of both staff and equipment in Alexandria. Most noticeable, perhaps, was the shortage of nursing staff in the British hospitals. This was overcome as the campaign developed, but, initially, British hospitals were fortunate to be able to use members of the AANS to fill the gaps.

Kum Kale: *Non il y en a un peu*

As part of the overall plan for the invasion of the Gallipoli Peninsula, General Sir Ian Hamilton had also drawn up plans for a diversionary attack on the Asiatic coast facing the beaches of Cape Helles. He had arrived at this conclusion because he was concerned that the proximity of the Asiatic coast meant that field guns could have hampered his planned landings at Helles. He therefore assigned the diversionary attack to the French forces commanded by General Albert D'Amade and sent the appropriate instruction to the general on 20 April.[33]

Thus, it was on 25 April that the part played by the French in the initiation of the Gallipoli Campaign was to create a diversionary landing on the Asiatic side of the Dardanelles at Kum

---

31 TNA: WO 95/4309: War Diary, 87th Field Ambulance, 30 April.

32 Macpherson, *History of the Great War: Medical Services*, vol. 1, p.366. See also comments by Sister Elsie Tucker of the AANS (Australian War Memorial (AWM) AWM41/1053: [Nurses Narratives] Sister E J Tucker), who served on the *Sicilia* for a time before the landing and estimated the accommodation to be closer to 400.

33 Aspinall-Oglander, *Military Operations*, vol. 1, Appendix 6.

Helles: A Solid Mass of Dead and Wounded 85

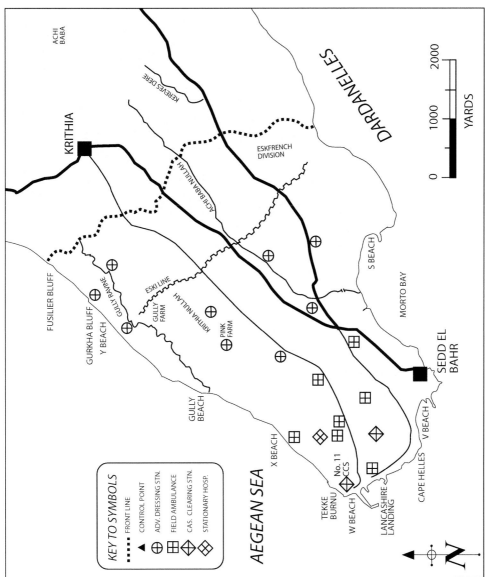

The Medical Services at Cape Helles – final situation. (Terence Powell after Macpherson)

86   The Fight for Life

Kale. In carrying out the diversions, they were also protecting the right flank of the main land-ings taking place at Helles and Gaba Tepe. The landing was undertaken by the colonial brigade of the 1st French Division of the *Corps Expeditionnaire d'Orient*. In particular, the three battal-ions of the 6th Mixed Colonial Regiment were used to spearhead the French action with other regiments, including the colonial brigade of the same division, held in reserve ready to assist the landings at Helles. Accompanying the 6th Mixed Colonial Regiment was one battery of 75's field guns, one section of engineers and one field ambulance of the brigade under Major Joseph Vassal.

The purpose of the attack as a diversionary manoeuvre meant that it had limited objectives. The main objective was to capture the town of Kum Kale and the adjacent village of Yeni Shehr. All of the action was to be contained on the north-western side of the Mendere River, that is, between the river and the Aegean Sea.[34] The timescale for the diversion was also limited and was dependent upon the successful landing of the British forces on the peninsula when all the French troops were to be re-embarked, abandoning any gains, to become a part of the larger-scale action on the peninsula.

The medical arrangements for the landing on the Asiatic coast fell largely under the direc-tion of the SMO of the 6th Mixed Colonial Regiment, Major Joseph Vassal. The arrangements included for the use of the field ambulance to form dressing stations and collecting posts and the evacuation by sea of the wounded from the fighting. Major Vassal was commanding no less than 21 MOs who were involved in the landing that morning. It was these men, together with suffi-cient stretcher-bearers, who were to operate the field ambulances and dressing stations. Vassal had at his disposal three transports that were converted hurriedly to hospital carriers – namely, the SS *La Savoie*, SS *Vinh Long* and the SS *Ceylan* from the five transports used to carry the troops that day.[35] These ships, ocean liners converted to auxiliary cruisers, were the troopships that had carried the soldiers to the landing, but, as soon as the troops were disembarked, they were to act effectively as CCSs since they were to treat wounded and evacuate them as quickly as possible to a single hospital ship, the *Duguay-Trouin*, which was standing off the landing beach fully prepared and ready to receive the wounded.

At the time of the landing, Major Vassal was on board the transport *La Savoie*, from which the ambulance had been landed. While all on board were trying to watch the progress of the landing at Kum Kale, he was making every effort to ensure that the transport was ready to accept the wounded from the shore:

> The establishment of a hospital on board the *Savoie* presented the greatest difficulties. It seemed an almost hopeless task in any case to prepare and make sanitary a transport in which thousands of men have been living crowded together for weeks. And when it had to be done in the middle of a battle, the difficulties can be imagined. Everybody declares that the wounded can be attended to – *after*. There is not time just now, and all hands are required for other services … At half past 8 I caught sight of a colleague who was only just up and was still in slippers … The autoclave ought to be at work

---

34   George H. Cassar, *Reluctant Partner: The Complete Story of the French Participation in the Dardanelles Expedition of 1915* (Warwick: Helion & Company, 2019), p.106.

35   The other ships involved that day were the *Carthage* and the *Theodore Mante*. See also Aspinall-Oglander, *Military Operations*, vol. 1, p.258.

without delay. We have to sterilize all the bedding, 500 sheets, 2,000 towels … I want the crew's quarters evacuated. The men cannot be disturbed, there are no orders for that – it is not possible.

It is exasperating. I open the portholes and say, 'If in ten minutes a clearance is not begun everything shall be thrown into the sea'.

Nearly all the cabins for wounded are still occupied by soldiers. I have them evacuated (by force when necessary) and place a guard over them …[36]

It is clear from Major Vassal's account that, at least from his standpoint, the wounded likely to occur from the landing and their treatment were very much an afterthought for the majority of the officers on board the transports. Nevertheless, through persistence, he was able to set up an operating theatre in the hairdressing salon of the *Savoie*. This was considered a suitable room because it had hot and cold running water, basins and a number of useful cupboards and shelves. As a result of his work, the ship was converted to a 200-bed and 300-hammock transport for wounded in a matter of hours. It has to be assumed that the difficulties encountered by Vassal on the *Savoie* in preparation for receiving wounded were similar on the other two transports standing off the coast for similar use that day. It is probable that they were in a worse position since they would not have had the benefit of the SMO for the landing on hand to deal with the issues that arose and who was, in Vassal's case, quite forceful in getting his arrangements sorted out. It was fortunate that Vassal had persisted in his work, for it was not long before wounded began to arrive from the shore. At 11:00 a.m., the first boats returned from the shore, carrying casualties for treatment. One of the first to be treated was a Russian sailor of the cruiser *Askold*, which had been bombarding the shore along with the French warships.[37] By 1:00 p.m., the makeshift hospital was in full swing, as convoys of wounded in small boats were towed from the shore to the waiting ships, and this continued throughout the afternoon:

From twilight on the 25th till the first rays of dawn the next day we are leaning over wounded in an atmosphere of blood, of groans and of indescribable horrors. We did not stop for a single minute.

The wounded still come in. They are mounted on the deck from the bottom of the boats, and form a long line of stretchers. We are able to put six wounded at a time on the big tables of the children's playroom of the *Savoie*.

The wounds of the night are, nevertheless, frightful. A sergeant major comes back to us only to die. His chest was crushed by shrapnel; and for a moment we saw his heart, almost bare, still beating. There is a Senegalese with his head torn, a foot missing and three fingers of his hand gone. Another black waiting his turn on a chair is asked '*Beaucoup malade?*' '*Non il y en a un peu.*' The doctor looks. Both his legs have been torn off by a shell.[38]

Whilst Vassal was organising the care of the wounded on the *Savoie*, on shore, the battalion MOs had established a collecting post and dressing station 'at the south east angle of the old

36 Anon., *Uncensored Letters*, pp.53–54.
37 Anon., *Uncensored Letters*, p.51.
38 Anon., *Uncensored Letters*, pp.56–57.

88   The Fight for Life

castle'.[39] Here, the wounded were carried by 'sublime stretcher-bearers', received their first attention and, if necessary, were dressed before being moved to the tows that would take them to the waiting transports.[40] Although the three transports involved seem to have been reasonably well equipped with a ship's hospital on board, the transports only acted as clearing stations for this landing since, as soon as it was possible, many of the wounded were removed to the waiting *Duguay-Trouin*, the hospital ship that had been assigned to this part of the French operations. Major Vassal inspected the hospital ship, which was carrying 430 wounded, mostly from the 6th Colonial Regiment, during 26 April and saw the casualties that had been delivered from the other transports. Once this ship was filled, it sailed for Alexandria, where the casualties were dispersed in the hospitals that had been arranged for French troops in and around that city.

Throughout the night of 25 April, fighting continued between Kum Kale and Yeni Shehr. The Turks made a number of local counterattacks, but the French troops held the ground that they had won without pressing further to the capture of Yeni Shehr: 'The morning rose on a memorable scene. Before us corpses were piled up for a space of 200 to 400 metres along the front. The long stretch of broken ground was coloured red with blood.'[41]

The French operation had been a success. They had succeeded in creating a diversion and, in so doing, had effectively protected the flank of the landings on the beaches of Cape Helles. By midday, General d'Amade, commanding the French force, felt that, without significantly more men, there was little to be achieved by holding his forces on the Asiatic coast at Kum Kale. He met with Hamilton on the *Queen Elizabeth* and requested that he be allowed to re-embark his force and land at Helles. This was agreed, and, in the early hours of the morning of 27 April, aided by significant naval firepower, the French soldiers were re-embarked and were then deployed at Helles to support the landing and the beachhead made by the 29th Division. Whilst the diversionary attack should be seen as a success, in that it had achieved its aims, it had not come without significant cost. The SMO stated that there was a total of 167 men killed, 459 wounded and 116 missing – giving a total number of casualties of 742.[42] The *Official History* gives the French casualties as 778, whilst those admitted by the Turks were 1,730.[43] For his part, Vassal recorded that 119 casualties had been treated on board the *Savoie*, which suggests that each of the other two transports set aside for this purpose handled somewhat more than that. Nevertheless, it appears that the medical provisions put in place, albeit under some haste as the landing took place, had worked well. Furthermore, the transfer of the wounded from transports to the *Duguay-Trouin* must have operated well since, a day later, the troops who had disembarked from the transports were re-embarked on the ships that had handled their wounded.

The French began arriving on the peninsula on 27 April when two battalions landed on V Beach. General Hunter-Weston, commanding the British forces at Helles, was planning the next move after he had stabilised his line subsequent to the 29th Division landing. The plan was to capture the town of Krithia and was to rely on the participation of the French force to attack and hold the right flank of the attack while Hunter-Weston moved his forces across the town in a sweeping manoeuvre that would bring him in front of Achi Baba and ready for a subsequent

---

39   Anon., *Uncensored Letters*, p.66.
40   Anon., *Uncensored Letters*, p.46.
41   Anon., *Uncensored Letters*, p.67.
42   Anon., *Uncensored Letters*, p.72.
43   Aspinall-Oglander, *Military Operations*, vol. 1, p.263.

assault on that Turkish position. He had hoped that this could be accomplished soon after the landing phase had been completed, but he was compelled to wait until he had sufficient French forces at his disposal, and this could not be so until 28 April. The French Metropolitan Brigade was earmarked for this assault and, in particular, the 175th Regiment. The medical arrangements were not dissimilar to that following the landing at Kum Kale, except that, since there was to be a longer involvement in this area, both field ambulances of the brigade were landed and established dressing stations, collection posts and clearing stations appropriately. The evacuation of wounded from the peninsula used the same approach as at Kum Kale, but the hospital ship *Duguay-Trouin* was, by this time, on its way to Alexandria and was replaced, probably by the hospital ship *Charles Roux*. The ensuing battle was not a success and resulted in heavy casualties for both the British and the French, totalling approximately 3,000, of which about one-third were French, many of whom passed through the hands of the staff of the *Service de Santé des Armées* on their way to evacuation to base hospital in Egypt.

4

Anzac: Landing Up Over Our Knees in Water

The plan for the Australians to land on the peninsula was to split the force into two parts: the covering force and the main force. The covering force, Brigadier General Sinclair-MacLagan's 3rd Brigade, was to land in three waves. The first 1,500 troops were to be taken to within two miles of the shore by three battleships and then landed in 12 tows. The battalions were to be split up: 500 men from each of the 9th, 10th and 11th Battalions would land in the first wave. The rest of these battalions, plus all the 12th Battalion, would land in the second and third waves. Seven destroyer towing ships' lifeboats would bring a second wave of 1,250 men through the battleships to within 100yd of the shore. Once the second wave had landed, the lifeboats would be used to bring ashore the third wave, also 1,250 men, at 5:30 a.m.

The 3rd Brigade's four battalions would strike quickly to the left and right. The 9th Battalion, after landing on the right, was to send two companies to clear Gaba Tepe; the other two were to head for Anderson's Knoll at the seaward end of the third ridge (Gun Ridge). The 10th Battalion was to land in the centre, capture the Turkish guns on 400 Plateau, which was part of the second ridge, then cross Legge Valley and occupy Scrubby Knoll on the third ridge. The 11th Battalion was to land on the left and seize Chunuk Bair at the top of the third ridge. The 12th Battalion was to be in reserve, and the artillerymen would take their mountain guns to 400 Plateau.

The main force, consisting of the 1st and 2nd Brigades, was to arrive from Mudros on eight transports. It was planned that these would approach the shore around 5:00 a.m. Four of the transports were to anchor and transfer their troops to the battleships' 12 tows. The other four were to transfer their troops onto the seven destroyers as soon as these had landed the covering force. If all went well, the three brigades and the mountain guns would be ashore by 9:00 a.m. The 2nd Brigade was to press on past Chunuk Bair and take Hill 971. It would protect the left flank by holding the line along North Beach to Fisherman's Hut. The 1st Brigade was to be the reserve of the main force.

The careful planning for successive waves of troops to transfer between transports, battle-ships, destroyers and tows sadly went all wrong as the 12 tows made their approach to the shore. Exactly what happened has been a matter of conjecture, but, certainly, the naval officer in charge of the right-handed tow was happy enough in maintaining his direction but was perturbed to see the tows, each some 150yd apart, veering off to the left. Eventually finding just himself and the nearest tow to him heading in presumably the correct direction but not wanting to land in

Anzac: Landing Up Over Our Knees in Water 91

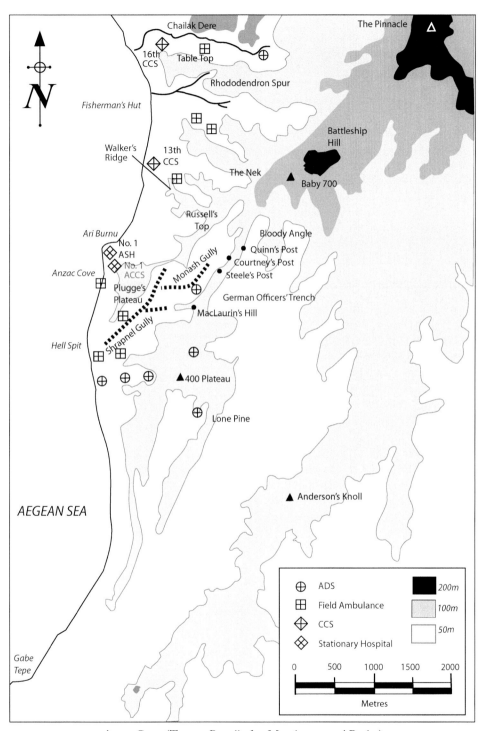

Anzac Cove. (Terence Powell after Macpherson and Butler)

isolation from the flotilla, he decided to veer left. In so doing, he crossed the bows of the other tows, and their leaders picked up this movement and also veered off to the left before straightening out and making for the shore. It was the man in command of the flotilla, Commander Dix, who sensed something wrong and exclaimed, 'Tell the Colonel that the damn fools have taken us a mile too far north'. They had in fact landed in a tight formation at the distinctive knoll at Ari Burnu.[1] Reasons for the error included ignorance of a 'northerly current'; the navy crews mistaking Ari Burnu for Gaba Tepe; the battleships possibly anchoring too far north and simply confusion over Braithwaite's written instruction to Birdwood, dated 13 April, referring to the landing being '… on the beach between Gaba Tepe and Fisherman's Hut'. Birdwood was to see the 'hand of Providence' having directly guided the flotilla to a beach having such steep cliffs that the landing force was almost immune from shell fire. The reality was that the tight landing formation spread around the knoll led to a hopeless mix of the landing battalions. It was not the time to wait and regroup. The Turks, expecting but not knowing the exact location of the landing, allowed the first boats to shore before subjecting the invading force to rifle and machine-gun fire. The heavily loaded troops had little option but to get out of the boats, into the water, wade ashore and rush across the beach to get under the shelter of the nearest cliffs before advancing up the cliff.

Under the strictest of orders that, as the covering force, they were to advance at all speed in order to protect the main force, the troops advanced.[2] The 3rd Infantry Brigade war diary records, '4:45 a.m.: advance pushed out, 6:00 a.m.: Brigade considerably mixed but roughly in order, 9th, 10th, 12th 11th from right. 7:00 a.m. Reorganising to push on. 8:10 a.m. Counterattack repulsed. 2nd Brigade put in on right, 1st Brigade right and left'.[3]

There were thousands of men scrambling up the steepest of hills covered with scrub composed of small stout bushes of prickly oak, waist high, that presented its own special obstacle. Progress was slow and tortuous as men grabbed at the roots to haul themselves up the slope or used their bayonets to give purchase on the steep hillsides. The edge of a plateau became visible as dawn approached and was an added incentive to get to the top of the hills. The wounded had little option but to slide down the hill until, perhaps, brought to a halt amongst the scrub. The first men arrived at the edge of the plateau to see their first Turks running back from a trench close to the edge. The forward edge of the cliff offered some shelter, and, as more and more men arrived at the top, the near edge of the plateau was secured.

There were heavy Turkish counterattacks throughout the day, but fierce resistance by the brigade – supported by the New Zealand Brigade, which had landed with the main force, a mountain battery and ship fire – repulsed the enemy. At 6:00 p.m., the order came to dig in for the night, and Turkish attacks continued but again were met with spirited resistance from the Australians and New Zealanders.

It has been suggested that the landing at Anzac was not accompanied by '… Field Ambulances of any kind'.[4] This would seem to be a misrepresentation of the facts based on the evidence from

---

1   Charles E. W. Bean, *Official History of Australia in the War of 1914–18: The Story of ANZAC* (Sydney: Angus and Robertson, 1940), vol. 1, see Map No. 10 following p.250.
2   Bean, *Story of ANZAC*, vol. 1, see Map No. 11 following p.256.
3   AWM: 4/23/3/1: War Diary, 3rd Infantry Brigade, Part 1.
4   Harrison, *Medical War*, p.187.

the war diaries of the medical units. During the landing phase of the operation, the following medical units were immediately involved:

- 1st ACCS
- 1st AFA
- 2nd AFA
- 3rd AFA
- 4th AFA
- New Zealand Field Ambulance (NZFA).

However, at least for some of these units, it was only part of the unit that landed, as bearer subdivisions were landed while tent subdivisions remained on their transports, providing assistance to those wounded coming off the beaches later in the day.

The effects of the landing were eventually to be felt farther afield. On 29 April 1915, Sister Bessie Pocock, a sister in the AANS stationed in Cairo, was to write in her diary, 'Report says Australians terribly cut up landing. Germans [sic] had forts on hill – mowed them down as they landed – know nothing yet – many killed and many wounded.'[5] At this stage, the truth of the landing was not known in Egypt, and few, if any, of the wounded had reached Cairo and the No. 2 AGH where Sister Pocock worked. For the medical units involved, the landings were to be just the beginning of their work.

The 1st AFA had landed as directed on the morning of 25 April when a bearer detail of three officers and 112 other ranks had landed in the midst of heavy fire at 9:30 a.m. Amongst this group of bearers was Private Thomas James Richards, who commented:

> … landing up over our knees in water from the rowing boats into which we had been transferred from the *Scourge*. As we were landing a shrapnel shell burst 150 yards away and threw a shower of bullets into the water – rather a pretty display! Twenty minutes later with stretchers we were climbing the steep, rough hills looking for wounded, but it was 1 o'clock when I got my first case and from then until 6 o'clock I had fully twenty dressing to do.[6]

In the 2nd AFA, a similar number of men landed with the attacking force by 1:00 p.m. The tent and transport subdivision of the unit remained on board the transport *Mashobra* and, later in the day, returned to Lemnos, where it remained out of the fighting for three days.

Meanwhile, the 3rd AFA Bearer Division, commanded by Captain Douglas Murray McWhae, had arrived at the landing site aboard the HMS *Ribble* along with a company of the 12th Battalion that was to be part of the covering force:

---

5   AWM: PR05050, RCDIG0001389: Transcript of Diary of Mary Ann 'Bessie' Pocock, 1914-1918 (Vol. 1), 29 April 1915.
6   AWM: 2DRL/0786, RCDIG0001478: [Transcript] Diaries of Thomas James Richards, Vol. 2, 25 April 1915. Richards was later commissioned and served with the 1st Battalion. He was awarded the Military Cross (MC) in 1917.

94   The Fight for Life

The disembarkation into the tows was made under rifle fire and two men were wounded on the torpedo boat and left behind. The unit disembarked into two boats of second tow about 5 am. Capt McWhae with C Section was in one boat and Capts Fry and Buchanan with A and B Sections in the other. Landing was affected under heavy shrapnel and rifle fire and several casualties occurred. The boat parties in two groups took shelter from direct fire under the sand bank at back of the beach and were shortly after enfiladed by a party of Turks along the curve of the beach. Fortunately, their hits were not many and about twenty minutes later the enfilading party were driven back by a further landing party. For another hour it was impossible to do more than attend to our own wounded as heavy sniping was coming down on our position. The coast then being moderately clear the men were set to work improving shelter to make collecting posts and attending to and bringing in wounded from nearby. Officers and sergeants then went out with squads not needed at collecting posts and scoured the vicinity along the shore and up over the hills as far as possible. Our fighting forces were largely composed of scattered groups at the time so a thorough and systematic search was impracticable. Wounded were dressed and taken back to the collecting posts. By midday when the officers returned to the station about 100 cases had been collected. About 1.30 [p.m.] the left flank was retiring and it appeared that the position of our collecting post was in danger. The wounded were quickly evacuated to the main beach, the final patients being embarked on a boat sent by the ADMS for the purpose. On the main beach till late in the evening officers and men were assisting the 1st Clearing Hospital in dressing and evacuating wounded to the Hospital Ships. At the end of the day our casualties were reported 2 killed, 18 wounded and 4 missing.[7]

The 1st ACCS had come ashore between 10:00 a.m. and 12:00 p.m.:

On reaching beach were allotted a position for establishing casualty clearing station. The number of casualties waiting to be treated was great and they came so quickly that nothing more than first aid could be done. Cases were evacuated to Hospital Ship *Gascon* which carried 350 severely wounded cases and Transport *Clan MacGillivray* which was to take lightly wounded.

Cases were loaded into boats and transported to ships by Navy. The whole clearing hospital staff worked splendidly throughout the day and most of the following night. Owing to pressure of work and necessity of keeping the beach clear (in event of having to retire) it was impossible to keep a record of all cases treated. I was especially instructed by the ADMS 1 Aust Div, Col Howse, to evacuate as rapidly as possible. About 700 cases passed through hands of the clearing hospital.[8]

The 1st Australian Division had made a landing and had established a tenuous beachhead from which operations could proceed. Fighting had been heavy, and the work of the field ambulances had been very intense. In the 1st AFA, the bearers continued their work until midnight,

7   AWM: AWM4/26/46/4: War Diary, 3rd Australian Field Ambulance, 25 April.
8   AWM: AWM4/26/62/1: War Diary, 1st Australian Casualty Clearing Station, 25 April.

carrying wounded back from the firing line. At that point, the CO split them into details, which allowed not only for the work to continue but also for some short periods of rest for the men in their camp immediately above the beach. For Private Richards, the work continued to be hard:

> A fellow came along and asked me to go up and fix up his pal whose foot was shot. With a stretcher, Watts and I went only 100 yards along the valley. The bush was too thick and the water-worn track too rough that we discarded the stretcher and proceeded on all fours up to the firing line trenches upon which our fellows had been driven back. Here was a poor devil with his heel and sole of foot blown away, and although in great pain he was what might be considered cheerful. I cut his boot off and dressed the foot. Bleeding was not heavy. Now the trouble was to get him away with rifle fire pinging overhead and through the bushes within a foot of us. This safely done the way out was awful but my patient skidded down the steep side on his hands and seat while I went forward holding the limb. In the bottom of the gorge, I got him on my back and made good progress but as the foot started to bleed heavily, I had to put a ligature on to the artery at the thigh. Fully two hours had passed before we got back to the boats taking wounded aboard the transports, and he bore up wonderfully well.[9]

All day, men and equipment were landing on the beaches that were to become known as 'Anzac'. During the late morning, the transport *Gosler*, carrying the NZFA, arrived off Gaba Tepe and shortly began disembarking to the destroyer *Foxhound*, which was to carry them closer to the shore before actually landing from tows as had the rest of the attacking force. Major E. J. O'Neill of this unit was the first New Zealand medic to arrive with a party of bearers, and he was immediately dispatched by Colonel N. Manders, the acting DDMS, to Plugge's Plateau to provide medical cover for the fighting that was taking pace there.[10] O'Neill found that he could not establish a dressing station at the plateau because it was so exposed and eventually set up a collecting post on the seaward side of the plateau. Here, in some dead ground, he was able to start the work of attending to the wounded coming from the fight a little above him. O'Neill's team worked continuously over the following hours, as wounded continued to come down the steep slopes from the firing line.[11]

At first, the 1st ACCS coped well, but, in the confined space, it had been allotted that there was no room to retain patients for any length of time, and it was soon necessary to evacuate as many as possible. This was the desire of the ADMS, Colonel Howse, but it was not to prove as easy as he would have hoped. The planning for the landing had accepted the need to evacuate wounded from the beach, and, at Anzac, one hospital ship, the HMHS *Gascon*, had been provided and one so-called 'ambulance carrier' or transport. The first of these vessels was to take seriously wounded, while the transport was to take only light cases. Howse accepted that he needed to wait until all infantry that were to land would take priority, but, at 1:00 p.m., he took it upon himself to make every effort, since all infantry had landed by that time, to get

---

9   AWM: 2DRL/0786, RCDIG0001478: [Transcript] Diaries of Thomas James Richards, Vol. 2, 25 April.
10 Major Eugene Joseph O'Neill was awarded the DSO for his service at Anzac on 25–26 April.
11 Carberry, *New Zealand Medical Service in the Great War*, pp.39–40.

wounded off the shore.[12] It is at this point that there were problems. It had been anticipated that there would be space to sort the wounded, but, in the event of the overall failure of the attack, the space was lacking, and the sorting was not thorough. This was compounded further by the lack of small boats to take the wounded off the increasingly crowded beach. This all meant that a large number of lightly wounded men were sent to the *Gascon* whilst more seriously wounded were sent to the transport. It was recorded that the *Gascon*:

> Moved out of Mudros at 1.30 am and arrived at Gaba Tepe about 7 am. The Australians and New Zealand contingents were being landed in boats under fire from the shore. Kept receiving wounded all day until towards evening the accommodation of the ship having been taken up, the ship left for Mudros Bay with 547 wounded including 23 officers.[13]

The *Gascon* was meant to carry 492 casualties, and, thus on its first journey from the peninsula, it was carrying more than had been intended. However, as the campaign developed, this situation worsened as problems over numbers of hospital ships continued. The impact of the landing was very clear to Sister Elsie Tucker, one of the seven members of the AANS serving on the *Gascon*:

> Shells bursting all around, we are off Gaba Tepe. The soldiers have commenced to land, there are Men-of-War and Transport Boats in every direction around us, an occasional shell burst quite near us. The wounded commence to come on board about 9 am, four die in the first boat that comes over, the patients just pour into the wards; from barges and boats. The majority of patients have first aid dressings and quite a number of the boys are soaked through; the RAMC and Indian orderlies between them get the men's clothes off and I start straight away at dressing; I'm responsible for about 76 patients in the ward and about 40 which I have on mattresses on the fore-deck. With the assistance of a medical student, we get through all the dressings by 2 am, have quite a number of compound fractures which I put up temporarily and apply pressure in other cases where necessary hoping that Colonel Hugo will soon finish the officers and get down to my ward, but we hear that he is working hard in the theatre so I dress in with many anxious looks at the paler faces down the long lines of bunks, in fear that haemorrhage might pass unnoticed. Several times I go back along the lines of dressing and find a dressing saturated and to apply more dressing and pressure. The boys are bricks, they smoke on, and patiently wait their turn, they think the old ship is heaven after the peninsula. All this time we can hardly hear ourselves speak with the banging which is going on outside. The ship shivers with the extra heavy reports, but we are much too busy to think of what is going on, even forget we haven't had a meal, till the steward says there is a cup of tea in the pantry sister – about 6 o'clock. The last dressing is finished about 2.30 am and the men are nearly all sleeping. Matron comes into the ward and absolutely bundles me off to bed; at 5.30 am up and in the ward again; the orderlies look after the feeding of the patients; we can't attempt to wash them or make their beds. I commence straight away at dressings and go on solidly until

---

12 Butler, *Official History of the Australian Medical Services*, vol. I, p.143.
13 TNA: WO 95/4145/1: War Diary, HMHS *Gascon*, 25 April.

10.30 pm. There are 557 patients on board and only 7 nurses so that we can't attempt to do anything else for the men except their dressings, it nearly breaks your heart to see them lying there looking hot and dirty and not be able to sponge them and make then comfortable.[14]

The *Gascon* sailed for Mudros that evening, but it was not able to disembark any patients and had to wait there throughout the following day before receiving orders to sail for Alexandria, where it disembarked 535 patients on 29 April. There were more than 20 deaths during the voyage, perhaps, in part, caused by the long delay waiting at Mudros Harbour for orders to proceed to Alexandria.

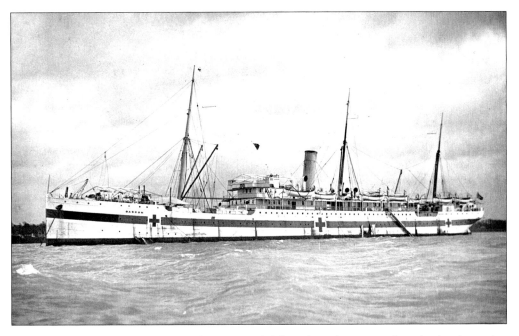

The HS *Gascon* was a regular transport for the wounded from Anzac but was used at other beaches as the need arose. (AWM: H18949/4)

At Mudros, No. 1 and No. 2 ASHs were unprepared for an influx of wounded from the peninsula. In the case of No. 1 ASH, this was partly because they were in the middle of evacuating the sick whom they had been tending on the island since their arrival there in March. The hospital was awaiting the arrival of the *Guildford Castle* to allow its evacuation to Alexandria. On 24 April, it was eventually able to evacuate 229 cases on the transport *Osmanieh* but had already been instructed to make itself available for the sick from the ships in the harbour at Mudros. As such, No. 1 ASH took no part in handling casualties from the landing at Anzac or the days immediately after.[15]

---

14 AWM: AWM41/1053: [Nurses Narratives] Sister E J Tucker.
15 AWM: AWM4/26/70/3: War Diary, No. 1 Australian Stationary Hospital, April 1915.

98   The Fight for Life

No. 2 ASH had embarked on the *Hindoo* on 20 April at Alexandria 'for unknown destination' and arrived off the island of Lemnos at 8:30 p.m. three days later. The hospital remained on the transport and, on 25 April, received orders to supply medical staff to departing transports:

- HMTS *Lutzow* – three officers and 23 others
- HMTS *Ionian* – three officers and 23 others
- HMTS *Clan MacGillivray* – one MO and 16 others
- HMTS *Seang Choon* – 15 other ranks.

This was clearly an effort to provide the transports with medical staff who would be employed once the ships were unloaded at the peninsula and took on wounded from the fighting. Unfortunately, the order had arrived too late, for three of the transports had already left for the peninsula by the time the men were organised to leave the hospital. Only the *Seang Choon* received the 15 other ranks to help the MOs of the RAMC who were already on board. Sergeant Roy Rowe was in the party that was supposed to staff the *Clan MacGillivray*:

> Our unit was divided today into 4 parties, each party to go on a transport. Captain Haynes, myself and 15 men were in one party. Our party and another one left the SS *Hindoo* for our respective transports at 6:30. Our party returned after a ride all-round the harbour. Our boat had not waited for us but had gone on to the Dardanelles with a lot more ships.[16]

The *Hindoo*, carrying the remainder of the hospital, left Mudros harbour at 7:00 p.m. on 25 April and sailed to the mouth of the Dardanelles but remained more or less uninvolved for three days while it waited for orders – the ship had effectively become lost to the communications of the higher staff, and it was not until 29 April that the ship was ordered to Gaba Tepe.[17] The loss of this ship and its hospital and staff for this period was to have a considerable impact on the evacuation of the wounded from Anzac. On 29 April, the ship was ordered to Gaba Tepe, where half the hospital, under Major George Walter Barber, was transferred to the *Devanha*, which had come alongside and treated wounded on that ship until it was filled and moved away from the area.[18] Finally, on 1 May, the remainder of the hospital, under Major Bernhard Trangott Zwar, was transferred to the *Minnewaska*, where a hospital was opened and wounded treated.[19]

In a similar manner, the *Hindoo* was also carrying No. 16 BSH, and this unit was also uninvolved in the opening moves of the campaign at the peninsula since it, too, remained on the ship, anchored some four miles outside the entrance to the Dardanelles for three days. It was not until 3 May that the unit was to become involved in supplying staff for transports then evacuating wounded from Cape Helles.[20]

---

16   AWM: PR04297, RCDIG0000269: Diary for Roy Rowe, 1915-1916, 24 April.
17   AWM: AWM4/26/71/1: War Diary, No. 2 Australian Stationary Hospital, April 1915.
18   The HS *Devanha* had accommodation for a little over 500 patients and had been commissioned as a hospital ship in August 1914.
19   AWM: PR04297, RCDIG0000269: Diary for Roy Rowe, 1915-1916, 1 May.
20   TNA: WO 95/4357: War Diary, No. 16 Stationary Hospital, April and May 1915.

The landings had not been a great success, but the Australians and New Zealanders had held their ground and continued to look for advantage as 26 April dawned. It had been a close-run thing, for, on the night of 25 April, General Birdwood had wired Hamilton to ask for the re-embarkation of the troops based on the none too favourable information coming from the beaches. Hamilton replied that the hard part was over and now they needed to dig in to face any Turkish counterattack. Work of the medical units had continued all night, and they had been especially aware of the request for the re-embarkation, as their responsibility would have been, of necessity, to evacuate any wounded. In the 1st ACCS, the staff:

> Had beach completely evacuated by 3 am. Wounded continued to come in very freely all day, and the same difficulties experienced in getting them first aid and evacuation. The only position possible was open beach 20 ft by 20 ft in which to treat a huge number of cases many of great severity. We were also clearing for 2 divisions with a reduced staff and very little equipment, having only landed a small portion of our gear. Evacuated about 700 cases.[21]

The work continued through the day, as field ambulances did everything possible to bring in the casualties. They, too, had been well aware of the difficult situation as the night of 25 April passed, and, in the 3rd AFA, it was noted, 'At 3 am the Ambulance was raised under orders to re-embark and two stretcher squads went out and brought two wounded patients who were reported. The re-embarkation order was countermanded shortly after.'[22]

The field ambulances soon began their work again once the thought of re-embarkation disappeared. Their work was relentless as casualties were collected:

> At 4 am Capt Buchanan went out with four stretcher squads near the head of Long Valley, rendering first aid at the firing line, and sending back wounded. At 5 am Capt Fry followed up with four more squads, established a dressing station and worked further up the Valley. When parties returned later in the morning the dressing station was handed over to Capt Thomson. Capt McWhae then went out with the majority of the squads of B and C Sections. They were detained for a short time in the valley by heavy shrapnel and then went on to 3rd Brigade Headquarters, where they worked that day and through the night. Capt Fry went out shortly after with sixteen stretchers and collected wounded from the left flank of the 3rd Brigade and from Capt Thomson's stations. In the meantime, Capt Buchanan received a call to 1st Brigade Headquarters and went up with two stretcher parties and brought back wounded. Our men were now worked to a standstill and a message asking for assistance was received from 1st Brigade Headquarters. Applications was made to Major Stokes of the 1st Field Ambulance and Capt Wassell went out with a section of stretcher bearers accompanied by Capt Buchanan, as guide, and Capt Fry. On the way a call to the 3rd Brigade Headquarters was responded to and wounded evacuated. Our three officers returned

---

21 AWM: AWM4/26/62/3: War Diary, 1st Australian Casualty Clearing Station, 26 April 1915.
22 AWM: AWM4/26/46/4: War Diary, 3rd Australian Field Ambulance, 26 April 1915.

about 4 am. During the day our casualties were 1 killed and wounded, 1 man missing on the 25th turned up.[23]

Here, the reference to the 'Long Valley' is an early reference to what became known very shortly as 'Shrapnel Valley', and, from this account, it was clearly a well-deserved name. The following day, Captain August Lyle Buchanan formed a dressing station near the head of this dangerous gully and took the medical care right to the front-line troops.

The military side of the operation did not progress any better on 26 April than it had on the day of the landings. However, the expected Turkish counterattack did not materialise. The Turks had fought hard on the previous day, were every bit as tired as the attacking force and had no reserves in place for such a major undertaking. The overall weakness of the Turks at this stage had not been realised by the leaders of the force camped on the beach.[24] 26 April was marked only by an advance of the 4th Battalion to capture ground that it had surrendered the night before. Whilst they overcame the Turkish defenders, the ground recovered was swept with machine-gun and shrapnel fire. It was soon untenable, and the battalion withdrew to its starting line by evening. The tired ANZACs spent most of the day consolidating and preparing for the advance that they knew would be asked of them very shortly. During the day, the pressure of the medical services continued more or less unabated, and this was reflected by Private Richards, who wrote in his diary that he had not managed to get to bed until 2:30 a.m. on 27 April, as the calls on the stretcher-bearers of the field ambulances continued deep into the night.[25]

The Turks made their anticipated attack on 27 April with two new regiments that had recently arrived in the area. With the help of heavy fire from the warships in the bay, this attack was broken up and was overall ineffective except at the Nek, where the line was threatened and Brigadier General H. B. Walker and Lieutenant Colonel Braund of the 2nd Battalion organised a successful defensive line. Nevertheless, casualties continued to come away from the line to the field ambulances and the 1st ACCS: 'Pressure of work still kept up. The position of Casualty Clearing Station exposed to shrapnel fire … Evacuated 659 cases'.[26] The large number of cases cleared through the CCS also reflects the amount of work carried out by the field ambulances and their bearers. On 27 April, Private Richards, 1st AFA, recorded that the 'improvised wharf from which our wounded, chiefly, leave has been shell swept for half an hour at a time', undoubtedly increasing the difficulty in getting the wounded evacuated to the transports then waiting for them.[27] By this time, the HS *Gascon*, which had been assigned to the ANZACs, was on its way to Alexandria, and it was the role of the so-called 'hospital carriers' or 'black ships' to take charge of those evacuated from the beaches.

Some of the field ambulance stretcher-bearers did not work during the day because of their exposure to fire, and Private Richards recorded that they did much of their collecting during the hours of darkness. On 27 April, he began his work at 6:00 p.m., but shrapnel fire and 'stray

---

23   AWM: AWM4/26/46/4: War Diary, 3rd Australian Field Ambulance, 26 April 1915.
24   Charles E. W. Bean, *Anzac to Amiens* (Canberra: Australian War Memorial, 1968), p.118.
25   AWM: 2DRL/0786, RCDIG0001478: [Transcript] Diaries of Thomas James Richards, Vol. 2, 27 April 1915.
26   AWM: AWM4/26/62/3: War Diary, 1st Australian Casualty Clearing Station, April 1915.
27   AWM: 2DRL/0786, RCDIG0001478: [Transcript] Diaries of Thomas James Richards, Vol. 2, 27 April 1915.

bullets' drove him and his comrades into shelter. It was 8:00 p.m. before they finally reached the right flank of the beachhead, where, fortunately, casualties had been light that day.[28] This set the scene for the ANZACs at their landing site, as they were overlooked by the enemy in many places and all the ground could be subjected to shell fire more or less at any time. The careful selection of sites for dressing stations and hospitals was essential, and, even then, there was no protection from stray Turkish fire.

Throughout the following day, the ANZACs firmly established themselves in the hills and gullies above the beach, holding tenaciously to every piece of ground possible as they dug trenches and prepared defensive positions. The number of casualties fell as these measures were taken, but there were problems of collecting and clearing wounded, even when the Turks were not attacking. In the 1st ACCS, this was more about tiredness than anything: 'The Field Ambulance of RMLI landed and assisted in medical work alongside Casualty Hospital giving my staff a very much needed rest as they had been working about 20 hours a day since landing. Evacuated 225 cases.'[29] The work was endless, and continued fire from the Olive Grove (Beachy Bill) made life very uncomfortable for everyone while they continued work gathering and dressing the wounded:

> Dug outs of our camp site very knocked about by a new gun which has recently opened fire from the neighbourhood of the OLIVE GROVE. Our line has suffered fairly consistently from fire of the enemy. The condition of the men is fine although the work up and down these steep grades is very distressing. The number of casualties for the last two days is considerably less and therefore Transport is much reduced. All transport of the wounded to the Casualty Clearing Station on Anzac Beach is by stretcher – nothing else available.[30]

Added to the problems caused by the enemy fire was also confusion caused by the more or less unknown terrain in which both the infantrymen and medical personnel found themselves. This was a particular problem to the bearer parties of the field ambulances who traversed the area collecting wounded:

> At 6 pm the three sections of Bearers went out in three parties and evacuated collecting stations on the right flank and other stations in the centre. Right up to this time there was great difficulty in founding systematic work as the valleys in the area were intricate and at the time tracks were ill defined and difficult to recognize. Further, fighting units were intermixed and split up and few could give directions to the location where help was required.[31]

By the end of the month, just five days after landing on the peninsula, the ANZACs were getting to grips with their new environment, and the medical arrangements were still evolving,

---

28   AWM: 2DRL/0786, RCDIG0001478: [Transcript] Diaries of Thomas James Richards, Vol. 2, 27 April 1915.
29   AWM: AWM4/26/62/3: War Diary, 1st Australian Casualty Clearing Station, 25 April 1915.
30   AWM: AWM4/26/62/3: War Diary, 1st Australian Casualty Clearing Station, 30 April 1915.
31   AWM: AWM4/26/46/4: War Diary, 3rd Australian Field Ambulance, 26 April 1915.

particularly in the matter of evacuation to transport ships. On 30 April, Lieutenant Colonel Arthur Thomas White, officer commanding (OC) of No. 2 ASH, was ordered to meet with General Birdwood's senior administrative officer, General Carruthers, to discuss the matter of transport for wounded as it would affect No. 2 ASH. The outcome of the meeting was that half the unit was transferred immediately to the HS *Devanha* while the other half was eventually transferred to the HS *Gloucester Castle* with medical and surgical equipment.[32] The space on the beach was both crowded and exposed, and the hospitals did not escape. On 30 April, the recently arrived No. 4 AFA was forced by shrapnel fire to dig a new position for the tent in which they treated the wounded.[33] In the response to the firing, the NZFA, working on the left flank, lowered the Red Cross flag that marked their position above them because it seemed to be attracting artillery fire.[34]

The hospital ship assigned to the ANZACs, the *Gascon*, had left its station off Gaba Tepe on the evening of 25 April.[35] This did not mean that there could not be evacuation since the planning, such as it was, for the landing had allowed for a number of hospital carriers, or what became known as 'black ships' since they did not carry the internationally recognised white livery of the hospital ships, had been ordered to the assist in the evacuation of the wounded. The tent division of the 1st AFA was on the HMTS *City of Benares* on the day of the landing, and, on 24 April, as was recorded by Major R. J. Millard, this ship was readied for the action:

> In case of casualties on board, we are going to use the 1st Saloon forward and the 2nd Saloon aft as temporary dressing stations. If we do get a shell on board in the right place, we shall go off pop as we are full of gun cotton and ammunition for small arms and guns, but that is a very remote contingency I hope.[36]

Millard was correct in his belief that a shell was unlikely to cause them problems. Nevertheless, on the day of the landing, the *City of Benares* did come into service not long after the *Gascon* had left the area:

> About 9 pm we were hailed by a launch 'Can you take some wounded on board?' We made hasty arrangements and received 75 wounded, many very severe, whom we stowed as best we could in the forward troop deck on the tables, and in the 1st and 2nd class saloons. This kept us intensely busy until 3 am. About midnight came a fearful report that the attack had failed, retirement had been ordered and that every ship was to send all boats ashore at once to re-embark troops.[37]

---

32 Note that the War Diary of No. 2 ASH calls these ships 'troopships', but, according to Macpherson, the *Devanha* was equipped as a hospital ship, or hospital carrier, from 22 August 1914, and the *Gloucester Castle* had been likewise fitted since 22 September 1914. AWM: AWM4/26/71/1: War Diary, No. 2 Australian Stationary Hospital, 30 April 1915.
33 AWM: AWM4/26/47/5: War Diary, 4th Australian Field Ambulance, 30 April 1915. The 4th AFA landed on 27–28 April.
34 AWM: AWM4/35/27/2: War Diary, New Zealand Field Ambulance, 30 April 1915.
35 TNA: WO 95/4145/1: War Diary, HMHS *Gascon*, April 1915.
36 AWM: 1DRL/0499, RCDIG0000181: Typescript Extracts from Diary of Sir Reginald Jeffery Millard.
37 AWM: 1DRL/0499, RCDIG0000181: Typescript Extracts from Diary of Sir Reginald Jeffery Millard.

Major Millard was too busy to concern himself with worry about the possible re-embarkation, for he spent most of the next 24 hours handling the wounded that had arrived during the night. The *City of Benares* was not one of the ships assigned to handle casualties from the landings in the original plan, but, since it had some medical staff on board, it was able to largely cope and offer care to those in most need. Nevertheless, during those first hours, a number of the cases died on the ship.[38] By this time, the Turks were also beginning to range in on the troop carriers, and shells began to fall between the ships. Whilst there appears to have been little damage, the net result was that all ships were ordered to stand farther off the shore. The effect of this was to add to the difficulties in evacuating wounded from the beach, as the distance to the waiting ships was thus increased.

On 27 April, the work of the tent division of the 1st AFA was to change since the CO, Lieutenant Colonel Bernard James Newmarch, with Captain Hugh Poate and a party of 22 men were transferred to the *Itonus* to take the wounded from the *City of Benares* to Alexandria.

The rest of the tent division, including Major Millard, were transferred to the *Derfflinger* to carry out similar work:

> On the *Derfflinger* I found strenuous work going on. Wounded had been arriving in barges and boats for some hours and to cope with them were a RAMC Captain Edmunds, a naval surgeon from the *Canopus* and an elderly ships doctor from the *Cardiganshire*. I hastily took stock of the situation distributed my 10 men to their work and waded in at the dressings. There was no intermission in the stream of wounded and I worked on solidly all though the night and all next day stopping only for meals. It was fairly ghastly work as some of the injuries were terrible and we could not possibly get to them all.[39]

It should be noted that neither the *Itonus* nor the *Derfflinger* had been earmarked for the carrying of wounded, but, as can be seen from the Millard's account, the medical staff aboard both ships seem to have done all they could for the wounded that made it to their ships. The *Derfflinger* stayed on station until the following day, and the wounded kept arriving from the shore: 'Despite my protests they continued to crowd wounded on until noon (of the 28th) by which time we had taken about 590. Every nook and corner of deck and cabins was chock full, the men lying so close that one could hardly step between them.'[40] The *Derfflinger* eventually left the peninsula early on the morning of 29 April for Alexandria. The doctors continued 'strenuously working amidst the horrors', and about 30 men died during the journey and were buried at sea by the two military padres on board.

The hospital ships began arriving in Alexandria on 29 April,[41] closely followed by the transports, such as the *Derfflinger*, which arrived with its cargo of casualties on 1 May:

---

38 AWM: 1DRL/0499, RCDIG0000181: Typescript Extracts from Diary of Sir Reginald Jeffery Millard.
39 The SMS *Derfflinger* was a German passenger ship that was impounded at Port Said at the start of the war and used as a troopship during the Gallipoli Campaign. It was renamed the *Huntsgreen* in mid-1915. AWM: 1DRL/0499, RCDIG0000181: Typescript Extracts from Diary of Sir Reginald Jeffery Millard.
40 AWM: 1DRL/0499, RCDIG0000181: Typescript Extracts from Diary of Sir Reginald Jeffery Millard.
41 The HS *Gascon* arrived in Alexandria just before midnight on 28 April but did not disembark patients until 29 April. See TNA: WO 95/4145/1: War Diary, HMHS *Gascon*, and AWM: AWM41/1053: [Nurses Narratives] Sister E J Tucker.

104   The Fight for Life

Alexandria about 6.30 am a most blessed haven of refuge for out troubles are over now and our poor men will soon be in a hospital where they can be washed and properly fed and cared for. The disembarkation was managed excellently by the No 1 East Lancashire (T) Field Ambulance.[42] They began about 12.30 pm and by 8 pm had our ship quite clear. Most were sent in hospital trains to Cairo and others, more urgent cases, to hospitals in Alexandria. The hospital trains, painted white with Red Crescent and fitted with bunks and conveniences for feeding patients were run alongside the quay so that there was the minimum of trouble over the transfer.[43]

An indication of the conditions on the transport is given in the above account when Major Millard referred to the fact that the patients could be washed once they reached hospital. With over 500 casualties on board a ship that had been hastily prepared for casualties, there was scant provision for such care. The main purpose seems to have been to evacuate patients as quickly as possible.

Whilst the hospitals in both Alexandria and Cairo had been prepared to some extent for casualties from the campaign, they were almost as unprepared as were the hospital ships. Matron Ellen Julia Gould of No. 2 AGH at Mena House at Gizeh recorded:

When the landing [on] 25th April took place, we got 24 hours' notice to be prepared for over 1,500 beds. The Gezireh Palace, in addition to Mena House had to be prepared in this 24 hours.

The sisters available, 45, had to be divided. Ten with Sister Johnston, J Bligh, went with some orderlies and prepared Gezireh. Bands of Arabs cleared out the hotel property and scoured and swept, fatigue parties brought and unpacked equipment from [the] station, Sisters made beds and supervised arrangements generally. 850 wounded arrived that next evening at Gezireh and 600 at Mena. In two days, 12 sisters had to be brought from Mena. One sister for 150 at night was too much, although they managed it and, most ably assisted by orderlies succeeded where one could not have blamed much had they failed.[44]

Whilst Matron Gould was quite upbeat about the preparations for the wounded, it is clear from her account that it was all done in some considerable haste, reflecting, perhaps, a reactive approach to the handling of the casualties that had occurred on the peninsula during the landings. Sister Nellie Constance Morrice of the same hospital was less than happy with the situation. Sister Morrice had been in Cairo since January and had been in charge of a medical ward where she looked after cases of measles and so on that were arising in the army camps around Cairo:

The biggest tragedy was when the wounded came in after the Gallipoli landing. I got orders to evacuate all my patients and get ready for surgical cases. Again I had to

---

42   Part of the 42nd (East Lancashire) Division, which served on the peninsula from early May 1915.
43   AWM: 1DRL/0499, RCDIG0000181: Typescript Extracts from Diary of Sir Reginald Jeffery Millard.
44   AWM: AWM41/975: [Nurses Narratives] Principal Matron Ellen Julia Gould.

manage without help and when I requisitioned for surgical stores to have things in readiness was told I could have them by applying to the Matron in her office at 8 o'clock that night. I knew the wounded were coming in that day so I applied to the Theatre Sister, Miss Kellett, who saved the situation by giving me a large supply of sterilized dressings. The patients came in at 6 o'clock. We just seemed to muddle along, as it seemed so hopeless trying to treat surgical cases without any appliances. We had to use our own instruments – dressing trays etc.[45]

The general feeling in the hospitals seems to have been one of supressed excitement as the news from the peninsula began to filter through. Several nurses' accounts reflect their feeling as the first wounded arrived in Cairo: 'There was great excitement in the hospital when the first wounded arrived after the landing at Gallipoli. These were the less severe cases, anyhow, they provided plenty of work for the Theatre, but were principally the removal of foreign bodies. The patients invariably asked that the bullet should be carefully saved for them, which they treasured greatly.'[46]

Sister Hilda Samsing recorded in her diary for 29 April:

> Today our first wounded have come and two trainloads are here, another coming later tonight. All day everyone has been excited and busy. The news is sad and yet so proud … I hope we will be able to find room for them all. Mena Hospital started to move to Gezireh Palace today, so they won't be ready for some days so we will be crowded.[47]

The two trainloads that had arrived in Cairo in the evening of 29 April carried those men who had been disembarked from the *Gascon* in Alexandria earlier in the day, and, as Sister Kellett commented, they were the less seriously injured cases, though that was to change as the casualties increased and hospitals became filled in Alexandria. Nevertheless, in April, the numbers of wounded arriving at the two Australian general hospitals in Cairo were close to overwhelming them: 'The wounded have just arrived today. We have admitted over 100 today … we have beds everywhere in the hall and verandas. Tomorrow, we move to Gezireh. Two more trains are coming tonight'.[48]

To cope with this sudden influx on injured men from the peninsula, there was a rapid expansion of the hospitals, and, in Cairo, No. 1 AGH started its expansion by taking over the local amusement park, known as Luna Park. At first, there was limited requisition of the site, but, as the crisis for care and accommodation grew as April ended, more and more were given over to the wounded arriving in Cairo:

---

45 AWM: AWM41/1013: [Nurses Narratives] Head Sister N C Morrice.
46 AWM: AWM41/988: [Nurses Narratives] Matron A Kellett. At this time, Kellett was the theatre sister at No. 2 AGH.
47 The Mena House Hospital, part of No. 2 AGH, did not move to Gezireh Palace at this time. As a result of the wounded arriving from the Dardanelles, Mena House remained open for another six weeks or so before being absorbed into the rest of No. 2 AGH at the Gezireh Palace Hospital. AWM: PR85/374: Samsing, Hilda Theresa Redderwold (Sister, b.1871–d.1957), 'Diary of Samsing (1914-1918)', 29 April 1915.
48 Margaret O. Young (ed.), *We Are Here, Too: The Diaries and Letters of Sister Olive L. C. Haynes, November 1914 to February 1918* (3rd edition, South Australia: Margaret O. Young, 2014), p.39.

106   The Fight for Life

On Thursday [29 April] midday I was ordered to Luna Park to set up a Convalescent Station – Sister Heath to be in charge then myself and two staff nurses for day and two for night duty …[49] We arrived there to find the skating rink with 500 beds in it quite unfurnished. The Arab beds are made of cane … They are exactly like chicken coops and are terrible things to sweep and clean under. The skating rink had a wide gallery around it and this too was fitted with these beds.

Well, we sisters arrived about 2:30 pm and the patients started to arrive at the same time. Med[ical] went upstairs to Sister Nichols. Surgical on the ground floor. By 4:30 we had 300 patients. They were all convalescent from the Palace, a great number of them were stretcher cases and some had only been operated on a few days previously. The work of getting their beds made and assigned – keeping their diet sheets etc – was almost overpowering. At 4:30 wounded commenced to arrive, covered in blood most of them with half their uniform shot or torn away. We found then that 700 badly wounded had arrived. All cases who could walk were sent down to us. By night we had over 500 patients and only 3 nurses and two orderlies to cope with the work. The meals had to be got and the wounded were clamouring to be dressed. They had been wounded on Sunday [25 April] and had not been dressed since.[50] We had no guard to keep order. The Arabs were crowding round the door and when tea time came the men rushed the barriers and those who were strongest got the most tea. It was a wild beast show; men went to bed without any nourishment at all … None of the men got dressed that night. There was no pause in the admissions. They kept coming in, 7 at a time. Soon all our beds were full and new ones were being brought in and put in every available corner. There was no pack store and men had to put their kits under the beds. Most of the kits were covered and stiff with blood and were crawling with lice. The wounded had not had baths for six weeks. We only had provision for bathing them three at a time.

On Friday [30 April] we arrived to find the place in a turmoil. They had rushed the food at breakfast time and the temper of the ward was very ugly … Soon the ward began to have some order … By this time we had 780 patients – all pretty sick – and the place had become an overflow hospital instead of a Convalescent Station. That Friday I worked from 9 am to 5:30 and did nothing else but dressings and Sister Heath administrated in general and S Nichols looked after the med cases upstairs … I must have done 400 dressing that day, no pause for refreshments. Those wounded men had been injured during the landing. Now on Friday night others who had been on land from Sunday until Tuesday arrived … We are all suffering from shock. The wounds are terrible.[51]

The system of evacuation through the lines of communication that had begun with the RMOs in the front line and passed successively through the collecting posts, field ambulance and CCSs on the peninsula and thence through the hospital ships and transports had ended with the

49   Sister Annie Heath AANS.
50   This comment suggests that the men arriving at Luna Park had arrived on a black ship since, had they arrived on a hospital ship, it is most likely that they would have been dressed on the two-day journey from Gallipoli to Alexandria.
51   AWM: AWM PR02082, RCDIG0000976: Transcript of Diaries of Alice Ross-King, 1915-1919.

casualties being treated in the hospitals of Egypt. In the opening phase of the campaign, there was clearly considerable improvisation as the situation on the beaches changed and evolved. For the MOs and their men on the beaches, the care of the wounded was uppermost in their thinking. This was continued on to the hospital ships. However, there were deficiencies in the transport of the wounded from the battle zone, and the use of black ships to transport the wounded across the Mediterranean was, perhaps, the weakest link in the whole chain of evacuation. Whilst these vessels had been suitable for troop transport, not all of them could be easily converted to temporary hospital ships. It is clear from the account of Major Millard that much was done on some of the black ships to make them as suitable as possible for the transport of wounded, and, certainly in the case of the *Derflinger*, the presence of medical staff on board made the care so much better. Unfortunately, this does not appear to have been universally true of all the vessels used for evacuation, and, at least in some cases, there seems to have been minimal medical care available for some of the wounded taken off the beaches. Whilst there were deficiencies in the system as a whole, this reflects more upon the planning than upon the MOs and men of the field ambulances and the lines of communication. As a group, these men, and indeed women, did all they could to get the wounded away from the firing lines and to treatment as soon as possible. In some cases, this was not soon enough.

Even when the wounded reached the apparent safety of Egypt, there were still issues over accommodation, and, as illustrated by the nurse's comments above, the preparations were, at least in part, going on as the wounded arrived and in some cases, all but broke down under the strain of the large number of wounded arriving. The lack of organisation and, perhaps, the lack of discipline amongst the troops, as seen in Sister Ross-King's account, required considerable work by medical staff at all levels before the system was working efficiently. The development of the medical services in Egypt was a process that continued from before the time of the landing until well after the evacuation, as hospitals grew, expanded to new locations and, in some cases, moved to better sites. As the numbers of casualties requiring care grew so did the medical services, and, whilst this was more reactive than proactive, it did demonstrate the determination of all concerned to achieve the best outcome possible for the wounded in their care.

5

The Landings: Effectiveness and Criticisms

There has been much written about the ineffectiveness of the medical services at the time of the landings on the Gallipoli Peninsula.[1] Much of this may have some justification, but it is not sufficient to assume that the failure, if that is what occurred, was due to a single cause or, indeed, to a single person. It is also probably inaccurate to assume that, because everything did not work exactly to plan, the whole system failed. The information available to give the foregoing account suggests that, in the stress of battle, much was done to handle casualties as well as possible under very difficult conditions. There was much adaptation and compromise, for even the MOs recognised that their work should have been more efficient and organised, but there was, nevertheless, considerable effort expended on caring for the wounded as the landings progressed.

In his personal diary for 17 March, General Hamilton made it clear that some key figures of his staff, mainly the administrative branch, had not been able to join him on his hasty departure from London.[2] At that time, Hamilton did not know who his SMO was to be. However, on the basis that Surgeon General Birrell had not been appointed at the time of Hamilton's departure, this is hardly surprising. Birrell, newly appointed as DMS for the MEF, left England on 20 March to take up his position in Egypt. Thus, it is hardly surprising that Birrell was not included in any early discussions on the preparations for the campaign. However, the failure to include Birrell in the discussions on planning after his arrival in the area certainly throws an unfavourable light on the importance that Hamilton attached to his medical services department. Hamilton's continued failure to use the knowledge and experience of SMOs as he evolved his plans in the early weeks of April should be seen as a considerable oversight by the commander-in-chief of the MEF. This also reflects badly upon the structure of the British Army of the time, within which the medical services had been largely relegated to a subordinate role.

It has been suggested that the plan for campaign depended upon complete success or complete failure of the landing operations.[3] This is, perhaps, an overgenerous assessment since there was little consideration of the failure of the landings or, indeed, the campaign as a whole. If there

---

1   See for instance Butler, *Official History of the Australian Medical Services*, vol. I, and Michael B. Tyquin, *Gallipoli: The Medical War. The Australian Army Medical Services in the Dardanelles Campaign of 1915* (Kensington: New South Wales University Press, 1993).
2   Hamilton, *Gallipoli Diary*, vol. 1, p.18.
3   Butler, *Official History of the Australian Medical Services*, vol. I, p.111.

had been a need to re-embark troops alongside casualties from the fighting as a result of failure, there can be little doubt that the medical services would have struggled to cope beyond the stress in which it actually found itself at the time of the landing. There appears to have been one provision for a failed landing, and that was the allowance for a number of ships, to be used for casualties, to remain on station for 48 hours in case re-embarkation was necessary.[4] On the other hand, total success was necessary to allow the medical services to be able to work as intended in the formation of the plan. That is, field ambulances needed to land and establish themselves and their dressing stations and collection posts in order to work closely with the CCSs, which also needed to be established as soon as the fighting had moved away from the beaches. This was partially successful at Helles, but, at Anzac, although the units landed, the limited ground taken meant that the medical units were unable to function at full efficiency and that such requirements as sorting the wounded became impossible more or less immediately. This points to only a partial success, or indeed a partial failure, and none of the planning, military or medical, had made any allowance for this. This points to overoptimism by the planners, but it was not confined to the General Staff since this was the pervasive attitude amongst the officers and men of the landing force, as they consistently underestimated the challenge that was ahead of them.

There has been considerable discussion over the number of casualties that was allowed for and who made the decisions on that number. It appears that, at an early stage, the DGMS in London had warned that high casualties should be expected but had not assigned a figure to this. Initially, and in the absence of SMO input, the General Staff had relied on a figure of 3,000 casualties assessed by a major of the Royal Engineers and based upon the losses in the opening exchanges on the Western Front. Immediately, Colonel Alfred Ernest Conquer Keble, Birrell's DDMS, disagreed with this figure, calling it farcical. As a result of his input, a figure of 10,000 casualties was ultimately adopted in the planning for the campaign.[5] Whilst both the General Staff, in the form of Brigadier General Woodward, DAG, and the medical services took credit for providing for the 10,000 casualties, this does not mean that either had much idea of the manner in which this large number could be handled.[6] The adequacy of this number in the provision for the casualties that actually occurred is often clouded by later estimates of the numbers and even the dates upon which these casualties occurred.

Before considering the adequacy of the plan further, it is pertinent to consider the casualties that occurred during the landings and what dates define the action that can be classed as the landings. The landings occurred on 25 April, but the fighting to establish the beachheads continued over several days, and it is perhaps appropriate to consider the casualties between 25–30 April. This follows closely with those dates given by the *British Official History* and other published works but is different to that of the *Australian Official History*, which continues the landing phase to 3 May.[7]

The *British Official History* gives the total number of casualties between these dates (25–30 April) as 9,139 killed, wounded and missing for Anzac and Helles combined. The *Australian Official History* suggests a figure of 8,000 for Anzac, which is close to twice the figure quoted

---

4   Macpherson, *History of the Great War: Medical Services*, vol. 4.
5   Macpherson, *History of the Great War: Medical Services*, vol. 4, p.19.
6   Alexia Moncrieff, *Expertise, Authority and Control: The Australian Army Medical Corps in the First World War* (Cambridge: Cambridge University Press 2020), pp.23, 38.
7   Aspinall-Oglander, *Military Operations*, vol. 1, p.315; Bean, *Story of ANZAC*, vol. 2, p.1ff.

by the *British Official History* for Anzac and considers this to be approximately correct.[8] A more recent study gives a figure of 4,931 for the 1st Australian Division.[9] Similarly, a figure of 3,800 has been given for the casualties of the 29th Division during the fighting at Helles at this time.[10] This would seem to fall broadly in line with that of the *British Official History*.

If the figures of 4,931 for the casualties at Anzac and 3,800 for 29th Division are correct, then the two divisions together had 8,731 casualties. Two further divisions were also involved in the opening exchanges: the New Zealand and Australian Division and the RND. The latter, comprising only two brigades attached to the 29th Division, sustained significant casualties at Helles, as did the battalions that served alongside the Australians. The former was involved almost immediately, landing on 25 April. The figure of 8,000 suggested by Charles E. W. Bean for Anzac covers those from these two divisions, though for a period up to 3 May. If the casualties at Helles are taken as 4,931, then the total loss during the period of the landing is approximately 12,500. It should be remembered that a proportion of this number were killed in action and, as such, would not require treatment by the medical services or evacuation to Egypt. It has been suggested that the ratio of wounded to killed for the entire campaign was approximately 2:1, which would suggest that the overall number of casualties requiring treatment or evacuation from the landing was of the order of 8,000–9,000 cases.[11] This suggests that the allowance of 10,000 casualties made by the head of the medical services was adequate. However, even if this provision was adequate, the fact that the military operation had not gone to plan meant that the medical arrangements were also likely to be unable to function as required.

Another way of looking at the casualty figures for the opening phase of the campaign is by reference to the records of the Commonwealth War Graves Commission (CWGC). If it is assumed that the numbers recorded as fatalities by the CWGC are a fair representation of the losses, then, on the opening of the campaign (25–30 April), a total of 2,715 men were killed or died of wounds and are commemorated in Turkey and Egypt. This suggests that the total casualty figures were, perhaps, lower than those estimated by official sources, unless the ratio of wounded to killed was of the order of 4:1. This would then suggest that in excess of 10,000 casualties would need to be treated by the medical services. On the basis of the CWGC figures, it would seem that the estimates made by the official historians are somewhat larger than they ought to be.

The question of the number of casualties occurring at Helles and Anzac during the landing phase of the campaign is not readily resolved, if only because of the lack of reliable and accurate data. However, from the foregoing, it is considered that the total number of evacuations required from the peninsula during the opening phase of the campaign was no less than 8,000 and no more than 10,000. It is this figure that is assumed throughout the following discussion for the provision of the evacuation of wounded.

Once the battle had commenced, there was an immediate need to control the manner in which the wounded reached the beaches and, once there, how they were treated. This was to prove to be a considerable problem on crowded beaches where men and stores were being

---

8   Bean, *Story of ANZAC*, vol. 2, p.1ff.
9   Nigel Steel and Peter Hart, *Defeat at Gallipoli* (London: MacMillan, 1994), p.137. This figure appears to have come from Bean, *Story of ANZAC*, vol. 1, pp.536–37.
10 Robin Prior, *Gallipoli: The End of the Myth* (London: Yale University Press, 2009), p.108.
11 Prior, *End of the Myth*, p.242.

The Landings: Effectiveness and Criticisms   111

landed as the wounded arrived back on the beaches. There was, generally, no hope of any meaningful triage as MOs attempted to handle hundreds of casualties as men arrived, often slightly wounded, requiring treatment. The lack of control, and possibly lack of discipline, compounded the problems faced by the medical services. This was exacerbated because of the lack of complete success of the landing and meant that, although medical units landed, they were sometimes fragmented or separated from their equipment. Under these circumstances, it is remarkable that the medical services were able to provide any care for the wounded. However, the RMOs and field ambulances provided a considerable level of care, although suffering casualties themselves throughout the operation.

The CCS provides the first link in the chain of the lines of communication. This unit, as the name implies, should be clearing casualties as rapidly as possible to the next part of the lines of communication, that is, the stationary hospital. At Gallipoli, this required the removal of casualties from the beaches by means of barges and small boats to hospital ships lying offshore. This required a minimum of three things: first, the close cooperation of the naval and military arms of the operation, second, the adequate supply of both small ships, or boats, to carry the wounded and, third, an adequate supply of hospital ships. In general, this has been seen as the weak link in the whole of the treatment provided by the medical services and is probably the part of the operation that has received the most criticism.[12]

The original plan, allowing for 10,000 casualties, had allotted a similar number of hospital ships to Anzac and Helles and, likewise, a similar number of transports to take care of 'light' cases. The breakdown of control on the beaches, the lack of triage and the close attention of Turkish gunners meant that the medical services could not adequately evacuate the wounded either quickly or appropriately to the necessary ships. It was accepted by MOs that there was a need to ensure that all the troops were landed before any evacuation of wounded could occur. As the casualties rapidly grew, the beaches soon became so crowded, particularly at Anzac, that it became imperative that evacuation was not delayed. This was further hampered by the frequent lack of small boats and barges to transport the wounded to the waiting ships. Nevertheless, everything possible was done, for instance by the 1st ACCS, to ensure that casualties were removed from the beaches. Unfortunately, this often meant that badly wounded were transferred from the beaches to any ship available offshore and not necessarily to the hospital ship. It was estimated that, by the end of 25 April, the HS *Gascon*, standing off Anzac, had taken on board far more lightly wounded than serious cases, and this ultimately was down to the situation on the beaches that prevented triage. This has been criticised heavily over the years but without due consideration of the imperative of the MOs of the CCSs to evacuate from fire-exposed beaches to points of relative safety.[13] There is no doubt that the process could have been better, but, under the conditions of an almost failed landing, the medical services were adapting to the situation as best they could and handling large numbers of casualties. This was further exacerbated at the end of 25 April by the possibility that there would be a full-scale re-embarkation of the Anzac force, with the subsequent pressure placed upon the medical services to remove wounded from the beaches. This would not appear to be a failure, or breakdown, of the medical

12   Tyquin, *Medical War*, p.21ff.
13   Bean, *Story of ANZAC*, vol. 2, p.1ff.

services.[14] Rather, it would appear to be the near loss of control of the military situation around the beachheads.

A further aspect in the care of wounded, and hence the effectiveness of the medical services, that is sometimes overlooked was the experience and knowledge of the MOs. As pointed out by Butler, many MOs had little or no experience in military medicine at all. Some had been little more than general practitioners in country towns before the war. This is echoed in an account by Colonel Ryan, who served on a number of ships during the early phase of the campaign, as he pointed out that the MOs on the *Dunluce Castle* comprised a major and two other officers who were all general practitioners and 'who did not profess to have any previous knowledge of surgery'.[15] Military surgery and the wounds that were inflicted by modern weapons that were encountered early during the campaign were, at least for some, completely overwhelming. Whilst all the MOs were very willing to give care to wounded, any training received for the new soldiers, particularly of the AAMC, could have given little preparation for the casualties received after the landings. It cannot be possible to blame these officers for their inexperience, but, perhaps when taken as part of the whole medical arrangements, it is likely that it did not help the overall situation.

The distance to base hospitals, mainly in Egypt, at the time of the landing is also raised as an issue to show the inadequacies of the medical services. Even on a reasonably well-staffed and equipped hospital ship, the two-day voyage to reach Alexandria was difficult for the wounded. There was little done to alleviate this during the first weeks of the campaign, although a stationary hospital had been set up on the island of Lemnos just a matter of hours sailing from the peninsula. However, the conditions for treating seriously wounded on Lemnos were poor, with a lack of facilities and, in particular, a good water supply. This improved slowly, but, overall, Lemnos was not a good place for base hospitals, so there was little to be done except send casualties farther afield. As the campaign developed, this included sending wounded to Malta and even to Gibraltar and eventually England. The unsuitability of Lemnos and the distance that casualties needed to travel can scarcely be the fault of the medical services since they seldom get to choose the battlefield on which they are to serve. However, the medical services are required to work within the framework chosen by the General Staff, and, in that context, the early involvement of the medical services would appear to be crucial. This did not happen in the hastily drawn up plans for the Gallipoli Campaign.

Perhaps a crucial part in the problems that arose in the medical services as the landings took place was the pronounced, and prolonged, lack of communication. A lack of communication between the senior medical staff, that is, Birrell, and the General Staff resulted from the use of separate ships and almost complete dismissal of the medical staff, as the General Staff sought to control everything from their HQ on the *Queen Elizabeth*. The care for the wounded suffered as a result of this decision, which possibly arose because the medical services were looked on as a less important part of the whole operation. This has much to do with the overall structure of the army as a whole and the War Council in particular. It did not help the care of the wounded, but, again, it is difficult to point a finger of blame specifically at the medical services, though undoubtedly any weakness in its plan was exacerbated by this lack of communication

---

14   Harrison, *Medical War*, p.203.
15   AWM: 1DRL/0560, AWM2020.22.104: Wallet 1 of 1 – Interview with Surgeon-General Charles Snodgrass Ryan Regarding the Australian Army Medical Corps, 1919, p.5.

and ultimately control of the care of the wounded. Surgeon General Birrell was isolated on his ship, the *Arcadian*, was not even able to make contact with the senior divisional MOs during the landing and was essentially kept in ignorance of the conditions at a critical time. This also meant that the ADsMS to the divisions that landed on the morning of 25 April needed to make their own decisions and run the medical services at a critical time without reference to the hierarchy, and, indeed, this is what happened both at Anzac and Helles. Perhaps, without the initiative shown by these officers, the conditions would have been much worse.

To make matters worse, the communications between the Royal Navy and the General Staff seems to have less than ideal.[16] To some extent, it is feasible to say that the Royal Navy ran their part of the operation without particular reference to the army and vice versa. This translated to difficulties in obtaining transports when and where needed and in issues transferring wounded from the beach to waiting hospital ships. The responsibility of the MOs extended to the high-water mark on the beach, and, thereafter, the casualty became the responsibility of navy until such a time as the casualty was placed on a hospital ship or transport when responsibility returned to the army. The hospital ships, for instance, were staffed by military MOs and nurses, but the ships, and their movements, were controlled by the navy. It was within this framework that the medical services worked. If the navy could not, or indeed would not, provide barges and lighters to take wounded off the beaches, there was nothing a well-meaning MO, even an ADMS, could do about it. That this generally did not happen was as much because of the cooperation of the naval officers controlling the traffic on the beaches and the MOs rather than because of the communications at a higher level. The navy did it all could to get wounded off the beaches, but it was not always as smooth as had been planned.

It has been said that, during the later phases, there was little coordination of the medical services between the arrangements at the Anzac and Helles beachheads when it came to the disposal of wounded.[17] During the landing phase of the operations, it is difficult to see where there could have been much cooperation since the two areas were, and remained, separate battlefields. The closest cooperation, coordinated by the ADMS Anzac, between medical services at the time of the landing came when a part of the RND landed at Anzac on 28 April with the 1st Royal Navy Field Ambulance, commanded by Staff Surgeon Aloysius Francis Fleming. This unit was able to assist the 1st ACCS after it had been working non-stop since it had landed three days earlier.[18] On the other hand, when British and Australian troops fought side by side later, there was little other than ad hoc cooperation, as stretcher squads from each army assisted in the removal of wounded from the forward areas. This was, at least in part, more to do with the command structures within the divisions and brigades than it was to do with any specific planning or preparation issues, or indeed issues intending to keep the forces separate. Field ambulances tended to serve the brigades to which they were attached, so cooperation with other units would, of necessity, have been limited. However, senior medical staff did not properly consider the proper coordination of the medical arrangements of the brigades involved at the time.

To conclude, it is perhaps necessary to include all the various strands mentioned above when considering the care of the wounded during the landing phase of the campaign. Could the

---

16 Butler, *Official History of the Australian Medical Services*, vol. I, pp.164, 223.
17 Butler, *Official History of the Australian Medical Services*, vol. I, p.152.
18 Douglas Jerrold, *The Royal Naval Division* (Facsimile edition of 1923 edition, Uckfield: Naval & Military Press, n.d.), p.115.

medical services have been better prepared? Undoubtedly, they could have been, but so could every unit that took part. It was a hastily planned operation, and the results reflected that. However, it is also necessary to consider that a larger part of the issues arising was without the control of the medical services. Even an early involvement in the planning could not have changed the large numbers of casualties coming off the beaches, but it may have forced the General Staff to provide more, and better, transports to remove them. The medical services were required to work on a problem that was not of their making, and much of the work carried out was essentially adaptive and reactive as it sought to meet the needs of the fighting men. In some areas, such as the provision of medical staff on black ships, the services fell short, but, in other areas, such as the tending of wounded and clearing them from fire-swept beaches, they seem to have excelled. The latter is sometimes forgotten. The need to evacuate men from fire-exposed beaches meant that there was also a need to utilise unsuitable vessels, and, whilst there can be no doubt that some men suffered and died as a result of treatment on black ships, many were likely to have been saved by the prompt action of the MOs and the prompt evacuation from the beaches.

6

Myriads of Flies: Helles May–July

At Helles, the problems faced by the medical services in the weeks immediately following the landing were every bit as bad as they had been on that day. Beaches were crowded, wounded continued to be brought in by hard-working stretcher-bearers, and space for wounded on the beaches diminished rapidly. Despite such difficulties, the 88th and 89th Field Ambulance Tent Subdivisions established dressing stations in whatever limited space was available. This allowed some form of organised treatment to be given to the large numbers of existing casualties and those new casualties arriving onto the beaches resulting from the continued fighting as the troops tried to establish secure firing lines.

The crowding had an immediate effect on the 11th CCS at W Beach when it was ordered to move to a more sheltered site on 15 May but failed to find such a spot on an already overcrowded beach. As an expedient, the Royal Engineers prepared a shellproof trench capable of holding 20 stretcher cases in relative safety.[1] Nevertheless, the 11th CCS was soon busy pitching 8 Eight Person Indian Pattern (EPIP) tents. The station soon came under shellfire. It was necessary for the CO to ask the divisional HQ to prevent groups of men from walking on the skyline, which was drawing fire onto the CCS.

The arrival of additional medical units was welcomed but added to the overcrowding on the beaches. Amongst those units was the 108th IFA, which had arrived along with the 29th Indian Brigade and was attached to the 29th Division. Its CO, Major W. R. Battye, IMS, recorded the problem of getting ashore:

> … and after considerable delay and difficulty in obtaining a trawler the whole of the ambulance shipment of three sections with the exception of a few things, was trans-ferred to the trawler and with personnel aboard we were taken to V Beach at Sedd-el-Bahr which was reached after dark at 8 pm. Unloading began at once but was very difficult owing to the men being very tired from the disembarkation to the trawler, owing to the darkness, absence of lights and to the very narrow plank gangways joining the lighters which the pier. In the dark three persons including myself fell into the sea in full marching order! By midnight all the shipment was dumped on the beach and it was

---

1   TNA: WO 95/4356: War Diary, 11th Casualty Clearing Station, 15 May.

decided to stay there for the night instead of attempting to join the Brigade Camp at that late hour. Heavy firing from a battery of French 75's was going on within a few yards and about 1 am the enemy shelled the beach heavily with howitzer high explosive [HE].[2]

Those men disembarked from the *Dunluce Castle* spent an uncomfortable night of 1/2 May on V Beach, where they came under Turkish fire throughout the hours of darkness. Nevertheless, the three sections of the ambulance that had landed were ready for work, and, by 11:00 a.m., two bearer subdivisions were bringing wounded Gurkhas to the ambulance for treatment. At this early stage of their stay on the peninsula, Battye was acutely aware of the problems he and his unit were to face. He was unable to disembark his fourth section from the *Japanese Prince* and was unable to communicate with them because of the almost complete absence of small boats. Nevertheless, he received an order that a portion of his ambulance was to be sent to the *Ajax*, which was to operate as a temporary hospital ship for Indian wounded. It was 3 May when Battye was able to send two officers and 31 other ranks to the *Ajax*.[3] Battye subsequently arranged the transport of the wounded of the Indian brigade from V Beach to the *Ajax*:

> Arranged today for transport of wounded from V Beach to Hospital Transport *Ajax*. In order to ensure satisfactory working I accompanied the wounded the first time and personally supervised their transfer and shipment. From *Ajax* I went to the *Dunluce Castle* and collected all the sick (20 cases) there and transferred them to the *Ajax*. Embarking stretcher cases from a lighter in the open sea is difficult. With a wind blowing it will be dangerous.[4]

By this time, the Indians were in action along the western road to Krithia, and Battye placed an ADS, under Captain C. J. Stocker, to support the regiments in action. Subsequently, a further dressing station was required as the brigade moved forwards, and this was placed under Captain G. S. Husband, on loan to the unit from the 69th Punjabis for the purpose.[5] Over the following days, the dressing stations were improved as they became better established and familiar with the conditions and the wounded they were to treat.

Whilst the Indians were settling into their positions on the left of the line, the French forces were moving into position on the right of the line. They had begun landing on the peninsula immediately following their diversionary attack at Kum Kale so that, by the end of April, the French were in position once again to take the fight to the Turks. Major Joseph Vassal was the SMO with the 6th Colonial Regiment, which had landed on 29 April. By 3 May, Vassal had set up his dressing station at the base of Hill 200, and, there on the same day, he began receiving wounded: 'A crowd of wounded arrived – fearful sight … Morphine injections to all. Sent some of them to the rear on stretcher carriages and mule basket chairs'.[6] The 6th Colonial Regiment

---

2 T (TNA: WO 95/4272: War Diary, 108th Indian Field Ambulance, 1 May.
3 The *Dunluce Castle* was commissioned as a hospital ship on 5 July 1915; the *Ajax* was a temporary hospital ship for a short duration after the landing of the 29th Indian Brigade and was then returned to troop-carrying duties.
4 TNA: WO 95/4272: War Diary, 108th Indian Field Ambulance, 4 May.
5 Captain Husband was eventually transferred to the 108th IFA on 16 May.
6 Anon., *Uncensored Letters*, p.79.

had been sent to support the 4th Colonial Regiment, and Vassal's dressing station was kept busy dealing with the casualties from the action attempting to drive the Turks along the peninsula and away from the beaches. The French were ultimately responsible for their own evacuations, and, through a similar process found in the British sector, the wounded were taken to hospital ships and transports. Transport offshore relied upon the French Navy to provide necessary small craft in much the same way as from the British sector.

The 89th Field Ambulance, A and C Tent Subdivisions, transport personnel, stores, wagons, horses and mules landed at W Beach on 2 May. The bearers were soon busy collecting wounded in the valley between Main and West Krithia Road but were ordered to join the tent subdivision camp on W Beach located beside the 88th Field Ambulance. They set about establishing a camp laid out as well as the conditions and nature of the ground would allow. Latrines and soak-pits were constructed, and an incinerator was used for burning refuse, as general camp cleanliness was attempted. Ambulance wagons were not allowed to land; the workload on the 89th Field Ambulance stretcher-bearers was not eased until C Section opened an ADS at West Krithia Road on 3 May.[7]

On 9 May, Major Battye, 108th IFA, moved Captain Stocker's dressing station into Gully Ravine about halfway between the beach and the front line at the head of the gully, whilst Captain Husband's dressing station followed the brigade to a position a little beyond Pink Farm. The work of the ambulance was continuous, if not heavy, and made worse by the fact that Battye had not been able to bring his fourth section ashore since it was still playing its part on the *Ajax*. Since this meant that Battye was short of officers in the hospital, he brought Captain Stocker from the Gully Ravine dressing station to assist with the work at his newly established HQ on Gully Beach. This did not last long since, on the same day (14 May), Major General Cox insisted that the Gully Ravine dressing station should not be left without a British officer, and Stocker was returned.

A and C Sections of 87th Field Ambulance Tent Subdivision had remained aboard the HMT *Southland*, where they continued to care for the wounded evacuated from the beaches until 9 May, when they were finally disembarked. These sections were instructed to make their way to Gully Beach, but, even then, the party had to rely on the beach master's 'kindly act' of providing transport in the form of two cutters and a launch to reach their destination. The party struggled on a very narrow beach, 20yd wide from the water edge to the start of the cliff, to find room to set up camp. The problems continued as the transport carrying stores could not get nearer than one-and-a-half miles away, requiring the men to manhandle the stores under shell and rifle fire. Space was so limited that the latrines were constructed on top of the cliff overlooking the beach, where they were difficult to reach and were under enemy fire. Some days later, the Royal Engineers arranged some excavation of the cliff to provide more shelter for the unit.

Whilst this unit was establishing itself, further medical units of the recently arrived 42nd Division were also disembarking. As they disembarked, further confusion ensued as the transport carrying the 1/3rd East Lancashire Field Ambulance (ELFA) sailed away without warning, taking all the medical and surgical supplies with it. This meant that the unit was unable to carry out its work on the developing battlefield.[8] The 2nd Field Ambulance of the RND arrived on 14

---

7   TNA: WO 95/4309: War Diary, 89th Field Ambulance, 3 May.
8   TNA: WO 95/4314: War Diary, 1/3rd East Lancashire Field Ambulance, 10 May.

118   The Fight for Life

May at W Beach and made camp about one mile north of the 87th Field Ambulance, as medical units continued to arrive on the peninsula in support of the military effort.[9]

During this early period on the peninsula, the evacuation of the wounded proceeded under very difficult circumstances, as wounded were moved from the lines to the barely established field ambulances and the CCS. The evacuation from the beaches was dependent upon the Royal Navy to provide suitable small vessels in sufficient numbers capable of transferring casualties to the waiting hospital ships. Occasionally, evacuation came to a sudden halt, such as on 3 May. On that date, lighters were not available because the navy put them to use on 'supply purposes', which were considered to be of greater priority. At the same time, the fleet sweepers that were supposed to take and distribute the wounded from the lighters to awaiting ships were withdrawn for 'naval reasons'. Of necessity, the MOs complained to the admiral and beach master about the shortage of lighters, and they responded that evacuation from the beaches would not be possible for at least 48 hours. This would have created further difficulties for the wounded at the already overcrowded ambulances and at the CCS. However, it seems that, in this instance, the complaint had achieved its ends since, shortly afterwards, the 11th CCS was told that a small lifeboat and a fleet sweeper would be made available for evacuating the wounded.[10] Nevertheless, the overall lack of organisation and cooperation between the two services meant that only a limited evacuation was possible that day. Fortunately, the following day (5 May), normal evacuation procedure was achieved. Sufficient small boats were supplied by the navy to allow all cases to be taken out to the HMT *Ajax*.[11] However, as a temporary hospital ship without the livery of a hospital ship, it became a target for Turkish gunners. During 14 May, the ship was shelled heavily and, according to Battye, was hit about 20 times, causing a number of wounded to be hit again and a number of the crew to become casualties. This tended to highlight one of the issues in the use of unmarked temporary hospital ships: since they could be shelled, it was necessary for them to stand farther offshore, thereby increasing the distance and difficulty of the shore-to-ship evacuation of the wounded. The net result of the shelling of the *Ajax* was that it was sent to Mudros on 17 May and the 108th IFA was then forced to evacuate wounded by a minesweeper that collected wounded at W Beach once a day and transferred them to Mudros.

In fairness to the Royal Navy, the military demand for movement of troops and the calls to provide a service for the medical units posed considerable difficulty and conflict of interests. Such demands proceeded quite smoothly during quieter times, but the situation changed rapidly when troops were fully engaged during major attack. For instance, the 42nd Division was landed between 6–9 May, during which time casualties were occurring during the fighting of Second Battle of Krithia. These sudden calls to assist with troop movement and for boats to remove the wounded sometimes brought about the near collapse of the evacuation process.

This problem was well illustrated after the landing and the Turkish counterattack that followed. Colonel Yarr, ADMS 29th Division, estimated about 450 casualties had passed through the 11th CCS on 2 May. Although about 350 cases were evacuated to ships during the day, 30 cases had to remain overnight, as no ships were available later in the day. On 8 May, the overcrowding at the 11th CCS was made worse when the CO was ordered to retain cases 'for

---

9   TNA: WO 95/4290: War Diary, 2nd Field Ambulance, 14 May.
10   TNA: WO 95/4356: War Diary, 11th Casualty Clearing Station, 3 May.
11   TNA: WO 95/4356: War Diary, 11th Casualty Clearing Station, 4 May.

Myriads of Flies: Helles May–July 119

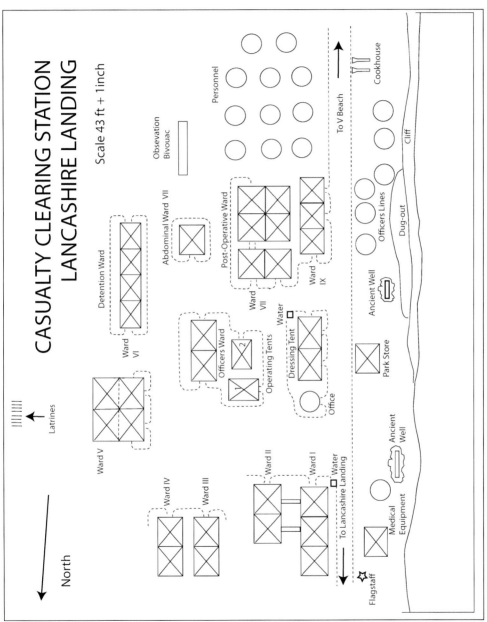

Layout of the 11th CCS at Helles in May 1915. (Terence Powell after War Dairy WO 95/4356)

the present' since ships were full. Colonel Yarr estimated that '… upwards of 10,000 evacuations to ships' were carried out by the 29th Division during the period 25 April–10 May.[12] This large number suggest that, in the first place, the medical services were working to the limit of their abilities and that there must have been a large number of vessels involved to take such large numbers from the beaches.

To complicate matters further, sudden changes in weather conditions could result in rough seas, making evacuation impossible. This often resulted in overcrowding at both the field ambulances and CCS, particularly during an attack. Under such conditions, ships, lighters and small boats were at risk of being swept ashore and embarkation piers destroyed, making evacuation hazardous and generally to be avoided. Situations such as these give an indication of the difficulties faced by both the military and the navy and the lack of organisation and coordination of these forces to enable them to balance the needs of evacuation of wounded from the peninsula with their other commitments to the campaign as a whole. Ideally, the DMS and his staff should have had their own transport to visit each medical unit along the coastline in order to provide overall leadership and for the medical services to have complete control of the availability of small boats such as lighters, trawlers, cutters, minesweepers and hospital ships. The prevailing difficulties of supplying material and equipment from Britain made this rather wishful thinking, but a case can be made that such medical demands should have been catered for, and this in itself shows the lack of authority of the medical services within the military chain of command.

General Sir Ian Hamilton, on 10 May, gave an account, as he saw it, of the difficulties when evacuating so many casualties to awaiting ships during a battle:

> A curious incident: during the night a Fleet-sweeper tied up alongside. Full of wounded, chiefly Australians. They had been sent off from the beach; had been hawked from ship to ship and every ship they hailed had the same reply – 'full up' – until, in the end, they received orders to return to shore and disembark their wounded to wait there until next day. The officers, amongst them an Australian Brigadier of my acquaintance, protested, and so, the Fleet-sweeper crew, not knowing what to do, came and lashed on to us. No one told me anything of this last night, but the ship's Captain and his officers and my own Staff Officers have been up on watches serving out soup, etc., and tending these wounded to the best of their power. As soon as I heard what had happened, I first signalled the hospital ship *Guildford Castle* to prepare to take the men in (she had just cast anchor); then I went on board the Fleet-sweeper myself and told the wounded how sorry I was for the delay in getting them to bed. They declared one and all they had been very well done but 'the boys' never complain.[13]

Unforeseen evacuation problems also occurred in the days immediately following an engagement. For two days (14–15 May), there were delays because the fleet sweeper was unavailable since it was being used to tow dead horses and mules, victims of enemy shell fire, out to sea. Problems were sometimes exacerbated by lack of planning on the beaches. A number of water

---

12   TNA: WO 95/4307: War Diary, 29th Division ADMS, 8 May.
13   Hamilton, *Gallipoli Diary*, vol. 1, 10 May.

troughs had been set up to water the mules and horses of the force just a little south of the 11th CCS. This soon caused congestion as animals were taken to the troughs, and this in turn prevented ambulance wagons and stretcher-bearers passing the spot to get to the beach. The CO of the 11th CCS coped by placing police on the road to divert traffic in an attempt to keep the route to the sea clear.[14]

The Second Battle of Krithia commenced on 6 May, and, during this action, A Section of the 89th Field Ambulance opened an ADS on Main Krithia Road. Over 100 casualties passed through the station on that day, and many had to be carried on stretchers over two miles to the CCS.[15] In the French sector, the medical services were heavily engaged in supporting the fighting in front of Krithia. Major Vassal's dressing station was busy:

> At 11 o'clock the attack. I went to the dressing station and a few minutes later a long line of wounded began to arrive. It went on uninterruptedly till 2 o'clock in the morning. Fusillade, cannonade, wounded.
>
> Sometimes they were very brave and watched the doctor's movements without gesture. Some felt themselves die. Blood, sufferings, cries, blood, groans. We bent over all these horrors and tried to do something … I could wish that there was no remembrance in my brain of those hours of blood and death. [16]

Vassal and his medics had little time to rest, for, the following day, the French were once again engaged: 'Soon our rest was interrupted by a long line of stretcher-bearers and the moans of more wounded. Here came a Lieutenant, there a Captain. Many of our men are wounded in the left hand.'[17] Here, Vassal was drawing attention to the self-inflicted wounds that were appearing amongst all the forces on the peninsula, but he stated, 'The moral is not so good', as an explanation for the wounds.

A further attack on 8 May lasted two hours, but failure to achieve the planned objectives brought about the end of the Second Battle of Krithia. Colonel Yarr, ADMS 29th Division, feared a very large number of casualties. He finally managed to get HQ to sanction the use of ambulance wagons to join the general service wagons and any other available mode of transport to assist bringing the casualties down to the CCS. Under this workload, Colonel Yarr feared a breakdown amongst the men of the ambulances and resorted to asking the Australian and New Zealand MOs to ask their troops to act as bearers. Staff Sergeant Corbridge, 87th Field Ambulance, told of the pressures during this time: 'Saturday 8th May. The infantry advanced which meant a long carry for the patients, about three miles. Spent rifle bullets and shrapnel flying around us. Lieutenant Seddon was hit by a bullet whilst walking by my side. Index finger right hand smashed. Awfully tired and weary, so are all the boys, lay down at 11.50 pm.'[18]

When the battle subsided, Major Vassal went forwards to inspect the battlefield and offer assistance where he could. The description that he gave of the Second Krithia battlefield gives an idea of the early fighting on the peninsula:

14   TNA: WO 95/4356: War Diary, 11th Casualty Clearing Station, 14/15 May.
15   TNA: WO 95/4309: War Diary, 89th Field Ambulance, 7 May.
16   Anon., *Uncensored Letters*, p.83.
17   Anon., *Uncensored Letters*, p.84.
18   MMM: PE/1/715/Corb.: Diary of Staff Sergeant Corbridge, 87th Field Ambulance, 8 May.

122   The Fight for Life

> Wounded everywhere. The killed lay in confused heaps which increases as you advanced … Some were in postures of attack, others of defence. A little soldier of the 6th had his hands behind him. He had been shot from behind, and his skull was blown to bits. The bodies were swollen and their uniforms were tight and narrow. It was awful! It might have been a drunken orgy – a sinister one![19]

Later the same day, Vassal returned to the beach to report to the chief officer of the *Service de Santé des Armées* and to explain the utter exhaustion of the men after days of fighting. He also used the time to search for drugs and other medical necessities – the battle had made a considerable impact upon the supplies at the regimental level in the French forces. Perhaps the one resource that was not readily replaced were the orderlies and stretcher-bearers who had been lost during the battle. Fortunately, up to that time, there had been no casualties amongst the MOs of the 6th Colonial Regiment.

Staff Sergeant Corbridge recorded more of the problems faced by the medical units at Helles during this period in the first half of May:

> 11th May. Terrific bombardment of the previous night caused a dugout, occupied by a staff sergeant and an interpreter, to collapse burying the two men. We had to dig them out and both were dead. After breakfast the Turks started to shell our position also the troops on W Beach about 3/4 of a mile further north, at our beach slightly wounded men were lying on the beach waiting to go on hospital ship were hit by shrapnel and badly injured also a Royal Garrison Artillery man was injured and a mule killed. It was a perfect hell but they fared worse at W Beach where 8 men were killed and 14 injured and no less than 76 horses killed or injured that they had to be destroyed outright. It was the worse shelling we have had and occurred just when we were beginning to think we were progressing well.
>
> We had Church Service on Thursday 13th May and the Chaplain was telling us it was Ascension Day, just as we were singing 'Fight the Good Fight' when CSM Smith of the SWB was hit by a bullet in the breast and fell mortally wounded.[20] Lieutenant Graham attended to him and I assisted to carry him to the Beach dressing station … These snipers hide in the cliffs etc covered with bushes and have sufficient food and water to last them a week or so.[21]

Advantage was taken of the relatively quiet times between 17–24 May to set up a number of forward medical stations and posts to support the advanced trenches. The ADMS 42nd Division received orders on 27 May for the 1/3rd ELFA, soon after its equipment had arrived, to open an ADS situated almost half a mile in the rear of the 1/2nd ELFA's ADS and immediately in front of an Army Service Corps (ASC) depot. Two days later, orders were received for this ADS to be converted to a main dressing station with an advanced post near the RND HQ in order to evacuate wounded from the remainder of the 42nd Division line along Krithia Road.

---

19   Anon., *Uncensored Letters*, p.88.
20   This possibly refers to Lance Corporal Sydney William Smith, 2nd SWB, who died of wounds on board the *Royal Edward* on 13 May. He is commemorated on the Helles Memorial.
21   MMM: PE/1/715/Corb.: Diary of Staff Sergeant Corbridge, 87th Field Ambulance, 13 May.

A wagon was to be used to evacuate wounded from the main dressing station to the 11th CCS on W Beach. To assist evacuation to the main dressing station, the unit set up an advanced post in a gully leading from the front line and a relief post at the RND HQ. Wounded from this divisional sector passed through these posts to the main dressing station and thence to the CCS.[22]

The problems of space for the medical units were not one that was easily solved, as they tried to accommodate the various units and the casualties coming from the developing trench warfare. In the French sector, Major Vassal was forced to move his dressing station that had served him through Second Krithia only to find that any suitable ground was at a premium and had seen some previous use such that 'Drastic disinfection was needed'.[23] However, at least according to Vassal, life was quieter at this time, but '… in the narrow space we occupy the "marmites" rain with pretty lively insistence'.[24]

From the time that the first troops landed, it was impossible to impose any form of sanitary control in the area. The emphasis was on getting troops, weapons of war, equipment, horses and mules on their way from the beaches towards the firing lines. Fouling of the beaches and hinterland was unavoidable and attracted swarms of flies much to the great discomfort of everyone. Furthermore, an inspection of the 89th Field Ambulance camp found many men infected with lice. A large zinc bath was found amongst the stores and used to boil all infected clothing. The clothing was then run through a water–cresol solution and allowed to dry in the sun. At the same time, new clothing was drawn from ordnance stores, and dugouts were cleaned and sprinkled with a cresol solution.[25] Nevertheless, the lice problem was one that continued throughout the remainder of the campaign.

Major Vassal was facing his own issues concerning sanitation: 'A very busy day – a few wounded but I was principally occupied with the hygiene of the district. I discovered that the water fountain, perfect until now, was running over Turkish corpses.'[26] The problems caused by the corpse-strewn battlefield was, by the end of May, becoming a big issue for the MOs across the peninsula, as they tried to organise and maintain good sanitation practices, often with very little result.

Supply problems continued through May. Colonel Yarr indented for 1,000 doses of anti-tetanic serum from No. 5 Advanced Depot Medical Stores but could only be supplied with 90 doses. This reflected upon the continuing emphasis on getting all the equipment of war ashore to the detriment of medical stores and, ultimately, the casualties needing them.[27]

Early in May, the first self-inflicted wounds of hands and feet began to appear at the dressing stations and field hospitals. These were often described as accidental by the soldier concerned, but, in most instances, this could be shown not to be the case. These men were reported to the provost and detained in camp to await court-martial and appropriate punishment. MOs were called upon to give evidence in such cases.[28] This put extra strain on the medical services and usually at a time when fighting was producing too many battle casualties.

---

22   TNA: WO 95/4313: War Diary, 42nd Division ADMS, 29 May.
23   Anon., *Uncensored Letters*, p.104.
24   *Marmite* is French slang for a large-calibre shell.
25   TNA: WO 95/4309: War Diary, 89th Field Ambulance, 24 May.
26   Anon., *Uncensored Letters*, p.121.
27   TNA: WO 95/4307: War Diary, 29th Division ADMS, 26 May.
28   TNA: WO 95/4356: War Diary, 11th Casualty Clearing Station, 6 May.

A conference was held on 30 May with Colonel Yarr and members of the RND and 42nd Division attending to consider the effects of the approaching hot weather. Among the subjects discussed was the proliferation of, and protection from, flies and the not unrelated topic enteric fever. The possibility of a gas attack was also discussed, which resulted in Colonel Yarr placing a divisional order to the ADMS MEF recommending masks be supplied that were dressed with sodium hyposulphite.[29] This issue was raised later that day with Sir Courtauld Thompson, a member of the Red Cross Commission, and he promised to cable Alexandria for War Office masks.[30] Considering that, at this time, there was the expectation of very hot weather, and with it an increased problem with flies, it is discouraging to note that the war diary of the 11th CCS reports that labourers were unavailable to clean the latrines. This had resulted in a rapid increase in the number of flies. An attempt to kill the flies was made at the CCS when two tents were sprayed with a cresol solution, but this proved to be unsuccessful.[31] It is also worth noting here that the problem with flies was never solved during the campaign; numbers did not decline appreciably until the weather changed during the autumn.

The expected warmer weather brought about its own specific problems. On 1 June, the 11th CCS reported being subjected to a '… very windy and dirty day resulting in a sharp increase in the number of the flies and dirt, a sufficient problem to make surgical operations impossible except those requiring urgent attention'.[32] The weather remained hot, with strong winds stirring up clouds of dust and yet more flies. The 87th Field Ambulance attempted to control these flies by spraying each tent with cresol and scrubbing floors with the same while each was evacuated of casualties. The north-westerly winds added another problem, as it became impossible to bake bread because of the dust getting mixed with the dough, which in turn had an adverse effect on the health of the men.

There was, at this time, little general appreciation of the need to observe the strictest control of sanitary arrangements, and this resulted in the 89th Field Ambulance appointing Staff Sergeant J. Corbridge, a sanitary inspector in civilian life, to take charge of its sanitary squad. Whilst these moves to improve conditions helped, it was to remain difficult to enforce good sanitary practice across the whole of the area. This was because of the constant movement of men to and from the front who continually fouled the routes they used. MOs could only control their limited areas of responsibility, that is, the hospitals and the immediate surrounds, and were frequently frustrated by the mess left by passing troops. This, of course, attracted large quantities of flies and with them came disease. The ADMS 29th Division was to record on 11 June that:

> … the beach area near to the 87FA Camp being invaded by the sudden arrival, without notice on 11th June of the 1st Lancs Fusiliers. These troops literally invaded the FA camp latrines, tearing down woodwork of same for firewood to light fires and digging out dugouts in and amongst the existing dugouts. On moving on, they left the camp and beach in a poor, badly fouled sanitary state.[33]

---

29 Gas had first been used against the Allies on the Western Front on 22 April at Ypres, see John Dixon, *Magnificent but Not War: The Second Battle of Ypres 1915* (Barnsley: Pen and Sword, 2003).
30 TNA: WO 95/4307: War Diary, 29th Division ADMS, 30 May.
31 TNA: WO 95/4356: War Diary, 11th Casualty Clearing Station, 30 May.
32 TNA: WO 95/4356: War Diary, 11th Casualty Clearing Station, 1 June.
33 TNA: WO 95/4307: War Diary, 29th Division ADMS, 11 June.

The CO of the 87th Field Ambulance expressed his frustration on the same day: 'There does not seem to be any particular reason for the sending of these men to our position on the Beach, which is already overcrowded: especially as there was ample room for their accommodation further up the Beach in a northerly direction it will be some days before the sanitary condition of the Beach resumes its normal state.'[34] Various attempts to improve the sanitary arrangements were tried. The 89th Field Ambulance made an improvement to the improvised box latrines introduced in May. Wooden biscuit cases, then readily available, had holes cut in the top to form a seat, and a lid was provided, with edges slightly everted to prevent flies getting in.[35]

The ADMS 29th Division acknowledged on 9 June the problems associated with such things as latrines, urinals and burial of refuse and of Turkish dead. He recognised that enormous numbers of flies occurred in certain sections of the trenches due largely to improper burial of refuse. No provision had been made, at this time, for efficient incineration of faeces, so it was necessary to dig a deep pit into which faeces were deposited on a daily basis as required. A covering lid was provided to keep out the flies. Latrines were introduced along Gully Ravine on 12 June. They were controlled and maintained by an NCO and 16 men from the regiments occupying Gully Ravine. These appear to have been successful, but moves to install similar latrines elsewhere in the ravine some days later were not. In addition to the problems of latrines, numbers of British and, to a certain extent, enemy dead lying just in front of the firing line could not be readily recovered. The prevailing north-easterly wind carried the smell from these decaying bodies into the trenches, making conditions very unpleasant. The ADMS admitted that there was no means of dealing with this directly but did give instructions for the free use of chloride of lime and a strong solution of cresol in order to mitigate the smell.

Lieutenant Ryan, RMO of the 1st KOSB, suggested three approaches for dealing with sanitation issues in his battalion's area:

1. Erection of a latrine frame and evacuation directly into the sea on the beach
2. The placing of the receptacle when full on a barge lighter taken out to sea and emptied
3. Establishing of a pail receptacle system on the side of the cliff, on a suitable platform, and the emptying of the pails into a properly made 'excreta pit' to be covered by four inches of soil three times daily.

Of these schemes, the third option was considered the most practicable under the circumstances and was recommended.[36]

Major Battye's responsibility included inspections of the trenches to ensure that there was a least some measure of control of the sanitation. In mid-May, he recorded that, overall, the trenches were 'fairly clean but the smell of corpses is offensive in some places'.[37] This was to be a continuing problem during the campaign, especially when the unburied dead became the breeding ground for the flies that soon appeared in large numbers. Although the trenches seem to have had some sanitation, the conditions in Gully Ravine were considered to be 'deplorable'.[38]

---

34 TNA: WO 95/4309: War Diary, 87th Field Ambulance, 11 June.
35 TNA: WO 95/4309: War Diary, 89th Field Ambulance, 8 June.
36 TNA: WO 95/4307: War Diary, 29th Division ADMS, 9–14 June.
37 TNA: WO 95/4272: War Diary, 108th Indian Field Ambulance, 17 May.
38 TNA: WO 95/4272: War Diary, 108th Indian Field Ambulance, 18 May.

126   The Fight for Life

Battye pointed out that this was largely down to the heavy fighting in the area since the landings, which had led to the neglect of normal sanitation procedures. Captain Husband was appointed sanitary officer to the brigade, and Major General Cox was approached to help provide sanitary police to help improve matters for the 29th Indian Brigade.

Despite all such efforts to maintain good sanitary practises, there was an outbreak of diarrhoea amongst the troops. The bacteriologist with the French force stated that there were no indicators of dysentery in the stools of affected men.[39] In an analysis of 23 cases of diarrhoea occurring from 12–30 June inclusive, the 87th Field Ambulance found the majority treated were returned to duty after an average of four-and-a-half days of treatment. In the majority of the cases, the cause was considered to be irritative enteritis. Some of the cases had definite sickness and vomiting for a day or two, but this did not persist. The main line of treatment was rest on stretchers with a sufficiency of blankets, occasional medium doses of magnesium sulphate, milk diet and biscuits instead of bread, which frequently contained a distinct amount of sand – a few cases got calomel. It was an observed by several MOs of the unit that, where a patient suffered with diarrhoea, it was sufficient to omit the bread ration and replace with biscuits for a day or two and that the diarrhoea, when not severe, quickly subsided. In some cases, the effects were more severe, such as the case of one man who fell into an immediate and very severe collapse and was found lying, semi-conscious on the floor of the latrine. He was taken into the sick tent at once and was immediately seen by the MO. He was found to be almost without a pulse, had a very drawn face and a cold clammy skin suggesting cholera. He was immediately treated by means of hot bottles, saline and brandy injections rectally, in medium quantity at frequent intervals, to which he responded very rapidly.

An adequate supply of water was absolutely essential for the work of the medical services and for maintaining the well-being of the troops in general, but providing this this was not without difficulties. The ADMS 29th Division commented on 9 June:

> Inspected water supply on the Nullah running from the firing area to Gully Beach and this, though sufficient, is limited in amount and had to be carefully organized. It is … surface water obtained from springs in the subsidiary nullahs and from the cliffs and by the means of shallow wells. The water is good but very hard. Larvae of mosquitos found in pools and small streams – pools are to be drained and the water kept running. It cannot be treated with kerosene owing to its being required by horses and mules.[40]

The 87th Field Ambulance appointed Private Manson, a water inspector for Liverpool Corporation prior to enlistment, to superintend the water supply. This appointment did not come too soon, as the unit was experiencing difficulty since it had only one usable water cart. Manson reported on a scheme, which included keeping 40gal of water in reserve, that provided a satisfactory solution. Furthermore, a new programme of sinking bores and providing covers for wells to prevent dust being blown into the well unnecessarily was recommended.[41]

Organising care for the wounded was often very difficult on the narrow beaches. Battye, 108th IFA, ordered that a number of terraces be cut into the cliffs near Gully Ravine in an

---

39   TNA: WO 95/4307: War Diary, 29th Division ADMS, 18 June.
40   TNA: WO 95/4307: War Diary, 29th Division ADMS, 9 June.
41   TNA: WO 95/4318: War Diary, 52nd Division ADMS, 27 June.

attempt to provide space and shelter from shellfire as far as was possible. There were also issues of poor communications between the units of the brigade and the field ambulances in the area. Battye's problems were increased because the 1/6th Gurkhas were on Gurkha Bluff with an aid post below on Y Beach. There was little communication between the aid post and the field ambulance, and, for much of the time, Battye relied upon the Royal Navy, in particular the surgeon on the HMS *Talbot*, to bring wounded to the field ambulance by sea from the aid post. Nevertheless, when Battye applied for a field telephone to help with this problem, he was told that there were none available on W Beach for his purposes. A day or two later, a telephone was installed for the joint use of the nearby 87th Field Ambulance and the 108th IFA.

The Third Battle of Krithia began on 4 June and demanded the full attention of the medical services. The 87th Field Ambulance was at Geogeghans Bluff, Gully Beach and Y Beach, the 88th Field Ambulance was at Main and Mid Krithia Roads, and the 89th Field Ambulance Tent Subdivisions, with attached bearers, was at an ADS out on West Krithia Road, 300yd short of Pink Farm. The 1/3rd ELFA was at Post H in Mal Tepe Dere, which had been converted into an ADS. The bearers had considerable difficulties during the battle because they were required to carry casualties for long distances. Under these circumstances, it was necessary to establish suitably spaced dressing stations. Three ADSs were established. The 87th Field Ambulance formed the first at Geogeghans Bluff, about three miles in front of Gully Beach, the second was also formed by the 87th Field Ambulance at Y Beach, about two miles from Gully Beach, and the third was formed by the 88th Field Ambulance about two miles up Gully Ravine.

At the 87th Field Ambulance ADS at Geogeghans Bluff, stretcher-bearers carried casualties 200yd down Gully Ravine and transferred them to awaiting horse-drawn ambulance wagons, which in turn made their way to Gully Beach. Walking wounded were encouraged to make their own way to the beach. This proved to be a successful method. At Y Beach, there was no suitable access for ambulance wagons, so evacuation was made entirely by the 87th Field Ambulance stretcher-bearers. A relay post was formed at Shrapnel Point about halfway from Y Beach and Gully Beach. Stretcher squads carrying empty stretchers from Gully Beach were to meet squads carrying casualties from Y Beach, and an exchange of stretchers took place. Despite being a relatively slow method of evacuation, this also proved successful. Ideally, the casualties at Gully Beach were transferred by small boats direct to hospital ship or fleet sweeper. Using this method, about 70 patients could be transferred in about one-and-a-half hours. The success of this approach was entirely dependent on a relatively calm sea, the condition of the pier and the availability of small boats, none of which could be guaranteed. The alternative was for the stretcher-bearers to carry casualties to the 11th CCS along the top of the cliff. This involved a steep climb for about 300yd before they made their way down to the 11th CCS. This could take up to four-and-a-half hours for the same number of patients to be evacuated. This was very wearisome for the bearers and added much discomfort for the patients. Walking cases had little alternative but to continue their walk, following the bearer's route as best they could to the CCS.[42]

The 108th IFA received its instructions on 1 June:

> This afternoon received instruction from the GOC Brigade that an advance is contem-
> plated shortly and arrangements are needed to push up advanced dressing station to

---

42   TNA: WO 95/4309: War Diary, 87th Field Ambulance, 3 June.

128 The Fight for Life

keep pace with advance of firing line. I decided to place an advanced dressing station at the site now occupied by HQtrs 14th Sikhs to deal with casualties on the right of our front line and the collecting post (and later a dressing post) at the present regimental aid post of 1/6th Gurkhas on Y Beach for the left of our line. In both cases wounded will be taken finally to the HQtrs of the Field Ambulance (108) for clearing to ship etc. Down the Gully I propose to assist by using my AT cart and if possible, borrow Ambulance waggons from the RAMC. In any case, if there are to be heavy casualties the naval arrangements for evacuating them from the beach will need to be greatly improved. I propose to see ADMS about this tomorrow.[43]

However, the planning was not straightforward. The 29th Indian Brigade had been reinforced by the Inniskilling Fusiliers and the Lancashire Fusiliers from the 29th Division in readiness for the attack. Shortly thereafter, the 1/5th and 1/10th Gurkhas arrived from Egypt and were attached to the 87th Brigade to replace those battalions moved to reinforce the 29th Indian Brigade. As far as the infantry assault was concerned, this was not a big problem since the brigade structure was not unduly disrupted. However, for the medical services, it was a little more complex, in so far as the wounded from the British battalions attached to the 29th Indian Brigade were to be treated by the 87th Field Ambulance as if they were part of that brigade. The Gurkhas attached to the 87th Brigade, however, were to be treated by the 108th IFA as if they belonged to the 29th Indian Brigade. This decision appears to be rooted in the differences in the way the field ambulances worked in this brigade and on the cultural, if not racial, differences that could be accommodated more readily in each of the relevant units.[44]

Battye set up an ADS part way along Gully Ravine and a collecting post near to the head of the ravine. An emergency dressing station was also set up on Y Beach to receive wounded from the RAPs in that area. The wounded from both Gully Ravine and Y Beach were to be taken to the main field ambulance, which was to act as a CCS for them. Battye needed to adapt his field ambulance since there had been no provision for the clearing of Indian wounded. In effect, this doubled the workload of the field ambulance, but there appears to have been little alternative. All of Battye's arrangements were also dependent upon the availability of suitable transport to evacuate the wounded from his makeshift CCS to hospital ships and transports.

During the first day and night of battle, a continuous flow of casualties, amounting to about 1,200, made their way to the 11th CCS. Small boats were used to transport about 120 cot cases and 515 walking cases via sweepers to awaiting hospital ships. Casualties continued to come into the 11th CCS; over the next four days, the 11th CCS handled 693 cot cases and 1,094 walking cases. Fortunately, calm seas allowed the mass evacuation of casualties, with the 11th CCS using 'Greek Coolies' and the Egyptian Labour Corps as stretcher-bearers to ease the situation. The operating theatre was fully engaged in treating head cases and fractures.[45]

A recurrent problem for the field ambulances was the shortage of stretchers at critical times during the fighting. On 4 June, as casualties arrived, each stretcher case was carried down the line of evacuation to the hospital ship using the same stretcher. These stretchers were supposed to be returned, but, most frequently, they were not. The number of stretchers at the

43   TNA: WO 95/4272: War Diary, 108th Indian Field Ambulance, 1 June.
44   TNA: WO 95/4272: War Diary, 108th Indian Field Ambulance, 3 June.
45   TNA: WO 95/4356: War Diary, 11th Casualty Clearing Station, 5–8 June.

field ambulances dwindled very quickly. The field ambulances were forced to send an officer out to the hospital ships to reclaim their stretchers, but it remained difficult to convince the ship's medical staff that they had to offload the wounded onto any available deck space and return the stretchers. If the officer was successful, the stretchers were loaded onto a returning boat as and when available. They were then unloaded at the beach and carried to an ADS, usually at some distance away. This process was further complicated during an engagement when there was little spare manpower available.

The 1/3rd ELFA struggled with transport on the first day of battle (4 June) – with only one service pattern wagon ambulance, one civilian pattern wagon and one general service wagon – but still managed to transfer all wounded to the CCS. It was found to be of benefit if orderlies marked all tallies at the ADS with an 'X', or similar mark, if further dressing was required at the main dressing station. The wounded were carried to horse-drawn ambulance wagons some distance behind, which then took them to Lancashire Landing. This approach did not work everywhere, as many cases were not similarly marked and were taken directly by Coast Road or Old Krithia Road by RND wagons to the CCS despite orders from the ADMS 29th Division.[46] In other words, the required attention in the field ambulance had been left out of the chain of evacuation.

The number of casualties arriving at the 11th CCS on the opening day of the battle was large, which meant that the sea conditions were all important to further evacuation and the efficient running of the CCS. The 11th CCS war diary indicates that a considerable number of cases were evacuated during the battle, which suggests that the seas remained calm throughout this critical time. However, some days later, on 10 June and for the two days following, a strong north wind and rough seas caused damage to the embarkation pier, which prevented any evacuations, so the CCS was required to hold wounded longer.

The 11th CCS recorded, 'In rough weather the clearance of sick and wounded is apparently impossible. The arrangements for embarking sick and wounded here inadequate and very bad. It has been represented repeatedly to Higher Authorities.'[47] The Royal Engineers did excellent work to get the piers in the best possible order but, all too frequently, saw their work of one day destroyed by the rough seas of the next. On 14 June, the 87th Field Ambulance commented that personnel of the Royal Engineers arrived to repair the pier but the condition of the sea was so rough that it prevented any work.[48] For the Royal Engineers, it was a continuing battle with the elements to keep the evacuation route open. When evacuations were impossible, the reality for the CCS evacuations was the likelihood of serious congestion at the hospital and overcrowding of the beaches, causing further discomfort for the wounded.[49]

On the right of the line, the French were engaged as part of the action of the Third Battle of Krithia. Major Vassal's regiment were in reserve. The French advanced against a strongly fortified Kereves Dere but made little progress. As the battalions of his regiment were called forwards, Vassal ordered an MO to follow each one closely, effectively carrying out the same job as an RMO in the British Army, to render assistance as needed. The operation failed at the cost of some 2,000 French casualties alone. Days later, after handling casualties continuously, Vassal's dressing station

46 TNA: WO 95/4314: War Diary, 1/3rd East Lancashire Field Ambulance, 4 June.
47 TNA: WO 95/4356: War Diary, 11th Casualty Clearing Station, 12 June.
48 TNA: WO 95/4309: War Diary, 87th Field Ambulance, 14 June.
49 TNA: WO 95/4307: War Diary, 29th Division ADMS, 12 June.

received a direct hit when 'A 77 shell landed in the middle of us', and he had a lucky escape.[50] Two men were killed outright, and two died in spite of the aid that a stunned, but otherwise uninjured, Vassal was able to give, of one he was to comment, 'The third had been caught in the hip by a splinter which had penetrated the abdomen, and another piece had grazed his head. He talked, but a fatal pallor slowly came over him.'[51] Vassal believed that he and his men had been fortunate, but it was clear to him that the brigade headquarters (BHQ) had been targeted by an 'avalanche' of shells, which had caused a number of casualties whom he had been unable to help.

The Turks responded to the attack on Krithia with a counterattack on 19 June. The 89th Field Ambulance worked most efficiently as a temporary CCS at Gully Beach and was able to evacuate 297 cases. The stretcher cases were carried up the steep climb to the top of the cliff before being transferred to awaiting motor ambulances. The four vehicles used were reported as running very well despite the state of the tracks and, perhaps, the general unsuitability of the vehicles. About 400 casualties came into the CCS during the attack, and, despite some heavy enemy shelling, 273 walking cases and 58 stretcher cases were sent off to fleet sweepers. A further 121 stretcher cases and 250 walking cases were evacuated the following day.[52]

As at Anzac, the hospitals at Helles were not safe from enemy fire. The 88th Field Ambulance dressing station, in the apparent safety of Gully Ravine, was exposed to enemy rifle fire, and, although casualties were infrequent, it was unsettling for the medical staff and wounded alike. The ADMS 29th Division, together with Major Dodsworth, Royal Engineers, requested permission to carry out work to make the hospital safe. However, for the personnel of the 87th Field Ambulance, the enemy fire was to cause casualties. Between 11:00 p.m. and 12:00 a.m. on the night of 15/16 June, Lieutenant H. Seddon was wounded in the left shoulder while lying asleep in his tent, and a wounded man already in the hospital was wounded for the second time in the abdomen. Later, the hospital was shelled, and two men were killed.[53]

Surgical procedures continued to be carried out as necessary, and the CO of the 87th Field Ambulance recorded, 'Amongst the cases received in the Station today was Lieut. Inglis (2nd SWB) who was suffering from a ventral hernia and perforation of the bowel due to a bullet wound. The perforated intestine was repaired, laparotomy performed and the intestine returned.'[54] In spite of the best efforts of the MOs at the 87th Field Ambulance, Lieutenant Rupert Charles Inglis died of his wounds at sea on 29 June and is now commemorated on the Helles Memorial.

During the last 10 days of June, the 108th IFA reported the increased number of sick arriving in the ambulance:

> There has been a good deal of abdominal indisposition, with diarrhoea and dysenteric symptoms among the British Officers of this and other Brigades. I think it is largely due to the myriad of flies which it is impossible to get rid of though every effort is made. For 2 days 2 of my officers have been [affected] in this way.[55]

---

50   Anon., *Uncensored Letters*, p.131.
51   Anon., *Uncensored Letters*, p.132.
52   TNA: WO 95/4307: War Diary, 29th Division ADMS, 19 June.
53   TNA: WO 95/4309: War Diary, 87th Field Ambulance, 16 June.
54   TNA: WO 95/4309: War Diary, 87th Field Ambulance, 28 June.
55   TNA: WO 95/4272: War Diary, 108th Indian Field Ambulance, 25 June.

This was a feature that was to become increasingly important during the summer, as increased sickness began to have a large impact on the whole of the campaign. To add to this problem, there were increasing issues over evacuation from its hospital on Y Beach. There was a small pier built there for this purpose, and this had been used during earlier operations; this was not to continue:

> The naval authorities absolutely decline to evacuate our wounded for us at Gurkha Beach, so they must perforce all come here to Gully Beach. The intervening beach road may be quite unsafe owing to shrapnel in which case the stretcher squads will have to try the much more difficult Gurkha Road over the hill and down the Gully Ravine where I shall have AT Carts waiting to meet them. If that hill road also proves not feasible the wounded will all have to remain at Gurkha Beach till dark and then be brought here. In that case I shall send another medical officer to the advanced dressing station for the day.[56]

This news was received by the 108th IFA a day before renewed operations along Gully Ravine and Gully Spur and could not have been considered in the best interests of the wounded that the ambulance knew it was going to have to evacuate as a result of the fighting. Battye, however, seems to have taken it in his stride, as he set about organising his ambulance for the coming operation:

The arrangement for today is:

> 4 Regimental aid posts under MO's and SAS's
> 1 Advanced dressing station and collecting station at Gurkha Beach with Captain Husband Captain Stocker and 16 stretcher squads.
> 2 Headquarters and tent division at Gully Beach to act also as Casualty Clearing Station, with Major Battye, Major Brassey, Captain Drake and Captain Rennie with 4 stretcher squads.
> As the distance from Gurkha to Gully Beach is 1 1/2 mile over very bad ground I arranged that every stretcher bearer on arrival at HQtrs with a case should be given a cup of hot tea and milk and 15 minutes rest before starting back again.[57]

On 21 June, the French forces mounted an attack in an attempt to improve their line by attacking the strong point known as the 'Haricot Redoubt' on the Ravin de Mort, a branch of Kereves Dere. Vassal's regiment was heavily engaged in the action, with the 176th Regiment on its left. The morning attack did not go well for the 6th Colonial Regiment, and it suffered heavy casualties including its colonel, Colonel Charles Augustus Paul Noguès, who was brought to the rear near to Vassal's dressing station:

> Half an hour ago Colonel Noguès, of the 6th Colonial, passed by on a stretcher. I was told and ran out to see him. Four men carried a little motionless figure dressed in

---

56   TNA: WO 95/4272: War Diary, 108th Indian Field Ambulance, 27 June.
57   TNA: WO 95/4272: War Diary, 108th Indian Field Ambulance, 28 June.

khaki. A white handkerchief covered his face. I raised it. His head was bound up in a red-stained bandage. His eyes, formerly so bright were dim, he was fearfully pale.

'Would you like a carriage?'

'Whichever shakes the least. I think I prefer the stretcher.'

I examined the strength of the stretcher-bearers. I added four more, so that they could change about and go more quickly. I sent orders to a doctor from a neighbouring post to accompany him … An hour later I was thankful to hear that the Colonel was safely on board the hospital boat *Duguay Trouin*.

The whole width of his chest was penetrated from left to right and from side to side. The wound in his head was less serious.[58]

Despite the losses, the French captured the head of the Ravin de Mort and took Haricot Redoubt. However, the redoubt known as the 'Quadrilateral' remained beyond their grasp. Nevertheless, the attack was hailed as a success by the French and reported as such by Hamilton to London.[59]

The day-to-day tasks of the French MOs continued as casualties arrived steadily at the dressing stations. At Vassal's main dressing station, the prompt action of a doctor saved lives when he carried a Turkish shell that had landed in the midst of 300 patients outside before it had the opportunity to explode.[60] The medics were not always so lucky, for one was killed and another seriously wounded when a shell completely destroyed the dugout in which they were sleeping.

In preparation for an attack on 28 June, the OC 87th Field Ambulance was directed to set up a dressing station at Gurkha Beach to take the casualties on the extreme right flank.[61] The pier at Gully Beach was improved, and the naval transport officer stated that he would give all the assistance possible to remove casualties from the beach by means of trawlers. The entire evacuation route from the right flank of the firing line to the dressing station near Pink Farm was inspected, and narrow trenches in places suggested difficulties for stretcher-bearers over the one-and-three-quarter miles involved. Working parties then set to work in the places identified to ensure that the passage was as good as it could be.[62]

Within the 29th Division area, three dressing stations were established:

- The first was about 200yd north of Pink Farm and about 50yd east of West Krithia Road by the 88th Field Ambulance and 1st Lowland Field Ambulance.
- The second was in Gully Ravine near the Indian brigade mule track by the 88th Field Ambulance and about 100yd farther up the ravine near the 89th Field Ambulance.
- The third at Gurkha Beach was formed by the 87th Field Ambulance and 108th IFA.

---

58 Anon., *Uncensored Letters*, p.137. Colonel Noguès survived the war and served in the Second World War. He died in 1971, aged 95.
59 Hamilton, *Gallipoli Diary*, vol. 1, p.158.
60 Anon., *Uncensored Letters*, p.139.
61 'Gurkha Beach' is the name by which Y Beach became known.
62 TNA: WO 95/4307: War Diary, 29th Division ADMS, 27 June.

The field ambulances were soon very busy, and heavy casualties saw the relief stretcher squads of the 89th Field Ambulance sent off to Gully Ravine at 7:00 p.m. At 10:00 p.m., with the sea too rough for evacuation, 20 bearers were required at Gully Beach to unload horse-drawn wagons and to carry the casualties along the steep hill route and thence to load motor ambulance wagons ready for evacuation of wounded to the 11th CCS at W Beach. No fewer than 296 wounded and 14 sick passed through the 89th Field Ambulance C Section Dressing Station in Gully Ravine during that day. Once the fighting on 28 June had commenced, it was soon clear that the 108th IFA would need to support the adjacent British dressing station. The conditions at the 108th IFA were described in some detail by Major Battye:

> When arrangements at headquarters were complete, I walked to Gurkha Beach to our advanced dressing station to see that all necessary preparations had been made. During this time a heavy artillery engagement was going on and the enemy were shelling the cliffs above Gurkha Beach along which troops were passing to the attack. Several British soldiers were hit by shrapnel. A little later a report came in that Lieut Cursetyi IMS MO 14th Sikhs had been hit by shrapnel on the hillside while attending to one of the British soldiers who had fallen near his dugout. As he was reported to be hit in the lung Captain Husband went to see him before allowing him to be removed. Soon After Lieut. Irvine, orderly officer to the Brigadier was brought in with a bullet wound in the head.[63] At this time a good many casualties due to the enemy's artillery among British troops were crowding in to the British Field Ambulance Dressing Station where the accommodation was very limited. The Indian Brigade had so far had very few casualties so at this stage I decided to offer our accommodation and services to the British Field Ambulance. Accordingly, a considerable number of British soldiers were taken in and treated and given refreshment. When our station however was full up a difficulty arose as the officer in command of the RAMC Dressing Station declined to evacuate his wounded until nightfall when he intended to do so by steam pinnace direct to hospital ship. This seemed to be a mistaken policy as the congestion was rapidly increasing. As it was imperative for me to empty my dressing station, I had just decided to send all the British soldiers away to the main Field Ambulance along the shore either walking or by our own Indian Stretcher Bearers when the RAMC officer i/c changed his mind and decided to evacuate and so solved the difficulty. By this time the enemy had ceased shelling to beach road to headquarters and it was safe for the evacuation of wounded. The dressing station was accordingly emptied of the British wounded and a few Indians and then more Indians began to come in about 4 pm.[64]

The following morning (29 June), the sea was perfectly calm, and there was a light wind, but it was a very hot day. Evacuation continued throughout the day, but, at about 9:00 p.m., a thunder-, lightning and rainstorm arose, making the sea so rough that evacuation had to be suspended. The 87th Field Ambulance, operating the dressing station at Gully Beach, evacuated a total of

---

63 Lieutenant Harold Irvine, 13th Worcestershire Regiment attached to Royal Munster Fusiliers, aged 29, has no known grave and is commemorated on the Helles Memorial.
64 TNA: WO 95/4272: War Diary, 108th Indian Field Ambulance, 28 June.

467 cases in the 24 hours between 9:00 p.m. on 28 June and 9:00 p.m. on 29 June. Conditions at Y Beach eased, and evacuation was then carried out into the early hours of the morning by trawlers, pinnace and cutters.

The 89th Field Ambulance worked throughout the whole night of 29 June. Over 150 cases were transferred to the 11th CCS at Lancashire Landing. The CCS at Gully Beach handled the rest of the casualties. The horse-drawn transport had worked for over 36 hours and drew special thanks from the CO for the splendid work carried out.[65] The wounded of 29th Indian Brigade and from the left flank had their own problems on 30 June. In the absence of transport by trawler, the wounded had to be carried from Gurkha Beach to Gully Beach, a distance of about one-and-a-half miles, around the coast over a heavy, sandy beach road.[66]

The total casualties suffered by the 29th Division, including the Indian brigade, as a result of the fighting of 28–29 June was 2,485. The ratio of killed to wounded was 1:3.7; killed and missing to wounded was high at 1:1.4. The ratio for stretcher cases to slight cases was at 1:4.2. The total number of cases evacuated from Y Beach during the last three days of June was 116 by trawler and 330 carried by stretcher-bearers. The 87th Field Ambulance recorded on 30 June that 4,600 had passed through the ambulance during the month.[67]

At this time, Major Battye was making one of his regular inspections in the forward trenches when:

> Two high explosive shells (? 9" howitzers) burst close to the trench behind us and little later when the bombardment became exceedingly heavy (the heaviest the Turks have ever fired at us) suddenly I was hurled into space and lost count of everything. I regained earth with a thud and a sudden consciousness of being still alive but with exquisite pain all over my body. I gradually opened my eyes to find myself in unknown ground and then bethought me of Captain Husband, whom I could see nowhere and feared he must have been killed. Presently far above me I saw his head appear from beneath a large mound of earth and gradually his whole body followed and he crawled out apparently very little worse for having been covered over and seemingly buried. I crawled up the hill to his side and ascertained that he was all right. Meanwhile the bombardment continued furiously and our men were prepared for an attack. Meanwhile a Gurkha Stretcher bearer reported to me that a medical officer had been killed in his regimental post. As soon as I was able to crawl, I got down to this aid post (sending Captain Husband back to his advanced dressing station) and found that Captain Reaney IMS MO 1/5th Gurkhas (FF) had been killed by a high explosive shell (his head had been blown away).[68] Captain Stocker (temporarily in m/c of the 14th Sikhs) had just arrived with Spot and I left him in charge of the combined regimental aid post (1/5th and 1/6th and 14th Sikhs) and returned slowly to headquarters. On my arrival at Headquarters Captain Drake was sent off to the advanced dressing station to relieve Captain Husband and with orders to send the latter to bed at once as

---

65 TNA: WO 95/4309: War Diary, 89th Field Ambulance, 29 June.
66 TNA: WO 95/4307: War Diary, 29th Division ADMS, 30 June.
67 TNA: WO 95/4307: War Diary, 29th Division ADMS, 30 June.
68 Captain Michael Foster Reaney, IMS, attached to the 1/5th Gurkha Rifles, commemorated in Pink Farm Cemetery, native of Reading, aged 37.

I considered it inadvisable for him to stay up at night treating wounded after the shock he had received.[69]

The fighting came to an end on 5 July when the Turks made a major counterattack that resulted in heavy casualties for the busy, overcrowded medical services on the beaches. The Battle of Gully Ravine had produced no appreciable territorial gain but had increased the pressure on the medical services as a whole, and, although perhaps better organised than previously, the services were stretched.

The 52nd Division had begun arriving on Gallipoli just in time for the action at Gully Ravine. Its final units arrived during the first week of July, and the division was called upon immediately to mount an offensive along the Achi Baba Nullah. This division, together with the RND, attacked along the Achi Baba Nullah on 12 July. The medical services were well placed to receive casualties. There were three field ambulances: the 1/1st Lowland Field Ambulance was on the line of evacuation on Kanli Dere, the 1/2nd Lowland Field Ambulance was in reserve, and the 1/3rd Lowland Field Ambulance was on the line of evacuation at Mal Tepe Dere. The evacuation of wounded was carried out by stretcher-bearers to a point 200yd north of the Water Towers. Horse-drawn ambulance wagons were waiting at this point to pick up the patients and to make their way to W Beach and the CCS.[70]

The CO of the 1/1st Lowland Field Ambulance was told on 11 July to report at RND HQ to discuss medical arrangements for the attack. It was agreed that two bearer subdivisions of the 1/1st Lowland Field Ambulance were to work with the 1st RND Field Ambulance from the RAP to Brown House. Here, they were to hand over stretchers and cases from the Achi Baba Nullah to the 2nd RND Field Ambulance dressing station at the head of the Nullah. Assisted by the 1/3rd Lowland Field Ambulance, the cases were then conveyed to wagons at Backhouse Post or at the RND ADS at Hill 200. Tent divisions of both ELFAs stood by ready to help in the RND main dressing station if called on.[71] The 52nd Division had a dressing station at Pink Farm, two ADSs at a half mile off the new bridge east of Sedd-el-Bahr to Krithia Road and at Brown House and a main dressing station on Sedd-el-Bahr to Krithia Road half a mile south of the new bridge. Ambulance wagons were unavailable during the attack, but the RND was detailed to carry out the evacuation of the wounded from these positions.[72] In addition to these preparations, the 42nd Division, on the left flank, had five dressing stations at Clapham Junction on West Krithia Road and two main dressing stations on the cliff 400yd south of X Beach. A further dressing station was set up on West Krithia Road. Four horse-drawn ambulance wagons were set apart for the use of the 42nd Division.

The 29th Division, involved in a demonstration on the left, had established dressing stations at both the upper and lower ends of Gully Ravine and two further stations at Gurkha Beach. They had nine horse-drawn wagons to be held in readiness by the 89th Field Ambulance at W Beach.

There were two lines of evacuation:

69 TNA: WO 95/4272: War Diary, 108th Indian Field Ambulance, 2 July.
70 TNA: WO 95/4313: War Diary, 42nd Division ADMS, 11 July.
71 TNA: WO 95/4319: War Diary, 1st Lowland Field Ambulance, 11 July.
72 TNA: WO 95/4313: War Diary, 42nd Division ADMS, Appendix 4, 31 July.

- Kanli Dere to ADS on West Krithia Road thence by wheeled transport on two roads (a) to the main dressing station on the cliff near X Beach (b) to W Beach
- Mal Tepe Dere to fork on Sedd-el-Bahr to Krithia Road thence by wheeled transport on two roads (a) to the main dressing station on West Krithia Road (b) to W Beach.

On the first day of the attack, the 52nd Division took over the naval lines and commenced to attack early in the morning. The responsibility for medical arrangements was in the hands of the ADMS RND, assisted by the 1st and 3rd Field Ambulances of that division. It was most fortunate that the sea remained calm during the entire time of the battle and allowed the evacuation of the casualties to proceed fairly smoothly. By 7:00 p.m. on the first day, close on 1,000 cases had been passed through the system. The casualties on the whole were described as 'not very severe, wounds of the limbs predominating'. The records of cases attended to were not kept separate and returned by RND medical units to their own HQ.[73] The 11th CCS was able to report a total of 596 cases evacuated to the HS *Ascania* by 3:00 a.m. on 13 July and a further 804 cases throughout the day until 9:30 p.m.[74]

However, not all had run completely smoothly. The ADMS 52nd Division made an urgent request to the ADMS 42nd Division at 3:25 a.m. on 13 July to send a bearer subdivision to help out, as wounded were reported to be causing congestion in the trenches. He estimated that the total casualty list on 14 July amounted to 1,805 all ranks. He also reported that the stretcher-bearers were becoming very much fatigued. The bearers of the 1/3rd Lowland Field Ambulance, in particular, were under heavy shell fire and indirect rifle fire, and several casualties had occurred amongst them. The greatest difficulty faced by the bearers was experienced when they were moving the wounded out of the advanced trenches at both flanks. A shortage of regimental stretcher-bearers, as a result of casualties, eventually had to be supplemented by ambulance bearers going forwards into the trenches beyond the RAP since all available men in the attacking battalions were required for holding and consolidating the positions gained.

The shortage of stretchers throughout the action was a problem. From the RAP down through the medical stations to the beach, there was a reluctance to remove wounded men from their stretcher unless there was another stretcher available. This is understandable but did little to assist the men moving casualties from the front. The problem was aggravated further when some stretchers became the worse for wear as the canvas ripped away from the carrying poles.

The fighting for the Achi Baba Nullah was over by 13 July, but casualties did not stop coming into the hospitals. The CO of the 1/1st Lowland Field Ambulance reported an unusual event on 15 July:

At 0530 a hostile plane dropped 3 bombs in neighbourhood of W Beach and shortly afterwards I was asked to send an MO to Supply Depot to attend to a man who had been injured. I went up and found that the injured man had been running for dugout but had been struck before he reached it. He had been near a pile of biscuit cases on which the bomb descended destroying both outer wood and inner tins. His right arm was shattered and Lt McGregor ASC had applied a tourniquet (untrained) to check

---

73   TNA: WO 95/4318: War Diary, 52nd Division ADMS, 12 July.
74   TNA: WO 95/4356: War Diary, 11th Casualty Clearing Station, 13 July.

bleeding from the brachial vessels which were torn. There was also a ragged wound in right by hypochondrium (superficial) and a puncture wound further round to the side. The man was laying much shocked in a shallow dugout. I cut away the shattered limb at middle of upper arm and dressed his wounds. He was immediately sent into No.11 CCS where I subsequently learned he expired in a couple of hours.[75]

The 11th CCS also continued to receive casualties. On 14 July, a large barge was used to evacuate no less than 361 casualties, mostly stretcher cases, to a hospital ship. One hundred and seventeen cases of sickness and light wounds were sent to Mudros. On 15 July, a further 81 cases were sent off to hospital ship and 370 to Mudros, which completely emptied the hospital.[76]

During the fighting along the Achi Baba Nullah, the French provided support on the extreme right flank of the line. Their objective was to carry the trenches in Kereves Dere. The fighting on 12 July was very heavy, and the French 1st Division suffered considerable losses. The CO (General Masanou), his chief of staff (Major Jacques Romieux) and others became casualties when a direct hit by a 105mm shell wrecked the 1st Division command post:

At half past eight an ambulance carriage arrived at our general headquarters. It brought back the body of Major Romieux, the most active and enterprising of all the Eastern Army. His skull was broken. A big bandage hid his wound … Captain Berge arrived in an ambulance carriage wounded in the head. He was with two or three other wounded men. I offered my services to him, but he only wanted one thing – to reach the hospital as soon as possible. The uneven and dusty roads are very painful for our wounded … four men carried into our general headquarters a wounded man on a stretcher. His face was hidden under a newspaper. I lifted it and found our General. His eyes were half closed and he recognized nobody. I had him accompanied to the hospital by one of our doctors. We are very much upset. General Masnou was all that was good and kindly.[77]

The fighting had captured further trenches from the Turks and most of the strong point known as the 'Rognon'. However, like the British troops on the left in front of the vineyard, the French forces were, by the end of the fighting, very weary and had suffered about 800 casualties. For the French 1st Division, it had been particularly hard, in that most of the divisional staff had become casualties very early in the fighting.

The problems that had been faced by the medical services during June had intensified during July. The weather remained extremely hot. The persistent wind ensured that clouds of dust entered every facet of the men's lives, including cookhouses, water supply and living quarters. On 22 July, the ADMS 52nd Division reported the persistence of a north-east wind from Achi Baba filling the camp and dugouts with dust.[78] This situation was not helped by unburied corpses between the firing lines, encouraging millions of flies to feed on the bodies and swarm through the trench lines, making any attempt by the men to eat any food near impossible.

---

75   TNA: WO 95/4319: War Diary, 1st Lowland Field Ambulance, 15 July.
76   TNA: WO 95/4356: War Diary, 11th Casualty Clearing Station, 14–15 July.
77   Anon., *Uncensored Letters*, p.137. General Joseph George Antoine Masnou died on 17 July at Malta aboard the battleship *Bretagne*.
78   TNA: WO 95/4318: War Diary, 52nd Division ADMS, 22 July.

138   The Fight for Life

At this time, the need to maintain the general health of the men was recognised. As just a part of this, the quality and supply of water was closely monitored by MOs of all the ambulance units and hospitals. Supply difficulties arose regularly, as men returning from the trenches often required more water than was available. This meant that, on occasion, water carts were filled from any source available regardless of quality with a consequent impact on the men's health. Once again, the MOs were powerless to control these actions, except in the immediate vicinity of their hospitals, particularly as water supply remained inadequate. Strategically placed intermediate tanks were filled with filtered water. The ADMS 42nd Division reported on 10 July the installation of water tanks and barrels in Kanli Dere above Clapham Junction and in three trenches on the north-east of the Nullah above Clapham Junction, where a direct water supply to tank from a spring was readily available. The water was sterilised and fed the latrines and places that had proved impossible for water-cart access. Petrol cans were used for water storage, and, when 150 were delivered to the 42nd Division, the ADMS remarked that, although they were very welcome, many more were needed.[79]

It was believed by MOs that much of the problem with cases of diarrhoea was caused by the sand and grit in both food and water. This meant that any filtration system was regarded positively, and the ADMS 52nd Division hoped that, with the introduction of storage tanks, there would be decrease in the number of cases of diarrhoea.[80] At this time, there was some thought given to the use of condensing systems for desalination of seawater to alleviate the water shortages. Whilst these were available on some ships, and eventually at Mudros, they were never operational on the peninsula.[81] In spite of the best efforts of all concerned, by the end of the month, the ADMS 52nd Division was reporting a '… gradual deterioration both in quality and quantity of the wells noticeable. No indications of deeper boring being attempted'.[82]

To add to this, there was an increasing worry over the men's diet. On 25 July, the ADMS 52nd Division was sufficiently concerned to express great concern, recording:

> This question of the men's rations is a serious one and I am certain the present dietary is having a deleterious effect on the men. Whilst there is no definite disease one notices a general listlessness and apathy amongst the troops all over the Division. The large number of diarrhoea cases adds to the urgent need for definite immediate steps being taken with regard to the general question of diet. These cases are not being sent sick to Hospital unless very bad or with temperature and the difficulties of treatment with present diet are very great. Further all general precautions (sanitary etc.) whilst they may be helping to reduce the actual number of cases now reporting daily, are certainly not producing any marked effect in this direction so that one is again forced into the position of regarding the dietary as unsuitable and my own opinion and that of my officers is that, with the precautions we have and are taking in regard to water supply and cleanliness of cooking places utensils etc. we are to get any definite improvements in health and tone of the troops we will best and most quickly do so by a liberal diet

---

79   TNA: WO 95/4313: War Diary, 42nd Division ADMS, 10–18 July.
80   TNA: WO 95/4318: War Diary, 52nd Division ADMS, 24 July.
81   Dixon, *Vital Endeavour*, p.404.
82   TNA: WO 95/4318: War Diary, 52nd Division ADMS, 31, July.

largely cereal and milk with tinned fruit and dried fruit in place of the largely meat diet we are at present getting.[83]

Whilst such recommendations may have had good intentions, they did not always get a sympathetic hearing, particularly where there were shortages of all kinds of stores for the continued campaign. The ADMS 52nd Division was informed by divisional HQ that there was nothing to be done for diarrhoea cases since such things as farinaceous foodstuffs were not available in sufficient quantities. The situation was exacerbated since there was also a shortage of medical comforts. This meant that men receiving treatment for intestinal issues of one sort or another had limited access to the diets considered necessary to assist their recovery.

The questions around the men's health were, by July, beginning to come to the fore. There had been considerable concern over the potential for an outbreak of cholera on the peninsula, particularly because of the poor sanitation and water supply. Throughout July, the medical services became engaged in the wholesale vaccination of troops against cholera. Although the serum was not, at first, as plentiful as MOs would have liked, steady progress was made, and the absence of the disease throughout the campaign possibly suggests that the vaccination programme had been successful.

Throughout the period since landing, every effort had been made by the medical services to improve the care of casualties. CCSs and field ambulances were better equipped, and experience in handling large numbers of casualties had improved the seaborne evacuation. Of course, the latter was still dependant on the availability of boats and hospital ships and on the weather conditions affecting the sea. On 1 July, the 11th CCS recorded that it '… transferred 60 cot cases and 12 sitting cases to the Hospital Ship *Nowra Eliya* [sic; *Neuralia*]. She was unable to take any more. Transferred 44 cot cases and about 100 sitting up to the Fleet Sweeper'.[84] In the days following, it appears that there was no hospital ship off Helles, and, for three days, the 11th CCS evacuated cases via fleet sweepers until the arrival of the HS *Dongola* on 4 July. The use of the fleet sweepers for evacuation was more established by July when they were acting as ferries to both Lemnos and Imbros, where, gradually, additional hospital facilities were being established. Of course, evacuation of wounded also relied heavily on the work of the Royal Engineers in maintaining piers and access routes on which to transfer more wounded. Nevertheless, there were days when rough seas prevented the transfer of wounded from the beaches to the hospital ships.

As mentioned previously, the care and evacuation of the Indian troops required different arrangements. Some of this fell upon the 110th IFA. For their part, the 110th IFA had rather less involvement in the operations on the peninsula. After arriving on Lemnos on 17 May, they had to wait a day for orders for them to staff the temporary hospital ship *Ajax*, where they were to begin taking on board casualties from the 108th IFA. The *Ajax* took on board 418 Indian wounded and 32 Turkish wounded prisoners of war (POWs) over the next week. The ship was then readied to sail, but, before departing, one section of the field ambulance was disembarked at Mudros with orders to form a small hospital for lightly wounded Indians who would not need evacuation to Egypt. The trip to Egypt was to be the only trip the field ambulance made on the

---

83   TNA: WO 95/4318: War Diary, 52nd Division ADMS, 25 July.
84   TNA: WO 95/4356: War Diary, 11th Casualty Clearing Station, 1 July.

Ajax, for, after disembarking the casualties at Alexandria, orders were received that it should join the troopship *Itonus* for the return journey. The unit reached Lemnos on 6 June and was disembarked to form a hospital for lightly wounded cases and POWs requiring treatment. The unit remained at Mudros for two weeks before further orders were received for it to join the HT *Seang Choon*, which was then acting as a temporary hospital ship. This transport was to act as hospital ship for Indians and Turkish POWs and was staffed by three sections of the 110th IFA. The other section of the ambulance remained at Mudros and eventually established a convalescent hospital for Indians. The convalescent hospital was staffed by British officers and Indian SASs, together with 117 other ranks, of whom 92 were bearers of the Army Bearer Corps (known as 'ABC men'). The hospital was designed to care for no more than 25 men, but, within a day of its formation, this had been exceeded. By early July, after receiving wounded from the HS *Neuralia* and the *Seang Choon*, it was caring for 253 sick and wounded.[85]

By the end of July, the *Seang Choon* had departed for Egypt, and, after discharging the cases at Alexandria, Major E. Bissett, the officer in charge of the medical staff on board, received orders to fit out the ship for an unspecified number of voyages to the peninsula. At this time, Major R. H. Price, OC 110th IFA, received information that the ship was to be converted to a permanent hospital ship. This, of necessity, would have to be completed in Alexandria following the discharge of patients and allowing for sufficient time before the transport was required on station at the peninsula or Lemnos again. The *Seang Choon* was back in Mudros on 3 August, and, although the work on its conversion had not been completed, it was ready to accept wounded. It appears that, although the ship continued to be used as a temporary hospital ship, it was never converted to a permanent hospital ship.

The attacks throughout the period from the beginning of May to the end of July had tested the organisation of the field ambulances and their procedures for evacuation to the CCSs. In general, aid posts, ADSs, relief posts and the main dressing stations were placed to support the fighting troops closely. Main dressing stations quickly moved casualties along the line of evacuation using ambulance wagons as far as was possible. Wherever possible, medical units supported one another as in the attack on Achi Baba on 12 July, when the 1st Lowland Field Ambulance of the 52nd Division supported the 1st Field Ambulance of the RND. This organisation and cooperation worked well during these attacks at Helles in spite of the large number of casualties that each attack produced. Overall, there had been an effort by the medical services to establish good care for the wounded, and later the sick, as the campaign proceeded. This was to be tested to the limits in the difficulties of the coming months.

As time went on, it was recognised that the men on the peninsula were always close to the fighting and subject to shell and rifle fire and that there was a need to find some sort of relief if at all possible. As part of this approach, orders were received on 19 July by the OC of the 89th Field Ambulance for the unit to embark at V Beach bound for Lemnos for a well-earned rest. The OC had received information that the facilities at Lemnos were extremely poor, and he pleaded with his ADMS to be allowed for the unit to take their rest on the peninsula. This was refused, and, after handing over all equipment and stores to the 41st Field Ambulance, of the recently arrived 13th Division, the unit sailed off on the SS *Abassiah*, arriving at Lemnos on the morning of 20 July.

---

85   TNA: WO 95/4272: War Diary, 108th Indian Field Ambulance, 6 July.

The CO's fears were very well founded. The camp commandant gave them only a general idea of where to camp, and, after being turned away from their first chosen suitable site, they eventually settled down behind some vineyards close to the 86th Brigade, which was also out of the line. They found there were no tents, digging tools or cooking utensils available and were asked to hand over whatever equipment and utensils they had brought with them. A field cooker, a few dixies, an axe and some spades were borrowed from a neighbouring infantry unit. Since they could not treat patients without the cover of tents, patients were sent to nearby stationary hospitals. The whole area allotted to the unit was filthy and with very limited, if any, areas specifically marked out for sanitary purposes. The open ground was fouled, and what shallow latrine trenches were available were entirely unprotected, with no screens or any other form of fly protection present. A persistent wind ensured dust and innumerable latrine papers being carried around the area. Under these conditions, it was not surprising that the OC felt the fly plague at Lemnos was five times as bad as that at Helles. The heat was far more intense than that at Helles, and the men were given the minimum physical drill and short route marches. It was with much relief that the unit was ordered back to Helles on 27 July and arrived at V Beach on 28 July.[86] Lemnos was not the best of places for rest, but, in later months, other units were sent there to the rest camp at Sarpi, and conditions improved a little. Nevertheless, Lemnos was always considered to be a difficult place to serve.

At the end of the month, Major A. U. McIntosh, Acting ADMS 52nd Division, was to report the following statistics for his division:

- Killed: 63 officers, 607 other ranks
- Wounded: 83 officers, 2,384 other ranks
- Missing: 40 officers, 1,277 other ranks
- Total: 186 officers, 4,268 other ranks.

These were casualties caused by the fighting since the division had landed, and the numbers take no account of the sickness that was, by the end of July, sweeping the peninsula.[87]

---

86   TNA: WO 95/4309: War Diary, 89th Field Ambulance, 28 July.
87   TNA: WO 95/4318: War Diary, 52nd Division ADMS, July.

7

Man with the Donkey: Anzac May–July

Following the landing at Anzac, the medical services needed to establish their various units on shore. For some, it was to be some weeks before they landed all their personnel at Anzac, as they provided medical staff for transports carrying wounded away from the peninsula. The 1st ACCS had been allotted space on Anzac Beach and, throughout May, had managed to carry out its work under adverse conditions and was often under artillery fire. The war diary for the unit records that, during May, it had evacuated no less than 4,895 casualties from the hospital. More than a quarter of these casualties occurred during the first four days of May as the CCS was establishing itself and coming to terms with the immediate battlefield conditions on Anzac Beach. It should also be mentioned that the unit was not up to strength because four MOs and nine men had been left on board their original transport, the HMT *Ivernian*, to give medical assistance to the wounded that this ship was taking away from the battle zone. Whilst staffed by the men of the 1st ACCS, the *Ivernian* made one trip to Alexandria, carrying 450 casualties. The medical staff was then transferred to the *Osmanieh* and made a further trip to Alexandria with wounded. It was 31 May before these men were able to join their unit at Anzac.

At this time, the 1st AFA was also operating as two more or less independent units with a bearer subdivision operating at Dawkins Point while the main body of the field ambulance remained at Brighton Beach. From the moment this unit had landed, it been subjected to enemy artillery fire, which added to the problems of continuing to care for the wounded. The beach-head was narrow and crowded, and, as a result, it was almost impossible to find shelter from the guns. The main body of the ambulance moved on 4 May to a new site '… on the southern side of Victoria Gully near the seashore – this is a far safer site than the original one'.[1] In spite of the difficulties, there seems to have been considerable desire of the men to carry on their job. In fact, 'Drivers Wetzel, P, 222 and Williamson, WA, 233 absconded from Alexandria to this unit and were here placed under arrest (open) pending sending back to their unit in Alexandria.'[2] This is, perhaps, an unusual occurrence, but it at least shows the determination of two men to be part of the operations at Anzac.

---

1   AWM: AWM4/26/44/3: War Diary, 1st Australian Field Ambulance, 4 May.
2   AWM: AWM4/26/44/3: War Diary, 1st Australian Field Ambulance, 26 May. Both men were members of the 1st AFA but appear to have been with the transport section, which had been left in Egypt.

The 2nd AFA had also been split, with the tent and transport subdivisions, four officers and 59 other ranks remaining on board the transport *Mashobra* to provide medical care as it, too, transported wounded from the area. The *Mashobra* sailed for Alexandria on 1 May where it arrived two days later. Here, the transport section was sent to Mex Camp, outside the city, where it was to remain, while the tent subdivision sailed again for Gallipoli. The subdivision remained afloat, serving on different vessels until it was landed at Anzac on 30 May, rejoining the 2nd AFA, when it opened a dressing station at Brighton Beach.

The 3rd AFA had landed in two parts, but all of it was ashore by the beginning of May encamped on Red Cross Hill, above Brighton Pier. Lieutenant Colonel Alfred Sutton explained the way that the work of his field ambulance was organised at this time and how the adjacent field ambulances distributed the work:

> Our stretcher bearers go out morning and evening and so to avoid double-banking and as no orders are issued, I arranged with No 1 and No 2 F Ambulance that we, No. 3, shall take charge of Shrapnel Valley and Death Valley opening off it and the valley where Capt Goldsmith is on our right flank nearer Kaba Tepe. This saves waste of effort for our work is very hard.[3]

Sutton also recorded the special general order of Hamilton of that day, thanking the stretcher-bearers for their work since the landings. For the 114 men and three officers of the 3rd AFA who were amongst the first men to land, this commendation was 'highly valued'.

It is noticeable from the records of the 3rd AFA how much of a problem the attention of the enemy artillery was to their work. Throughout early May, enemy shelling caused damage to the wards dug into Red Cross Hill as Sutton insisted that they were dug ever deeper into the hillside for increased protection:

> Heavy shrapnel all day, it blew our dugouts to pieces. Our hill was raked, our patients were killed and wounded and No 56 Pte H J Shepherd was wounded in the foot, No 28 Pte W R Baker was shot through the wrist; No 105 Pte G E Hone was shot through lip and cheek. The DADMS, Col Marshall, was shot in the ankle whilst he was in our camp and when I went to see him and fix him up a shell blew my dugout to bits.[4]

By 10 May, their site had become so exposed to shell fire that Sutton was forced to find a new position for his unit. It is clear from the war diary that Sutton was no happier with the new site in a gully nearer to Gaba Tepe, and, as they moved into the site the following day, the enemy '… rained shrapnel upon us and I found the new site untenable'.[5] Sutton eventually chose a site on a hillside at the entrance to Death Valley – 'It is bad but I had no choice' – and the 3rd AFA began to dig in again. During the following days of digging and preparing the site for the ambulance, the unit was shelled intermittently, which caused a number of casualties including Private Sydney John Penhaligon, aged 20, who died of wounds on 14 May aboard the HS *Gascon*.[6]

---

3   AWM: AWM4/26/46/5: War Diary, 3rd Australian Field Ambulance, 2 May.
4   AWM: AWM4/26/46/5: War Diary, 3rd Australian Field Ambulance, 6 May.
5   AWM: AWM4/26/46/5: War Diary, 3rd Australian Field Ambulance, 11 May.
6   No. 77 John Penhaligon of Brisbane is commemorated on the Lone Pine Memorial.

144   The Fight for Life

Whilst most of Sutton's unit was ashore, two officers and 91 other ranks were serving on five different transports, providing medical cover for the black ships. This situation appears to have been an attempt to man as many such ships as possible, although, in most cases, this was to prove to be inadequate for the number of casualties evacuated from the beaches.

It was the service of one man of the 3rd AFA that was to give rise to one of the legends of Anzac. That was the story of 'the man with the donkey', who was to become one of the heroes of the entire Australian war effort. The man in question was the English-born John Simpson Kirkpatrick, who served in the Australian Army as 'John Simpson'.

Simpson's journey to Gallipoli was just like that of thousands of his comrades. His unit reached Cairo in mid-December 1914, and there began the period of training that was to ready it for war. After a short spell on Lemnos, Simpson and his comrades landed at what was to become known as 'Anzac Cove' on 25 April 1915, and, from that day, two legends of Australian military endeavour arose. The first is the obvious legend of the Anzac Cove Landing, whilst the second is perhaps a lot less tangible – that of the man with the donkey. 'The man with the donkey' is said in Australia, even today, to epitomise the spirit of Anzac, and John Simpson was the man who, it is said, gave rise to that legend.

Simpson was considered to be ingenious by his mates, and he had not been ashore more than a few hours when he spotted the donkey and saw immediately the possibilities for carrying men down Shrapnel Gully. After carrying two particularly large men down on a stretcher, he saw a way of making the job easier and the journey quicker for the wounded. The donkey was described as 'a little mouse coloured animal no taller than a Newfoundland dog'. Nevertheless, the donkey proved to be a sure-footed companion for Simpson, as they went up and down the twisting valleys of the Sari Bair looking to help any wounded they could. The animal apparently responded to Simpson's deft touch and obeyed his direction readily, as it found its way up and down the gully often under fire. Simpson always spoke kindly and encouragingly to the animal. He did have a number of names for the donkey such as 'Murphy' and 'Duffy', though his favourite seems to have been 'Abdul'. On one occasion, he was heard to call the donkey 'Queen Mary' – supposedly after the great battleship! This, of course, has suggested that there was more than one donkey, and it is likely that Simpson did use more than one animal, but there is no record of any of the animals being killed during the journeys.

It has been recorded that Simpson worked all day and night, barely stopping to sleep or eat. On 1 May, 'No 202 Simpson acting on initiative uses a donkey from the 26th to carry lightly wounded cases and has kept up his work from early morning till night every day since.'[7] The legend was born. Simpson was now allowed to act as a more or less independent unit; he even stopped billeting with the Australians, preferring to take his rest when he needed it with the Indian Mountain Battery nearby, where he seems to have been readily accepted.[8]

A few days after he started this work, one soldier, Private P. G. Menhennett, who survived to tell his tale of the ride on Simpson's donkey was to record:

It was fierce and many of us were soon out of action and placed out of the line of fire for evacuation when possible. After a terrible night daylight eventually arrived and soon

7   Sir Irving Benson, *The Man with the Donkey: John Simpson Kirkpatrick, The Good Samaritan of Gallipoli* (London: Hodder & Stoughton, 1965), p.43.
8   The 21st Kohat Indian Mountain Artillery Battery. Curran, *Across the Bar*, p.283.

after came Simpson. Some of our cases were pitiful, but this cheerful digger had a word and a smile for them all. He came to me and asked me what was wrong and I told him I had been shot through the right leg just above the knee, he asked me could I walk. I told him I might have been able to a few hours before had I known the way down, but now it had got cold and stiff and I doubted my ability to do so. He re-bandaged my leg and helped me to his famous donkey. Two or three times on the way down he grinned at me and said 'That was a very nasty spot we have just passed. Jacko's snipers are wonderful shots. It doesn't do to loiter in such spots.' When you realize that he knew the extreme dangers to which he so constantly exposed himself in his self-imposed errands of mercy you can only marvel at the cheerful way in which he carried out his duties. He brought me to the Beach clearing station and when I thanked him, he smiled and said, 'Glad to help you'.[9]

The quiet courage of Simpson and the placid animal in his charge had a considerable impact on those around him as he journeyed up and down the gully hour after hour through the shell-torn days and often well into the night. Padre George Green commented, 'If ever a man deserved a Victoria Cross, it was Simpson. I often remember now the scene I saw frequently in Shrapnel Gully of that cheerful soul calmly walking down the gully with a Red Cross armlet around the donkey's head. The gully was under direct fire from the enemy almost all of the time.'[10] Simpson completed as many as 15 return journeys in a day to bring wounded men to the relative safety of the dressing station.

He became a familiar sight to the soldiers in that part of the peninsula, and men asked after him through the long days of fighting, wondering if he was still alive. They recognised all too clearly the perilous nature of his work – perhaps realising that even Simpson's astonishing luck could not continue. After a little over three weeks and transporting over 300 casualties down the slope, on 19 May 1915, Simpson was struck through the heart by a bullet and killed instantly. His mates buried him at Hell's Spit with a simple wooden cross bearing the words 'JOHN SIMPSON' and nothing else to mark the hero's departure. Colonel John Monash wrote to his HQ:

> I desire to bring under special notice, for favour of transmission to the proper authority, the case of Private Simpson, stated to belong to C Section of the 3rd Field Ambulance. This man has been working in the valley since 26th April, in collecting wounded, and carrying them to the dressing stations. He had a small donkey which he used, to carry all cases unable to walk.
>
> Private Simpson and his little beast earned the admiration of everyone at the upper end of the valley. They worked all day and night throughout the whole period since landing, and the help rendered to the wounded was invaluable. Simpson knew no fear and moved unconcernedly amid shrapnel and rifle fire, steadily carrying out his self-imposed task day by day, and he frequently earned the applause of the personnel for his many fearless rescues of wounded men from areas subject to rifle and shrapnel fire.

9   Curran, *Across the Bar*, p.284.
10   Benson, *The Man with the Donkey*, p.43.

Simpson and his donkey were yesterday killed by a shrapnel shell,[11] and inquiry then elicited that he belonged to none of the Medical Corps Units with this brigade, but had become separated from his own unit, and had carried on his perilous work on his own initiative.[12]

On 24 May, Lieutenant Colonel Sutton was to write in his diary, 'I sent in a report about No. 202 Pte. Simpson J, of C Section, shot on duty on May 19th 1915. He was a splendid fellow and went up the gullies day and night bringing down the wounded on donkeys. I hope he will be awarded the DCM [Distinguished Conduct Medal].'[13]

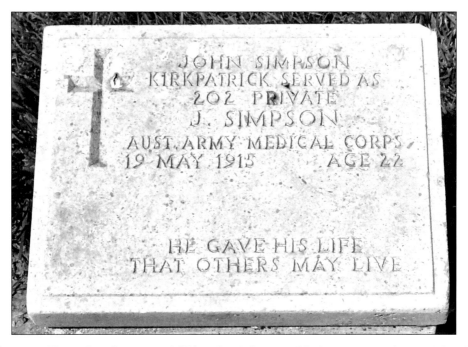

The grave of Private John Simpson, 3rd AFA, at Beach Cemetery. His bravery was used to symbolise the Anzac spirit. (Author)

On 1 June, he was to add, 'I think we will get the VC for poor Simpson.' By 4 June, he was having second thoughts: 'It is difficult to get evidence of any one act to justify the VC the fact is he did so many.'

Simpson did not receive any posthumous award, although he was mentioned in despatches. There would seem to have been plenty of evidence to demonstrate that he showed nothing but courage from the moment he landed at Anzac until his death. Possibly, some of the reverence and great respect his name has attracted over the years since the war is down to the fact

---

11 Monash was mistaken since the donkey was not killed.
12 Curran, *Across the Bar*, p.367.
13 Curran, *Across the Bar*, p.367.

that his bravery went almost unrecognised. But it is quite clear that Simpson saw what he did as nothing more than his job – he said so himself, and survivors of the war confirmed this fact. However, there are at least five statues remembering his service throughout Australia, and, in 1967, when the ANZAC Commemorative Medallion was issued by the Australian Government, the man with a donkey was chosen as the embodiment of the service at Gallipoli for the design. The first medallion was issued to Simpson's sister.

It was not only Simpson who was using a donkey to carry wounded during those early weeks on Anzac. In the NZFA was a group of bearers who also used donkeys for a few days at the beginning of May. One of them, Private James Gardner Jackson, was to bring their story to light over 20 years later when he wrote to the then Director of the Australian War Memorial (AWM), Major Treloar, in 1937. In the course of his letter, he wrote:

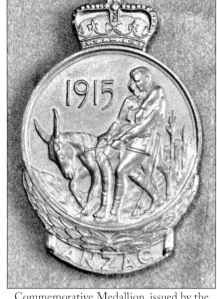

Commemorative Medallion, issued by the Australian Government in 1967. The obverse of the medallion bears a representation of Simpson and his donkey. (Author)

> I will place it on record, Sir that Simpson was the first man that I saw or heard of using a donkey for the evacuation of wounded on Gallipoli. I was struck with the idea and it seemed to me a jolly good idea, especially as he just took leg or foot cases where there was no fracture, as, although they could not walk, they were not wounded severely enough to justify a stretcher; especially in rushed times when a good number of badly wounded men were lying about.[14]

Jackson acquired a donkey and worked up and down Shrapnel Valley in the same way as Simpson, often coming in to contact with him as they carried their wounded to safety. There were three other New Zealanders of Jackson's squad who worked in the same way until their unit moved, it became impossible to keep the animals fed and the mode of transport had to be abandoned. One of the other men, Private Richard Alexander 'Dick' Henderson, was to become almost as famous as Simpson. On one occasion, Jackson met Henderson on the beach as he was returning with a wounded man and took his photograph. This photograph was to become the source of Horace Moore-Jones' painting 'The Man with the Donkey', which now hangs in the AWM and was originally identified as Simpson. Jackson's account is clear in naming Simpson as the first man to use a donkey for his work and points out that, although the New Zealanders copied the method, it was for no more than five days.[15]

14 Curran, *Across the Bar*, p.385.
15 Curran, *Across the Bar*, p.386.

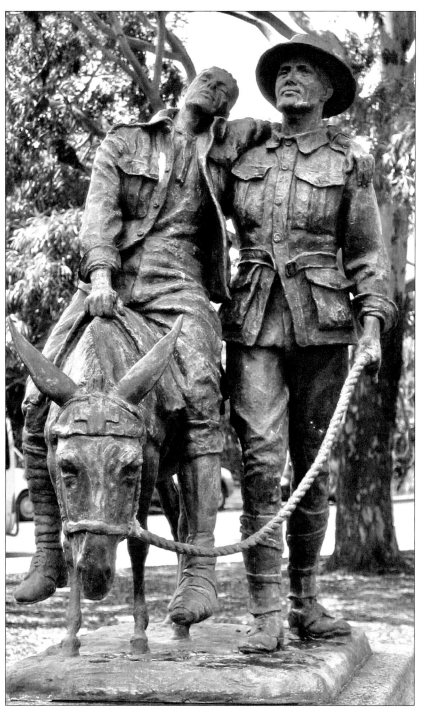

Bronze statue commemorating the ANZACs near the Melbourne War Memorial. It, too, uses the man with a donkey to convey the spirit and compassion of the Australian soldier. (Author)

At the end of May, Lieutenant Colonel Sutton was to make the following entry to sum up a month's service for his unit:

> My average strength for the month was 6 officers and 135 men. Stretcher squads have been sent daily to clear Walker's Road and Shrapnel Valley, never less than two squads are sent, they remain all day and are relieved at 8 pm by two other squads. These squads are marched by an officer who assists the Regimental MO when necessary. All squads are turned out whenever necessary and on instructions received from ADMS.
>
> A small hospital has been carried on in dugouts for the reception of cases who would be again fit for service in 48 hours. Our daily average for patients in May was 18. Details are shown in A & D books of the Corps and on a daily basis furnished to ADMS.[16]

Sutton's situation was not too different to other medical units on the peninsula at this time as they battled against shortages of men and equipment to maintain their hospitals and dressing stations. On the left of the Anzac position, that is, to the left of the 1st Australian Division, was the New Zealand and Australian Division. This division had established itself since the landings as best it could on the narrow beachhead. The 4th AFA, serving the 4th Australian Brigade, was facing similar problems to the other field ambulances, as the unit's camp came under regular shrapnel fire and the men sought methods of sheltering their hospital on the crowded beaches. From the outset, the unit had helped the 1st ACCS at Anzac Cove and provided bearer sections as needed throughout its divisional area. Soon, it was clear to the CO that casualties amongst his bearers would mean that this would become increasingly difficult. On 9 May, a 'Large shell fell on one of our men and killed him'.[17] Whilst there was only one man killed during the first days of May, there were at least 12 men wounded and one officer transferred to a hospital ship, mostly as a result of the Turkish shrapnel fire over the beach. A week later, the war diary records a sad incident when two bearers from the unit were carrying a wounded man back to the ambulance on a stretcher. A shell burst over the group, and both bearers were seriously wounded, one losing a leg whilst the man on the stretcher got up and ran for cover and was not seen again.[18] The shelling of the area was a daily occurrence, and, whilst probably not directed specifically at the hospital, it caused considerable problems. The 4th AFA lost its dressing station on 18 May when it was 'blown to pieces'. The Turkish attack on the Australian lines on 19 May brought more shelling over the hospital, but, during the fighting, the 4th AFA carried on its work. Bearers from C Section were ordered to go up to the cliffs directly behind the front line and to carry wounded halfway back down the steep slopes where bearers of A Section took over the job of carrying the wounded to the ambulance at the beach. B Section remained in reserve. This method was used to conserve the bearers as much as possible whilst still allowing the removal of those most in need from the forward areas. Other field ambulances adopted similar approaches. By the end of May, over 1,700 casualties had passed through the 4th AFA.

16 AWM: AWM4/26/46/5: War Diary, 3rd Australian Field Ambulance, 31 May 1915.
17 AWM: AWM4/26/47/6: War Diary, 4th Australian Field Ambulance, 9 May. The man killed was Private Cornelius Murphy.
18 AWM: AWM4/26/47/6: War Diary, 4th Australian Field Ambulance, 16 May 1915.

150   The Fight for Life

By 2 May, Lieutenant Colonel Begg and his unit, the NZFA, were working from a dressing station on the landing beach with four MOs and the tent subdivisions of A, B and C Sections of the ambulance. The bearer subdivisions were established in a further station behind the left flank of the divisional area. Lieutenant Colonel Begg reported the difficulties at this dressing station at the end of the week:

> As an instance of the work of the men, three days ago a twelve pound shell penetrated the Dressing Station and burst inside. At the time I was operating on a case assisted by seven or eight men. Not one of these left for a moment the duty on which he was engaged – even those holding the basins of lotions did not spill a drop. It is extremely difficult to select names for mention when all ranks worked so well. The chief difficulty the officers have is in restraining the men from taking too many risks. All ranks worked fearlessly under heavy fire for days on end.[19]

However, by the end of the second week of May, Begg was able to report on the surgical work that he was performing at the ambulance:

> Surgical Cases: Having a properly fitted up operating tent now I have been able to perform a large number of urgent operations. Assisted by Major Murray, I have performed a large number of laparotomies, resected portions of damaged intestine, sewed up intestinal perforations, arrested haemorrhage of the mesentery, liver spleen and kidneys and drained bladder wounds. In all cases I have been able to ligature ruptured middle meningeal arteries in three of which there was no perforation of the skull. Last night I had an interesting case in which a bullet entered the lower jaw on the right side below the canine fossa. The jaw was shattered and the bullet traversed the base of the tongue on the left side and lodged under the skin behind the sternomastoid on the left side of the neck. There was a large increasing haematoma on the side of the neck and increasing difficulty in breathing. On cutting down the neck we found both the lingual and facial arteries divided close to the carotid and were able to ligature then and stop the haemorrhage.[20]

There was also a pragmatic side to Begg, who recognised some of the more difficult issues that MOs, particularly RMOs, faced and recorded in the war diary:

> One point I would like to bring to your notice that frequently men who are obviously fatally injured – such as extensive brain lacerations – are sent down to the beach by the regimental medical officers. These cases die very quickly and it is unfair to the stretcher bearers to make them carry these cases sometimes over a mile over a rough road. It would be much better to make them as comfortable as possible where they are hit and bury them.[21]

---

19   AWM: AWM4/35/27/3: War Diary, New Zealand Field Ambulance, May 1915.
20   AWM: AWM4/35/27/3: War Diary, New Zealand Field Ambulance, May 1915.
21   AWM: AWM4/35/27/3: War Diary, New Zealand Field Ambulance, May 1915.

This was one of the hard facts of life on the peninsula: the MOs could not save everyone even with their best efforts. It is not known if this form of front-line triage was ever carried out and, if so, to what extent, but it is clear from Begg's note that it was something he wanted his MOs to consider. The bearers were clearly important in any field ambulance unit, and, again, Begg was clear on their importance in his unit:

> The almost invariable treatment used by Bearer Subdivisions has been to paint over the wound with iodine, and then apply the First Field Dressing carried by the wounded man, or, if necessary, the additional field dressing carried by the bearers for the purpose.
>
> Where haemorrhage has been severe, some method has been used to tourniquet the necessary artery. Splints have been improvised from anything to hand; rifles, bayonets, handles of entrenching tools, firewood etc. Equipment has been freely used for supporting bandages as also have putties, and for slings.
>
> Triangular bandages have been found of great value and should in our opinion be more widely provided and used by the bearer subdivisions and stretcher bearers (regimental). Where very apparent, pieces of shrapnel or dirt have been removed from wounds, but no attempt has been made to wash these. In only one case that has come under out notice in the field has there been an absolute indication for immediate operative interference. This was a case in which a shrapnel bullet had perforated the internal jugular and the trachea, and death was caused by haemorrhage into the air passages causing suffocation. Opening up the wound and dealing with the bleeding point would have given this patient his only chance; this was impossible as at the moment nothing was at hand.
>
> When cases have come into the hands of the tent subdivisions it has been found that, with a few exceptions, the first aid rendered by stretcher bearers of Regiments, bearers of Ambulances, and in many cases by comrades of the wounded men, has been of a very high standard.
>
> It has been noticed that much ingenuity has been used in improvisation.
>
> In some cases, it has not been considered necessary to interfere with the dressing before further evacuation, but in most cases, wounds have been re-examined and dealt with.
>
> Two methods have been used; to paint the whole area including the wound with iodine, after shaving the part where necessary, and secondly to paint the circumjacent area with iodine, and wash out the actual wound with 1 in 40 carbolic lotion. As these cases have passed out of our hands it has been impossible to express a first-hand opinion as to which is the better. Where bullets have remained in and are easily available these have been removed, generally under local anaesthesia. In other cases, they have not been interfered with being left for X Ray examination.[22]

The NZFA dressing station that had been established on the beach was soon tackling serious cases, and, by the end of the third week of May, Begg was able to report:

---

22   AWM: AWM4/35/27/3: War Diary, New Zealand Field Ambulance, 16–19 May.

> A very useful operating theatre has been set up by digging out and sandbagging … where an operating tent has been pitched. Thus, several trephining and abdomen sections have been carried through. In the later cases (bullet and shrapnel wounds of abdomen) the gut has been perforated but not torn across except in on case in which the bowel was severed. The immediate operative treatment of these cases gave them a very much better chance of recovery than they would have had if delay of getting them on the Hospital Ship had been permitted. In the trephine cases that occurred some in which the whole thickness of the skull was depressed or smashed up in others only the inner table. In many cases great splinters were split off the table with very little damage to the other. 2 cases of damage to the middle meningeal artery without apparent bone injury were dealt with.[23]

This was, to some extent, going beyond the remit of the field ambulance, which was essentially to patch up the wounded to be dealt with farther along the lines of communication. At Gallipoli, the need to use sea transport before the men could reach a fully equipped base hospital meant that there was some recourse to more unusual methods and to carrying out intervention at an earlier stage than perhaps would have been considered elsewhere. Begg would not have been alone in his attempt to give the wounded the best chance possible. Unfortunately, there is no record of how well the seriously wounded men who were treated in this manner fared once they had left the peninsula, though it is known that abdominal wounds tended not to do well after their removal from the beaches.

It is interesting to follow the evacuation of one of the wounded at about this time. Sapper Roy Howard Denning of the 1st Field Company Australian Engineers was wounded in action on 16 June by a shrapnel bullet that struck him in the back whilst working in the front line at Anzac: 'I felt a stinging blow that seemed to kink my spine and fell flat on my stomach. I was afraid to move. The most dreaded wound was a spinal wound.'[24] The RMO arrived on the scene almost immediately and told him that he was not to move until the stretcher-bearers had arrived, who then '… lifted me on to the stretcher and carried me down the rough winding path to the dressing station on the beach, where the stretcher was placed on two high trestles and became the operating table'.[25] Whilst at the makeshift operating table, the MO was able to extract the bullet from his back, after which 'I was rushed along the beach to a waiting barge, and placed alongside twenty more stretcher cases. A number of these men were in a very bad way, others with lesser wounds were delighted to have received their issue and to be able to get out of it.'[26]

From the barge, he was transferred to the fleet sweeper *Clacton*, which then carried him to the HS *Sicilia*, standing off the beaches. By the time that Denning arrived on board, the ship was near full, and it was not long before it was leaving the station at Anzac to be relieved by the HS *Gascon*. Upon arrival on the *Sicilia*, Denning was examined by an MO and ordered to be taken down two decks to a ward. Here, he saw other badly wounded soldiers, and he felt ashamed of

---

23 AWM: AWM4/35/27/3: War Diary, New Zealand Field Ambulance, 18–19 May.
24 Roy and Lorna Denning, *Anzac Digger: An Engineer in Gallipoli and France* (Loftus: Australian Military History Publications, 2004), p.22.
25 Denning and Denning, *Anzac Digger*, p.23. This possibly refers to the 1st ACCS, which evacuated 82 cases that day.
26 Denning and Denning, *Anzac Digger*, p.23.

his wound since, at this time, he was in no real pain and had little idea of how bad his wound was. In a matter of minutes, an Australian nurse came to his bedside, and, for the first time, he was aware just how dirty and sweaty he was after weeks in the trenches. The *Sicilia* was staffed by Australian nurses of the AANS under Matron K. Fawcett of the QAIMNS. For many of the men coming off Anzac, it was a pleasure, close to relief, when they realised that they would be nursed by Australian women. Denning was thoroughly washed, and his wound redressed. He was 'satisfied with life' and wrote, 'Strange old organization the military, while one is well, they make it as hard and tough as possible, but once a man is wounded they leave no stone unturned to add to his comfort.'[27]

The *Sicilia* reached Malta on 20 June, and Denning was disembarked and taken to a makeshift hospital set up in a gymnasium, as all the hospitals were full at that time. Shortly afterwards, he was transferred to what is termed the 'main hospital', which possibly means the military hospital at Cottenera. Denning remained at this hospital for about a month, but, with more and more casualties coming from the peninsula, all the beds possible were needed, and, to that end, there was an effort to move men back to duty or to one of the convalescent camps. Denning was sent to the St Andrew's Convalescent Camp, where he remained for a further few weeks, as the wound on his back had not fully healed. However, by this time, he was feeling guilty about being away from the unit, and he wanted to get back to Gallipoli. On 21 August, he volunteered to return to duty and reached Anzac via the base hospital at Mustapha in Egypt on 8 September, back with the 1st Field Company Australian Engineers. He was to remain on the peninsula until Anzac was evacuated on 20 December. It would seem that, at least in case of this wounded soldier, the whole evacuation procedure had worked well.

The work of the New Zealand Mounted Field Ambulance (NZMFA) was rather different to the other field ambulances of the New Zealand and Australian Division. In this instance, this unit did not leave Egypt until 15 May and was not officially attached to the division until that time. Its service to the wounded began aboard the transport *Galeka*, on which they had sailed for Gallipoli. By 19 May, this unit was treating wounded on board, transferred from the beaches at the height of the Turkish assault on the front lines. It was expected, at least by the CO, that the unit would land at Anzac on 31 May, and, although it was on board a minesweeper in readiness for disembarkation, it was sent back to the *Galeka* and eventually transferred to the transport *Ivernian* in Mudros Harbour on 2 June.[28] The unit was to provide medical staff for the *Ivernian*, which was then acting as a temporary hospital ship. Three days later, 1,266 wounded were embarked on the ship, and everyone, including the ship's company, were kept very busy. This black ship seems to have been ready to handle casualties in a much better fashion than some of those in the days immediate upon the landing, but 'As the ship was not registered as a Hospital Ship no Red Cross was flown. Had we been submarined the majority of the 1,266 could have done very little to help themselves.'[29]

The *Ivernia* and its wounded were directed to Malta, where it arrived three days later, and perhaps the quality of the care is reflected in the fact that, during the voyage, there were only

27 Denning and Denning, *Anzac Digger*, p.23.
28 The *Galeka* officially became a hospital ship on 22 June 1915, see Macpherson, *History of the Great War: Medical Services*, vol. 4, p.367.
29 Australian War Memorial (AWM) AWM4/35/26/1: War Diary, New Zealand Mounted Field Ambulance, 6 June.

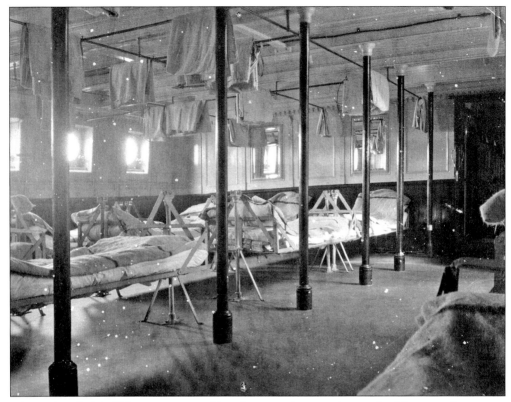

Officers' ward of the HS *Grantully Castle*. Note the screens hanging above each of the cots and compare with the ward on the HS *Sicilia*. (TAHO: NS669/14/1/5)

three deaths on board. During the voyage, the CO of the NZMFA made some observations for improving the care of the wounded:

1. I had a wooden cot made for lowering stretchers over the side of the vessel in the naval way, of the thickest and heaviest timber available. The weight steadied the cot in its transit and prevented its swinging and bumping the side of the vessel, as I have seen lighter cots do. It was made big enough to take two stretchers, or one with two attendant orderlies if required, or four less seriously wounded in a sitting or lying position.
2. One man lost his arm through the abuse of the tourniquet in the field. Only one, I am afraid, of several during the war. The tourniquet was not required and had not been removed. There is a most unfortunate tendency amongst men learning 'First Aid' to apply a tourniquet when there is no need.
3. Many wounds were bandaged much too tightly and gave rise to a considerable amount of unnecessary pain. I think this is largely due to the fact that the First Field Dressing is applied with a roll of bandages in each hand which tends to a tighter pull being taken on the bandage than when one hand only is used. The septic condition which prevails amongst wounds caused swelling and gives pain by tightening the bandage, undoubtedly, but I refer

particularly to wounds that were not septic and from which there was no possible fear of bleeding.[30]

The unit remained on Malta until 23 June, with some of its personnel doing duty at the Florian hospital there during its two weeks stay.

At the start of July, the NZMFA reached Lemnos and was transferred to the *Alnwick Castle*, which was prepared for wounded and, with 348 wounded on board, sailed for Alexandria. This unit was probably getting used to work on black ships by the time it arrived in Alexandria and transferred, again, to the *Minnewaska* for the return trip to Lemnos. Here, it was finally disembarked and set up camp on 14 July. Ten days later, the first three officers and 35 other ranks of the unit made their way to Anzac on the fleet sweeper *Hythe*, where it assisted the NZFA at Walker's Ridge with the evacuation of the wounded at that ambulance. Their arrival at the end of July should be seen as part of the general preparation for the August Offensive at Anzac.

Whilst the hospitals and field ambulances were getting used to their environment and generally handling the casualties as they arose, the enemy shelling remained a problem. At the start of June, the 1st ACCS was recording the use of sandbag walls to provide cover and of shelters to protect the men waiting for the boats to evacuate them. Nevertheless, the shelling continued to cause problems. One patient at 1st ACCS was killed on 14 June as a result of HE shells falling near the hospital. The patient was perhaps even more unfortunate since he, Stoker Frederick Upward of the HMS *Majestic*, had survived the sinking of his vessel only to die while receiving hospital treatment.[31] The shell fire continued to hamper evacuation as the jetties came under fire, and this was further compounded by a lack of boats and poor weather. It was not until 1 July that the 1st ACCS was able to move to a safer location, but, of course, at Anzac, no location could be considered entirely free from fire.

One problem that was increasing during the months from May to July was the plague of flies. Most units remarked on the problem:

> The fly trouble in camp is becoming very acute. Precautions are being taken in the way of burning used dressing and refuse but still the flies swarm round the supply depot in particular. The Clearing Station is also very much affected. I am sure much of the diarrhoea which is prevalent among the whole force is due to flies infecting the food.[32]

It did not take long for MOs at all levels to recognise the linkage between the growing numbers of flies and the increase in enteritis, diarrhoea and dysentery that was occurring in the troops across the peninsula:

> When one comes to consider medical cases, the story is different. No fewer than 141 cases entered as gastro-enteritis or enteritis have been dealt with at Anzac Cove besides a large number treated at the Advanced Dressing Stations – 10 at that in Monash's Gully. When the carelessness of the troops as regards sanitation is observed the wonder is not that these cases are so frequent but that the whole force is not cleared off the

---

30   AWM: AWM4/35/26/1: War Diary, New Zealand Mounted Field Ambulance, 6 June.
31   The HMS *Majestic* was sunk on 25 May.
32   AWM: AWM4/26/62/5: War Diary, 1st Australian Casualty Clearing Station, 19 June.

peninsula by an extremely serious epidemic. As regards use of latrines it is more rare that the reverse to see men cover their excreta even though a shovel is placed at the latrines for the purpose. Empty meat tins, bits of biscuit, food refuse from mess tins, tea leaves, jam tins etc are practically always to be seen thrown about – sometimes in heaps and frequently emitting a foul smell. Myriads of flies swarm over these plague spots breeding freely. In some cases, it has been observed that such conditions obtained for 2 or 3 days on end in spite of condemnatory reports by Sanitary Officers. Combatant Officers seem to take no care and less interest in seeing to the sanitary environment of the troops under their command. More than that combatant officers have frequently been observed to be themselves offenders against sanitary precautions. In some cases, notice boards placed at latrines have been removed for firewood every time they are put in position. Although the ambulances as units have nothing to do with the Sanitary Supervision of areas other than those on which Ambulance detachments are encamped yet the noticeable increase in sick passing through their hands seems to justify some comment on such an extremely important subject.[33]

The MOs and the attached sanitary officers were soon looking at a variety of methods to try and improve the overall situation and the fly problem in particular:

Flies are still in millions and it has been observed that almost pure Cresol is practically useless in keeping them down. Flies have time after time been observed swarming over an area that has a short time before been soaking in a strong solution of this disinfectant. In small areas kerosene has been (when obtainable) mixed with the disinfectant fluid and the result has been immensely better than without.[34]

As the heat of the summer increased so did the problems of the medical services, as the numbers reporting sick soon took on epidemic proportions. On 26 May, the DMS MEF reported to the War Office in London that there was little sickness on the peninsula and that enteric and dysentery had not been identified amongst the troops there. This was in error since the RMOs had begun to evacuate cases of enteric to Lemnos by this time and, a day or two later, No. 16 BSH had admitted cases to the hospital, closely followed by the unit opening a new camp to separate and treat all enteric cases.[35] The small number of such cases being diagnosed in late May and early June was to prove to be no more than the harbinger of a rapid spread of disease across the peninsula. Butler was to comment:

In particular, the conditions were those which in the history on war have commonly been associated with serious outbreaks of disease. A rapid deterioration in health, which was to play an important – possibly a determining – part in the campaign was the outstanding medical feature of this period; in all arms throughout June and July the wastage from sickness was in excess of the replacements and recovered 'casualties'.[36]

33   AWM: AWM4/35/27/4: War Diary, New Zealand Field Ambulance, Summary for Week 13–19 June.
34   AWM: AWM4/35/27/4: War Diary, New Zealand Field Ambulance, Summary for Week 27 June to 3 July.
35   Butler, *Official History of the Australian Medical Services*, vol. I, p.244.
36   Butler, *Official History of the Australian Medical Services*, vol. I, p.206.

The conditions to which Butler referred were those obtaining on the crowded beaches across the peninsula as the summer began and, in particular, to those at Anzac. To this overcrowding was to be added the increasing summer temperatures as the summer heat began to build. By July, the midday temperature was between 28–30 degrees Celsius in the shade at Anzac as everyone began to feel the difficulties of crowding and lack of water.[37] Lieutenant Colonel Carberry of the NZMC considered that, by July, the numbers of sick reporting daily were turning Anzac into 'one big hospital'.[38] The conditions were worsened for the men by their relatively poor diet, which was at best monotonous and at worse more or less ineffective at maintaining general health. On top of these issues was the more intractable problem of the number of flies that began to appear. From the second half of May, war diaries and personal accounts make mention of flies, as their number grew to plague proportions: 'Few more terrible plagues can have afflicted British troops than the flies on Gallipoli. In May, by comparison there were none. In June they came by armies; in July by multitudes.'[39] It was in this plague of flies that the source for much of the disease on Gallipoli can be found. Of course, flies, on their own, do not provide the whole of the problem. For there to be 'multitudes' of flies, there must be suitable feeding and breeding grounds for them to prosper. This was provided at Anzac, and Helles, where the crowded troops lived in relatively insanitary conditions and consequently cheek by jowl with disease. At Helles, things were better than at Anzac, for the 29th Division had a sanitation unit and sanitary discipline was good. At Anzac, however, the sanitary squads were improvised in the first instance by using one officer and a small number of men from the 3rd AFA.[40]

At the time of the landing at Anzac, there were no sanitary arrangements, and men were allowed to use the water's edge as a latrine.[41] This was a situation that could not be allowed to continue, and each divisional area, two at Anzac at this time, was called upon to begin more formal arrangements for sanitation. This led to the men of the tent division of the 3rd AFA being taken from the ambulance for sanitary work and inspection on 4 May. In the first instance, the work was to consider the preparation of shallow latrine pits and the protection of such limited water sources as were available at Anzac. The shallow pits presented problems since they needed to be sited in spots that were not under enemy fire, always difficult at Anzac, or they simply would not be used by the troops for whom they were intended. Each time a pit was used, it was the responsibility of every man to cover the waste with a layer of soil. This simple action seems to have been difficult to enforce, and regimental officers often did not grasp its importance. This was, possibly, one of the first issues in the whole of Anzac developing poor sanitary conditions. By mid-June, shallow pits were abandoned, but deep pits did not provide any better solution to the problem as flies took advantage of the insanitary conditions:

> During the first few days at Anzac, I did not see a fly; there were practically no grazing animals, the country sparsely populated, and it was cool. About the third week I

---

37   Carberry, *New Zealand Medical Service in the Great War*, p.63.
38   Carberry, *New Zealand Medical Service in the Great War*, p.64.
39   A. P. Herbert, *The Secret Battle* (Oxford: Oxford University Press, 1982), p.45. Herbert served as a sub-lieutenant with the Hawke Battalion in the RND.
40   Butler, *Official History of the Australian Medical Services*, vol. I, p.229.
41   AWM: AWM4/35/26/1: War Diary, New Zealand Mounted Field Ambulance, Sanitary Report 25 April to 17 May.

noticed a few flies. Being interested in this subject I looked around for breeding places and came on the 'refuse pit' of an Indian Mountain Battery. It had been covered over lightly with soil. At the surface of the soil were pupae and digging down a few inches, I found larvae in enormous numbers. I reported this and suggested larger supplies of disinfectant, particularly blue oil. The flies increased rapidly and by May 19th small flies (*Musca domestica* and *Musca homolyia*)[42] were very numerous, also large flies, bluebottle and green bottle.[43]

Sicknesses were soon to follow, and these became a major problem, particularly those that were broadly termed 'gastrointestinal'. At first, these were simply described as 'diarrhoea' by MOs. RMOs sought to treat such sickness in their aid posts close to, or even in, the front-line system of trenches. There was an attempt to keep battalions up to fighting strength, and both COs and RMOs were reluctant to see men sent away from their units for what, on the face of it, was a relatively minor complaint. It was not considered what the effect upon manpower would be if the sickness was rather more serious or more infectious. It was not until the second half of May that RMOs began to think that there were other gastrointestinal complaints arising in the front-line soldier. However, by the end of May, medical units, such as the 1st AFA, were beginning to recognise the link between increased sickness and the proliferation of flies.[44] By mid-June, the NZFA was reporting that the '… cases of diarrhoea are suspected typhoid and rapidly increasing'.[45]

The relationship between flies, insanitary conditions and the health of the troops may be obvious, but the linkage, perhaps, needs some clarification. By mid-July, the strength of the battalions was perhaps 25 percent lower than establishment, and much of the wastage was down to disease, mainly dysentery and undifferentiated 'enterica'.[46] Dysentery of two varieties was identified in men evacuated from the peninsula. In the first instance was bacillary dysentery, caused by *Shigella dysenteriae*. This bacterium has one form of transmission, that is, the faecal–oral route: 'It is particularly important to armed forces because it renders fighting men non-effective and increases the burden on the Medical Corps.'[47] The disease is generally caused by poor sanitary conditions and poor hygiene practices, is compounded by overcrowding and, although caused by contaminated food, is often waterborne. *Shigella* also causes the release of toxins into the blood stream, which can cause damage to the kidneys and eventual renal failure.

The second type of dysentery, also found in troops at Anzac, was amoebic dysentery. In this type, an amoebic cyst passes into the gut via the mouth as a result of poor hygiene. The cyst is not affected by stomach acids, but, upon entering the alkali environment of the small intestine, it dissolves and releases the cells responsible for the amoebic dysentery. These, in turn, form a cyst that passes out of the gut, and so the life cycle is continued. The fly can act as the vector of

---

42   *Musca domestica* – the house fly.
43   Account by Captain A. H. Tebbutt, RMO of the 4th Battalion AIF, and quoted in Butler, *Official History of the Australian Medical Services*, vol. I, p.238.
44   AWM: AWM4/26/44/3: War Diary, 1st Australian Field Ambulance, 26 May.
45   AWM: AWM4/35/26/1: War Diary, New Zealand Mounted Field Ambulance, Summary for Month 20 May to 19 June.
46   Carberry, *New Zealand Medical Service in the Great War*, p.65.
47   Lucian A. Smith, 'Shiga Dysentery', *Journal of the American Medical Association (JAMA)*, 130:1 (1946), pp.18–22.

the pathogens for both types of dysentery and thereby acts as the connection between the poor sanitation, in the form of poor latrines and maintenance, and the food that was difficult to store and keep away from the swarming flies. Flies swarmed over everything on the peninsula, and open latrines provided suitable breeding grounds, as indeed did the bodies of the slain in no man's land, whilst the daily ration of food was not far from the men at any time and were an obvious attraction to the flies. Under these conditions, it was but a short step from good health to debilitating disease and possibly death.

Added to the problems associated with dysentery was that caused by enteric fever or undifferentiated typhoid fever. Once again, the fly acts as the vector for the pathogen *Salmonella*. The bacterium has only human carriers and is again spread through the faecal–oral route, which also stems from the poor sanitation and hygiene issues. This was to become a major problem as the campaign developed through the summer, and, of course, the problem was exacerbated by the summer heat. Lieutenant Colonel Carberry of the NZMC summed up the problems: 'The distance from the bases and the lack of pathologists and prompt notification of infectious diseases, bacteriologically diagnosed, prevented earlier diagnosis of the dangerous cases of typhoid, paratyphoid and dysentery which were treated at RAP's and permitted to remain as a further source of infection.'[48]

Although the fly problem was well recognised, it was not handled as readily as perhaps it could have been. The recommended treatment for the breeding grounds of the flies was to use a 1:10 dilution of creosol in water to be sprayed liberally and frequently over the areas. MOs noted that this was an ineffective treatment and applied to the DMS for other preventative measures, such as petrol or 'blue oil', but this was refused with the suggestion that fly papers were to be used instead. This showed to the men on the ground how divorced from the situation across the peninsula the DMS had become. This recommendation was treated with little more than contempt by the officers and men facing the daily battle against the ever-increasing fly population.[49]

In addition to the problems of dysentery and enteric that were emerging in the early summer, there was a cholera scare. This was, in part, because of the lack of suitable diagnostic methods on the peninsula to identify the disease. When the suspected cases were diagnosed as bacillary dysentery, there was something of a sigh of relief from the MOs. Nevertheless, cholera precautions were put in place, and vaccinations were commenced for troops on the peninsula. Indeed, all the 29th Division at Helles were vaccinated against cholera. When the sick eventually reached Egypt, they were screened bacteriologically in an effort to ensure that cholera was not introduced to the existing large hospital population. It was not until the end of July that a pathology laboratory was established on Lemnos, and, whilst this was a useful addition to the facilities immediate to the peninsula, it was perhaps too late. By the end of July, the problem associated with gastrointestinal disease 'was quite out of control'.[50]

As an example of the prevailing conditions at Anzac during this period, it is useful to consider the situation at Quinn's Post during June. At the beginning of the month, the New Zealanders had relieved the Australians at Quinn's Post. On 9 June, the position was taken over by the Wellington Battalion, commanded by Lieutenant Colonel William Malone. Malone was to

---

48   Carberry, *New Zealand Medical Service in the Great War*, p.61.
49   Butler, *Official History of the Australian Medical Services*, vol. I, p.240.
50   Butler, *Official History of the Australian Medical Services*, vol. I, p.249.

remark that he had been given the command of 'a dirty, dilapidated, unorganized Post'.[51] He immediately set about cleaning it up since he saw the condition of the post as unhealthy and un-soldierly and felt that there should be both cleanliness and organisation, which would assist in maintaining better sanitary conditions. Captain Thomas Ritchie, RMO of the Canterbury Battalion, was appointed sanitary officer for the post and given the job of cleaning up the post and the approaches along Monash Valley. His job was not easy. The Australians had buried their dead, often in shallow graves, all over the area, making no effort to collect the bodies into one spot. The bodies provided breeding grounds for flies, and Ritchie set about covering these bodies as far as was possible with lime. The random burials had also polluted the groundwater, limited as it was, of the entire area, and Ritchie found it very difficult to impress upon the thirsty troops that it should not be drunk. Ritchie set up latrines, and men were encouraged to use them rather than fouling the ground. Efforts were made to control the disposal of food waste and empty bully beef tins since this was also recognised as providing breeding grounds for flies. Soon, the post, or at least the Wellington's lines, was described as very clean. It was not without result, for the Wellington's sick list was the shortest of the division, which went some way to justifying the work that had been put in to clean up the post and the obsession of the CO. Furthermore, it demonstrated that, at least to some extent, the filthy conditions of the trenches could be alleviated, if not completely solved.[52] Unfortunately, this exercise in good housekeeping was not repeated throughout the Anzac area.

At the end of July, one of the brigadier generals at Anzac called a conference of his RMOs in an attempt to assess the overall condition of the troops in his command. The MOs could offer little comfort when they reported:

1. The general health of the troops and their physical condition is below normal and getting progressively worse.
2. No further steps can be suggested to improve the hygienic and sanitary conditions other that change of bivouacs to a fresh unused site.
3. The principal symptoms of sickness are: gastric derangement, bronchial affections, loss of weight, rapid pulse, dilation of the heart.
4. Predisposing causes: irregularity of rest and meal hours; restricted dietary as regard variety; heat, dust and flies.[53]

This can hardly have been good news for an officer attempting to prepare his command for a major offensive in a matter of a few weeks.

However, for all the work the medical services were doing, there was considerable concern amongst senior officers about not only the overall condition of the troops but also the quality of some of the men and their overall state of health. Problems that should have been picked up at an early stage in the service of some were exacerbated by the arduous conditions on the peninsula:

---

51   Peter Stanley, *Quinn's Post: Anzac, Gallipoli* (Crow's Nest: Allen and Unwin, 2005), p.101.
52   Stanley, *Quinn's Post*, p.106.
53   Carberry, *New Zealand Medical Service in the Great War*, p.65.

I was watching the embarkation of sick and undesirables today at the pier. They are a degenerate looking lot in appearance and it seems a marvel how they passed the medical exam in the first instance. They are the crowd who break their dentures or lose them – have glasses and break them … and undiscovered hernias. Certainly, the original medical exam should be more strict and searching. Too many men [use] this shorter exam to enable them to get away. We are better without them but they put the country to a lot of expense [from] which they gain the cheap glamour of 'having been to the front'.[54]

Whilst this observation may not have been universal amongst MOs, it is quite clear that, during the early summer months, the health of the troops began to deteriorate quite rapidly. Clearly, if the men had not been in the best physical condition to begin with, then their deterioration was likely to have been more rapid. This put additional strain on everyone in the medical services, which was, at times, struggling to cope with large numbers of battle casualties. The problem associated with sickness, and that of the plague of flies, did not diminish until well into the autumn, and, by that time, the overall condition of all troops on the peninsula could only have been considered to be poor.

During the three months between the landings and the August Offensive, the medical services had established themselves in a number of sites across Anzac. They had adapted to the difficult conditions and shortages of medical equipment and sometimes drugs to provide a reasonably efficient process of treatment and subsequent evacuation for both sick and wounded. There is no doubt that it could have been better, and the war diaries of the units concerned often point directly to problems such as the loss, or shortage, of staff, shortage of boats for evacuation and the lack of sufficient protection for the hospital from persistent, if not directed, shelling on most of the sites. Nevertheless, the services worked to provide the best medical cover for all the men at Anzac, and, for many, they provided the difference between life and death.

The work of the men of the medical units was not always recognised by the men they served and cared for, though perhaps the work of Simpson is an exception to this, so it was probably a morale boost for all of the 1st ACCS when Private Mawer Douglas Cowtan was awarded the DCM, recorded in the war diary of 21 June, for his work during the first days of the campaign. The citation for his award runs as follows:

On 25th April and subsequently, for distinguished conduct during the landing opera-tion in the neighbourhood of Gaba Tepe. He was indefatigable during the first four days in giving and carrying water to the wounded and his unswerving courage under fire was invaluable in its effect. The work of the Casualty Clearing Station was carried out under great difficulties and was very heavy.

Private Cowtan's award was officially gazetted on 5 August, at which time he was also mentioned in despatches. However, the CO of the unit was to note in the war diary that, although the award was deserved, the behaviour of Cowtan was no different to at least 'a dozen other men of

---

54   AWM: AWM4/26/47/8: War Diary, 4th Australian Field Ambulance, 5 July.

162   The Fight for Life

the unit'. There is no doubt that the CO was pleased with the conduct of the men of his unit, and he commented further that it was an exception 'to find any shirking'.[55]

It is easy to assume that the work of the medical services was relatively easy when there was no major offensive or enemy action. This would suggest that the time between the landing and the August Offensive was a relatively quiet time. It has already been noted that the 1st ACCS evacuated 4,895 cases during May. In June, there was a sharp decline when the hospital evacuated 2,951 cases, but the constant level of close-quarter fighting and bombing in the trenches above the beaches did not let up. During July, a month that saw no major engagement, the 1st ACCS evacuated 5,460 cases. This was the cost of holding the line at Anzac.

After three months on the peninsula, the various units of the medical services could have been considered experienced and were probably about as ready as they could be for the planned offensive. They had established routines to enable the wounded to be cared for and, in conjunction with the lines of communication units, had a ready and workable system for the evacuation of casualties. Any breakdown in the latter was seldom as a result of fault of the shore-based units since insufficient boats and inclement weather played a much larger role in this element of the medical services and were, essentially, out of their control. The units went into August capable of dealing with the problems of the battlefield; however, few would have guessed the magnitude of the problems that the August Offensive would cause.

Not all the medical units that were involved in this phase of the operation were on the peninsula. It had been the original plan that two stationary hospitals would be landed shortly after the beaches had been cleared. This plan was soon abandoned because the beaches were not cleared as effectively as hoped. This meant that, although there were medical staff available, they could not be landed, and No. 1 and No. 2 ASH medical staff were used for at least part of May to staff black ships and give assistance to the wounded in whatever way was possible. Eventually, during May, stationary hospitals, both British and Australian, were established on Lemnos, but, before that happened, there was considerable work for those staff assigned to work on the transports. One officer of No. 2 ASH, Major Bernard Traugott Zwar, left a clear idea of his thoughts on the black ships when he wrote to Colonel White, his CO:

> In your capacity of senior Medical Officer in the Australian Medical Service of the L of C, I desire to bring before your notice certain conditions that obtain on the temporary hospital ships at present used for conveyance of sick and wounded.
>
> This communication is based on the personal experience in the conveyance of wounded gained
>
> 1.   As Officer in Command of a temporary hospital ship from 3rd May.
> 2.   As medical Officer assisting on a temporary hospital ship from 21st May to 3rd June.
> 3.   As a Medical Officers giving assistance on a temporary hospital ship when travelling as a patient from Lemnos to Alexandria from 21st to 23rd June.

---

55   AWM: AWM4/26/62/5: War Diary, 1st Australian Casualty Clearing Station, 21 June.

Attention is directed to the fact that Transports whose decks have recently been occupied by Mules or horses are still being used for the transport of wounded without such decks having undergone efficient cleaning or disinfection.

The personnel to look after the wounded and sick is still quite deficient in Officers, Nursing Sisters and Orderlies. It is, in consequence, impossible for the wounded and sick on these transports to receive the amount of surgical, medical, nursing and general attention that they should get. The result is a state of affairs which is hard to conceive. It does not seem possible to obtain a keener impression of the horrors and suffering of war in any other area of the service than on the temporary hospital ships.

It is pointed out that there are at present, particularly at the Base, Medical units the service of some of whose Officers, Nursing Sisters and Orderlies cold be dispensed with without endangering the present efficiency of these units.

It is urged that as many of these Officers, Nursing Sisters and Orderlies should be placed at the disposal of the proper authorities for duty on these temporary hospital ships.[56]

Major Zwar wrote this letter from No. 1 AGH in Egypt on 25 June. Zwar made a case for more medical staff for black ships based on his experience. Unfortunately, things did not immediately improve, but there was a general effort to place more medical staff on the transports to assist wherever possible. Zwar had clearly seen some of the worst conditions, but, by the very nature of the vessels used, some were better than others, and some were better staffed. During 3–12 May, Zwar had served on the HMHS *Gloucester Castle* until his party was transferred to the HMTS *Franconia*, on which he made a return trip to Alexandria.[57] The *Gloucester Castle* was equipped as a hospital ship, and this would suggest that Zwar's opinions were based on the time that he spent on the *Franconia* or on the unknown ship on which he was evacuated to Egypt. Nevertheless, the situation on the transports was not all that was wanted or expected by the MOs, particularly where more seriously wounded men needed to be transported. This was a situation that changed but slowly throughout the early summer months, and periods of battle added to the stress brought on the transport system, which further slowed down improvements.

---

56 AWM: AWM4/26/71/1: War Diary, No. 2 Australian Stationary Hospital, Appendix 3, May 1915.
57 The *Gloucester Castle* was launched in 1911 with a tonnage of 7,999 tons and a top speed of 13 knots. It was taken into service as a hospital ship from 24 September 1914, carrying a compliment of eight MOs, 10 nursing sisters and 41 RAMC orderlies. See Macpherson, *History of the Great War: Medical Services*, vol. 1, p.366. The *Franconia* was a Cunard liner of 18,150 tons with a top speed of 17 knots. It served as a troopship from early 1915 until it was sunk on 4 October 1916.

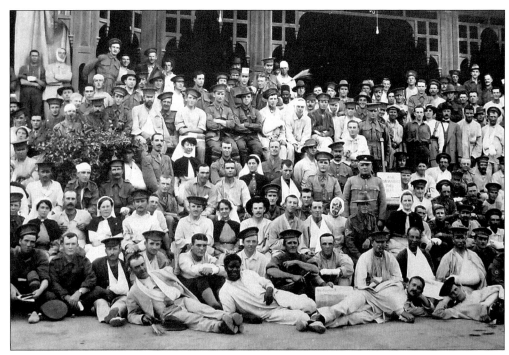

Some of the first casualties to reach Mena House (No. 2 AGH) in Egypt, taken during May 1915. These men are 'walking wounded'. Matron Nellie Gould is seated near the front and to the right. (NSW State Library: Irene Victoria Read Papers, pictorial material and relics, 1839–1951)

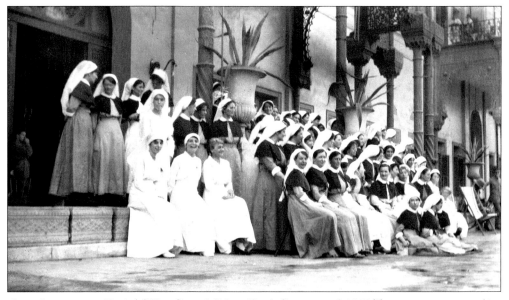

Australian nurses at No. 2 AGH at Gezireh Palace Hotel, Cairo, in mid-1915. The senior nurses seated in the first row are Matron Nellie Gould (slightly forwards) and (to her right) Sister Julia Bligh Johnson. On the other side are seated Sister Jean Miles Walker and Sister Maude Kellett. (AWM: J06857)

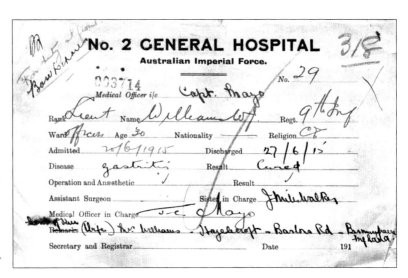

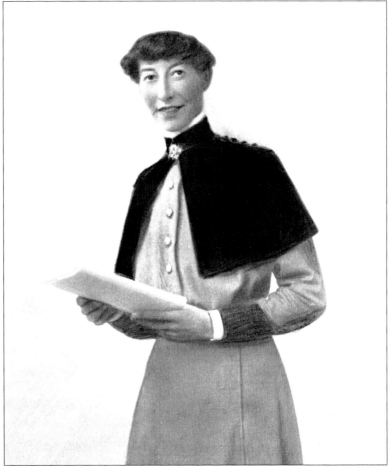

Patient's record card from No. 2 AGH. The patient Lieutenant John William Williams, 9th Battalion Australian Imperial Force (AIF), had been admitted for neurasthenia (later to be known as 'shell shock') and gastritis after service on the peninsula. The MO in charge was Captain John Christian Mayo, and Sister Jean Miles Walker was the sister in charge. (Courtesy of the National Archives of Australia (NAA): B2455, Williams W. J.)

Matron Jean Miles Walker, AAN in 1918. In 1915, as a sister, Matron Walker had served at Mena House and on the HS *Gascon* during the Gallipoli Campaign. (AWM: H19428/2)

8

We Had Nothing for Them: Hospitals on Lemnos

The island of Lemnos was, at first, considered to be an ideal location for a forward base for the Gallipoli Campaign. To this end, it had been considered suitable by GHQ, and it was looked at in this light by the arrival of Colonel A. C. Joly de Lotbiniere Royal Engineers, who was asked to report on its suitability as a base. By 12 March, the day that Hamilton was appointed commander-in-chief of the MEF, Joly de Lotbiniere was able to report that the island was not suitable for such use. He based his argument largely on the lack of potable water on the island and on the fact that there were no suitable wharves or infrastructure to handle the requirements of a base for thousands of troops. Joly de Lotbiniere was an experienced hydraulic engineer and had spent years in India developing hydroelectric schemes.[1] At the time that he made his survey of Lemnos, he was General Birdwood's chief engineer. Despite Joly de Lotbiniere's reservations, the 3rd Australian Brigade was despatched to Lemnos as the detached force and was to remain there until the land campaign commenced when it became the covering force for the division for the landing at Gaba Tepe. Whilst it was clear to the detached force that the water supply was an issue, since most of it was supplied from the transports that had carried it to Mudros Harbour, the island was to become crucial to the campaign as part of the lines of communication, including the development of hospitals, which continued more or less until the evacuation of the peninsula.

The development of hospital facilities on Lemnos largely reflects the development of the campaign as a whole and the number and type of casualties arising from the actions on the peninsula. The hospitals were to suffer, to a greater or lesser extent, from the lack of water as warned by Joly de Lotbiniere, but, in spite of that lack, a total of 13 hospitals of various kinds were developed by the British Empire medical services, with further hospital arrangements also developed by the French Medical Corps. These hospitals were supported by base depots medical stores and later by the development of large convalescent depots, which also fell under the remit of the medical services.

---

1   Colonel (later Major General) A. C. Joly de Lotbiniere was responsible for the design and construction of the Cauvrey Power Scheme for the Mysore Government and the Jhelum Hydroelectric Installation for the Kashmir Government. Both were completed before the Great War when he was serving as a major in the Royal Engineers. See Lieutenant Colonel E. W. C. Sandes, *The Military Engineer in India* (Chatham: Institution of Royal Engineers, 1935), vol. 1, pp.47–50.

The hospitals all developed around Mudros Harbour, an obvious choice since the harbour was the point of arrival of all the casualties arising on the peninsula and where there was good natural protection. In the first instance, the east of the harbour, around the town of Mudros, was developed, and, later as the campaign developed, hospitals were sited on the west of the harbour. The first hospital to arrive at Mudros East was No. 1 ASH, which arrived as part of the detached force on or near 12 March. At this stage, the work of this hospital was geared to the treatment of sick amongst the 3rd Australian Brigade and the crews of the ships gathering in the harbour in preparation for the start of the campaign. There was enough sick to keep this hospital busy in the run-up to 25 April, and, indeed, there were attempts to evacuate all the sick before the landings took place. This did not happen, as the medical cases were added as quickly as they were removed. This meant that No. 1 ASH spent the first months of the campaign handling sick cases despite the large number of battle casualties arising on the peninsula.[2]

The lack of success that had not been anticipated of the landings was to have an influence upon the manner of the development of the hospitals on Lemnos. The concept had been that, as soon as the troops had moved off the beaches, the CCSs and stationary hospitals of the attacking force would be landed and establish suitable accommodation for wounded arriving from the fighting, which should have been, by that time, some distance away. That this did not happen probably reflects upon the overall planning for the campaign and not upon the medical services themselves. At the time of the landings, the medical units were as a ready as any of the other arms involved but were subject to the vagaries of the landings, in so far as, without the ability to set up their hospitals, there was a limited impact that they could make upon the overall situation.

As an example of the work of a stationary hospital in the early stages of the campaign, it is useful to consider that of No. 15 BSH. This hospital had embarked at Avonmouth on the *City of Edinburgh* and the *Dongola* on 16 March 1915 to take part in the campaign. The hospital arrived at Alexandria at the end of the month and went into camp for a little over two weeks before embarking on the *Hymettus*, bound for Lemnos, where it arrived on 20 April. At this stage, it was expected that the hospital would land on the peninsula immediately after the capture of the beaches, and, in readiness for this, the hospital was divided into four groups so that, on 22 April:

> 3 officers, 20 NCO's and men embarked on the SS *Aragon*,
> 1 officer, 20 NCO's and men embarked on the SS *Californian*,
> 4 officers, 32 NCO's and men embarked on HMT *Dongola*,
> 1 NCO and 11 men sent to assist at No. 1 ASH.[3]

All the hospital stores were loaded onto the *Dongola* in expectation that they would be unloaded on shore at the peninsula as soon as the landing had succeeded. It was to be a month before the hospital personnel were recombined and all the hospital stores landed. However, when that happened, the hospital was established on Mudros East on 22 May. During that month, the hospital had not been idle – there had been plenty for it to do. For instance, the party on the

---

2   AWM: AWM4/26/70/3: War Diary, No. 1 Australian Stationary Hospital, April 1915.
3   'Diary of Service with No. 15 Stationary Hospital on Lemnos during the Dardanelles Campaign, June 1915-Jan 1916, and in East Africa, May 1916-Jan 1917', *Welcome Collection*, <https://wellcomecollection.org/works/yfvzvc4a>, accessed April 2021.

Dongola began receiving wounded almost immediately and, by 27 April, had set up an operating theatre on board, eventually with three operating tables, to handle the serious cases.[4] At this time, the *Dongola* was what was to become known as a black ship. That is, it was a troopship that had never been intended to have a primary use as a hospital ship, though it had been allotted to the 29th Division for the accommodation of casualties. The *Dongola* was classified as a 'hospital carrier' from 25 May, and, from an account of No. 15 BSH, it appears it was refitted as a hospital ship in Egypt and returned to the peninsula as such during July 1915.[5] No. 15 BSH, or at least part of it, remained on the *Dongola* during the landings, discharging cases to hospital ships as they became available, and, on 4 May, left for Alexandria with 570 cases on board, though 52 of the casualties died before reaching port.[6] On its conversion to a hospital ship, the *Dongola* had accommodation for 475 cases. The *Dongola* was not the only transport to become overcrowded, as every attempt was made to remove wounded from fire-swept beaches.

The experience of No. 16 BSH was similar. It had embarked at Avonmouth on 21 March and sailed to Alexandria. After being held at Alexandria for more than two weeks, it embarked on the *Hindoo* for Lemnos in readiness for duty at the Cape Helles beaches. Unfortunately, the *Hindoo* became disconnected from the action, for, with a lack of communication, the ship more or less disappeared for three days. Nevertheless, when it received orders, on 29 April, they proceeded to Gaba Tepe to disembark No. 2 ASH, which was also on board.[7] Eventually, No. 16 BSH was ordered to transfer to the *Alaunia* to establish a hospital, and it was on this ship that the hospital commenced its work for the campaign. The hospital reached Mudros on 17 May, where it was disembarked over the following days to establish a hospital on site next to No. 15 BSH on ground that had previously been a French camp.

By this time, it was clear that there would be no rapid advance from the beaches, and a number of hospitals began to arrive at Mudros East to assist with the treatment of casualties. By early June, the following hospitals were established:

- No. 1 ASH (transferred to Anzac in early November)[8]
- No. 15 BSH
- No. 16 BSH
- No. 24 British Casualty Clearing Station (BCCS)
- No. 2 ASH (transferred to Mudros West on 4 August)
- No. 110 IFA
- No. 24 British Field Ambulance, C Section, Indian Establishment.

Also established at this time were No. 5 Base Depot Medical Stores and, shortly afterwards, the Mudros East Convalescent Depot.

---

4   'Diary of Service with No. 15 Stationary Hospital', <https://wellcomecollection.org/works/yfvzvc4a>, accessed April 2021.
5   Macpherson, *History of the Great War: Medical Services*, vol. 1, p.367; 'Diary of Service with No. 15 Stationary Hospital' <https://wellcomecollection.org/works/yfvzvc4a>, accessed April 2021.
6   'Diary of Service with No. 15 Stationary Hospital', <https://wellcomecollection.org/works/yfvzvc4a> (accessed April 2021).
7   TNA: WO 95/4357: War Diary, No. 16 Stationary Hospital, 29 April.
8   Macpherson, *History of the Great War: Medical Services*, vol. 4, p.42.

In addition to these medical units, Mudros East was also the site of the 3rd Australian Light Horse Field Ambulance (ALHFA) between 27 June and 3 August. This unit, together with the 2nd ALHFA, had been stationed at Anzac for a month prior to removal to Lemnos. However, in a move to create space in the narrow beachhead at Anzac, these two field ambulances had been taken off the peninsula.[9] The work of the 3rd ALHFA on Lemnos was summed up by its CO:

> In the period on this island, we have treated 889 patients in hospital, sick and wounded, but this has been done under much difficulty as neither extra tents nor adequate equipment for so many over our normal capacity could be obtained at first from the Ordnance Store Ship and full feeding equipment was only procured shortly before closing [the] hospital. Much difficulty was met in obtaining means of transport to the store ship and getting stores from it in under a few days. The absence of staff medical officers on shore caused difficulty at times as access to the headquarters ship was often difficult and involved so much waste of time. Medical comforts were plentiful and rations easily obtained and great help was afforded by the liberal supply of Red Cross materials from the local branch of the British Red Cross Society.[10]

The CO of the 3rd ALHFA was voicing some of the concerns that dogged the organisation of the island as a hospital base and that were to increase as the campaign developed. As for the 2nd ALHFA, it did not land on Lemnos but was posted to serve on SS *Ausonia*, a hospital carrier, for one trip to Alexandria and thence to Malta. The return trip to Alexandria was aboard the SS *Karroo*, where the field ambulance was then ordered to the HS *Formosa* to return to Mudros on 5 August. The following day, the field ambulance was posted to Anzac, where it remained until the end of the campaign.[11]

As the campaign developed so did the calls upon the medical services. As the Mediterranean summer reached its peak, there were increasing numbers of casualties caused by dysentery, diarrhoea and enteric. The swarms of flies on the peninsula had been identified as the cause of the spread of these diseases, but great difficulty was encountered in dealing with this problem effectively, as the measures recommended by the sanitary officers were often seen as hardly worth the effort.[12] Nevertheless, it was clear to the medical services that the surge in cases of gastrointestinal disease that occurred from August onwards was caused by the more or less uncontrollable swarms of flies both on the peninsula and Lemnos. Tens of thousands of sick occurred monthly, and these largely unexpected casualties put an unexpected strain on the medical services.[13] In addition to this issue, it had been recognised in the early summer that, if there were to be any success in the fighting, there would need to be a new offensive with fresh troops. This was to result in the August landings at Suvla Bay and the associated fighting on the peninsula, particularly at Anzac. It is, perhaps, as a direct consequence of these two strands that more

---

9   AWM: AWM4/26/40/1: War Diary, 2nd Australian Light Horse Field Ambulance, May 1915.
10 AWM: AWM4/26/41/1: War Diary, 3rd Australian Light Horse Field Ambulance, May 1915.
11 AWM: AWM4/26/40/1: War Diary, 2nd Australian Light Horse Field Ambulance, May 1915.
12 Butler, *Official History of the Australian Medical Services*, vol. I, p.356ff.
13 During the three months between August and October, a total of 94,012 casualties were evacuated from the peninsula, and, of these, 57,168 were as a result of sickness. Butler, *Official History of the Australian Medical Services*, vol. I, p.375.

170   The Fight for Life

hospitals were sent to the Mediterranean area and particularly to Lemnos. All reasoning against using this island for extensive troop accommodation, particularly the shortage of water, had been set aside, as the need for hospital accommodation and supporting units took immediate precedence. Many of the almost 100,000 casualties arising between August and October were evacuated through Mudros, and the need for hospital accommodation was critical throughout these months.

As discussed above, the area around the town of Mudros had been developed into a centre for hospitals. These were under the nominal control of ADMS Mudros East. From August, a similar development was to be witnessed on the opposite side of the harbour, where, in time, they were to come under the control of an ADMS for Mudros West. The first hospital to take its place on Mudros West was No. 2 ASH. This hospital had been on Lemnos for two months when it was ordered to move from the eastern side of the harbour to the new area on the west designated for hospitals often referred to as 'Turks Head'. This move was completed by 4 August, and, shortly after, the hospital was receiving patients in its new location.[14]

A day later, No. 3 AGH arrived in its transport in the outer harbour at Lemnos. No. 3 AGH was the last of the Australian general hospitals to depart Australia for service in the Gallipoli Campaign. The hospital embarked on the transport *Mooltan* in Sydney and departed on 15 May 1915, though 'Of course, we had no idea to where we were going'.[15] At this time, the CO of the hospital was Colonel Thomas Henry Fiaschi DSO, a Boer War veteran then aged 62, and in charge of the nurses was Principal Matron Grace Wilson. It is interesting to note that Colonel Fiaschi's wife also served with this unit, but, because of the restrictions imposed by the Australian Government on the service of married women, Mrs Fiaschi served under her maiden name as Sister Amy Curtis.[16]

There was considerable anticipation that No. 3 AGH would join the other Australian general hospitals that were, by that time, well established in Egypt. However, after passing through the Suez Canal, the *Mooltan* proceeded directly to England, where it was disembarked on 27 June 1915. As the hospital was now in England, everyone then expected that the hospital would be sent to France for service on the Western Front. In due course, orders for France were received, but these were more or less immediately countermanded and replaced by orders to proceed to Lemnos. This should probably be seen as a result of the developing plan for the August campaign on the Gallipoli Peninsula, as government and military hierarchy sought to bolster the medical services after both the perceived and actual shortfall of April and May. The officers of No. 3 AGH departed from Devonport on 12 July 1915 on the *Simla*, which was also carrying medical stores.[17] By this time, there was little doubt as to its final destination or what part it would be expected to play when it arrived. The nurses of the hospital did not leave until 19 July and were divided between two rather overcrowded transports, the *Themistocles* and the *Derfflinger*, the latter of which had been renamed the '*Huntsgreen*' by that time. Both were troop-ships and carried soldiers as well as medical staff. For instance, the *Huntsgreen* had embarked the 10th Middlesex and the 5th Welsh, as well as half of the nurses of No. 3 AGH. Of the 5th

---

14   AWM: AWM4/26/71/2: War Diary, No. 2 Australian Stationary Hospital, August 1915, Part 1.
15   AWM: AWM41/1045: [Nurses Narratives] N F S Smith.
16   This was his second marriage in August 1914. Colonel Fiaschi's son, Piero, also a medical practitioner, was already serving overseas with the 1st ALHFA by the time his father left Sydney.
17   AWM: AWM224/407: Narrative of Colonel J. A. Dick.

Welsh, Sister Smith was to say that '... they looked like devils, sang like angels', and, at least for one Australian sister, the trip towards war was made memorable by a rendering of 'Men of Harlech' by these tough territorial soldiers from the mining valleys of South Wales. Meanwhile, the transport *Ascot*, carrying all No. 3 AGH equipment, left Britain separately on 12 July, and this was to cause problems later on.

Although there seems to have been some forethought in sending another general hospital to the Mediterranean theatre, it was perhaps too late for the major offensives of the campaign. Furthermore, it was considered suitable to send the hospital personnel on three ships with the officers and men travelling on different vessels to the nurses while the hospital equipment was transported on yet another. It was perhaps too much to hope that both staff and equipment would arrive at the same place at the same time.

The ships carrying the nurses coaled at Malta on 26 July and then proceeded to Alexandria, where they were disembarked on 30 July. The officers and men of the hospital had sailed direct to Lemnos, where they had arrived on 29 July.[18] However, for the nursing staff, there seems to have been some delay since it was not until 3 August that the nurses were embarked upon the HS *Dunluce Castle* for their trip back across the Mediterranean to Lemnos.[19] The *Dunluce Castle* had just completed disembarkation of casualties from the peninsula, and the nurses were put to work '... to make beds for patients on the return journey'.[20] The ship was largely empty, and the nurses on No. 3 AGH were accommodated in one of the wards and were '... made most comfortable'. It was to be their most comfortable accommodation for some considerable time. The *Dunluce Castle* arrived in Mudros Harbour early on the morning of 5 August, and the nurses were immediately faced with a problem that was totally out of their hands and control. The equipment for the hospital had not arrived, and, at that time, no one was sure where it was or when it would arrive. As a result, the nurses were not allowed to disembark immediately. The following day, the nurses were transhipped to the HT *Simla*, a hospital depot ship anchored nearby, where they were to wait on what has been described as a 'dirty ship' until they could disembark.[21]

That same evening, six of the nurses were called upon for duty on the HS *Formosa*, a French ship flying the French flag that was destined to pick up casualties from the Suvla Bay landings that had occurred that day.[22] The ship was placed in readiness to receive wounded by the Australian nurses, together with four MOs of the RAMC and a number of their orderlies. A small theatre was also prepared.[23] Although the *Formosa* arrived on station early on the morning of 7 August, it did not begin to receive casualties until 5:00 p.m. This appears to have been a result of the fact that the ship was flying a French flag and was, therefore, ignored by the medical teams evacuating casualties from the shore. As soon as the ensign was hoisted, the casualties began to arrive: 'We were receiving wounded all night and terrible wounds they were – the majority of these were ten days [sic] old, fly blown and septic.'[24] For many of the casualties,

---

18 Butler, *Official History of the Australian Medical Services*, vol. I, p.286.
19 The HS *Dunluce Castle* came into service on this voyage on 6 July.
20 AWM: AWM41/1045: [Nurses Narratives] N F S Smith.
21 AWM: AWM41/1065: [Nurses Narratives] Sister Louise E Young.
22 According to Macpherson, *History of the Great War: Medical Services*, vol. 1, the *Formosa* was in service from 26 June 1915, so this voyage was unlikely to have been its first to the peninsula.
23 AWM: AWM41/998: [Nurses Narratives] Sister I G Lovell.
24 AWM: AWM41/998: [Nurses Narratives] Sister I G Lovell.

172   The Fight for Life

the delay in treatment was to cost them a limb, if not their lives. It was this group of wounded on the *Formosa* who were to become the first patients of No. 3 AGH. The nurses remained on duty on this British-run French ship for three journeys, collecting wounded from Suvla and Anzac. Whilst the first load of casualties had been transported to Lemnos, the later casualties were transferred to larger ships for direct transport to Alexandria. This probably reflects the overall readiness and capacity at Lemnos in general and No. 3 AGH in particular. The six detailed nurses were returned to their unit on 15 August '… after having had a very busy but happy time'.[25]

Whilst the officers and men of No. 3 AGH had landed as soon as they arrived, the lack of equipment had meant that there was little that they could do to set up the hospital. However, on 7 August, Colonel Dick recorded:

> By dint of hard work on the part of the CO the hospital site has been pegged out and some marquees erected which had been obtained from a small ordnance store, and from various sources, for the reception of patients. Bell tents (Double Circular) are being erected for nursing staff. Also, some for the male personnel. The place of the hospital has been made out upon the site which is upon Turks Head, and has frontage to the inner harbour.[26]

Two days later, the hospital was admitting patients when 200 sick and wounded arrived first thing on the morning of 9 August.

The nurses remained on the *Simla* for a while before the first group was allowed ashore after dark on 8 August. Sister F. Howitt was amongst this first group:

> We arrived at Lemnos in the middle of the night on a tug, and, as there was no accommodation, we slept on the ground for that night. We had absolutely nothing as our equipment did not arrive for three weeks. We went on duty at six o'clock the next morning and we found there was no water for washing. When the patients came in, we had nothing for them and had to tear up sheets and towels etc to wash and bandage them with. We had to use sanitary utensils to wash them …[27]

On 9 August, the rest of the nurses, along with Matron Grace Wilson, were disembarked. Before reaching the camp, they were to take part in one of the most ridiculous pieces of military theatre of the whole campaign, as they followed a soldier, Corporal Monks, playing bagpipes to their camp:

> … when we were all off the lighter, we were told to get in line and then to form fours and I must say we made a hash of the job. We had forgotten whether the odd or even numbers moved so to be on the safe side we all moved.

---

25   AWM: AWM41/998: [Nurses Narratives] Sister I G Lovell.
26   AWM: AWM224/407: Narrative of Colonel J. A. Dick.
27   AWM: AWM41/1072: Kellett Interviews, Sister F. M. Howitt.

We Had Nothing for Them: Hospitals on Lemnos   173

Finally, we got in some sort of order and marched! Matron and Colonel leading. We passed several bell tents. Some dogs barked and some men cheered, never laughed which we thought nice of them.[28]

They marched to the site chosen for the hospital on a slope overlooking the harbour on West Mudros: 'There was no vegetation whatever to be seen and at one period or another it seemed to have rained stones as they were everywhere. Bell tents had been erected – two sisters to each tent. Weeds and stones were disposed of and the unpacking began.'[29] Getting the hospital in order was urgent, and no easy matter, for sick and casualties of the August fighting on the peninsula had already started to arrive at the site before any of the nursing sisters had disembarked:

The patients arriving all right and here you have a picture of them on the ground with a tarpaulin and blanket under them and then over them and not a stitch of clothing on them after cutting off their gore soaked and dirty uniform and washing them and preparing for the theatre, which we did in bed pans, they being the only vessels holding water to be procured or borrowed at that time.[30]

The accommodation for the wounded cannot be considered to have been basic – it was far worse than that. Some shelter began to appear as marquees were found and put up, though, as one nurse stressed, it was only the top of the marquees since there was no time to put on the sides of the big tents. There was no proper operating theatre, no dressing room and no basic hospital equipment such as bed pans and bandages. Some of the casualties were lucky to get a mattress, although this was on the ground, and the patients were wrapped in blankets. This was considered uncomfortable for the patients and very difficult for their medical care and nursing. It was the best that could be achieved by the members of No. 3 AGH under the circumstances and in the absence of their own equipment. There was nothing else that could be done, and everyone tried to carry on in the most adverse conditions by some improvisations and ingenuity:

To wash them, and they were all longing for a wash, we had to use salt water and any utensil we could find. I washed my unfortunate patients with sea water out of their own small Dixie! And then gave then rice and tea from the same article. Though soap was not much use we used our own and I remember tearing up old blouses for cloths and towels.[31]

This was not the best start for No. 3 AGH. Sister Aitken recalled that many of the sisters were forced to wash in the sea, but this 'was not the cleanest', as it was becoming polluted by the ships in the harbour, and was probably not ideal for washing casualties from the peninsula.[32]

It was late August when their equipment arrived, and, for the intervening three weeks, the members of No. 3 AGH had to cope as a functioning base hospital with all it could scrounge

28   AWM: AWM41/1045: [Nurses Narratives] N F S Smith.
29   AWM: AWM41/937: [Nurses Narratives] Margaret Aitken.
30   AWM: AWM41/1065: [Nurses Narratives] Sister Louise E Young.
31   AWM: AWM41/1045: [Nurses Narratives] N F S Smith.
32   AWM: AWM41/937: [Nurses Narratives] Margaret Aitken.

from the surrounding units. For those three weeks, the general hospital was less well equipped than the forward field ambulances that it was designed to serve. It was not only lacking basic medical necessities, but the supply of food was also bad. It was never enough and always of poor quality. No doubt, everything possible was done by the staff to ensure that the patients had enough, but the nurses, at least, were grateful to the Royal Navy officers on the ships in the harbour who sent food to supplement their diets or invited them to dinner aboard vessels such as the HMS *Cornwallis*. With the arrival of the equipment, everything improved in the care of the casualties, and, over the following weeks, No. 3 AGH became firmly established, efficient, clean and thoroughly well run. The arrival of the equipment was greeted '… with loud cheers, the boat with the hospital equipment arrived at last. Marquees were speedily erected over the patients, canteens opened and the outward structure of No. 3 AGH came in to being'.[33] The weeks of difficulties had passed, and, although it has to be wondered how such an appalling situation could have been allowed to develop, it is a credit to all members of the staff of No. 3 AGH that it survived the trial and continued to serve casualties throughout the rest of the campaign.

The Australian hospitals were followed in quick succession by other hospitals during the first three weeks of August. Arriving at the same time were No. 1 and No. 3 CSHs. These hospitals had both embarked at Southampton on the HS *Asturias* on 1 August. They arrived in Alexandria with all personnel and equipment on 11 August. After a three-day delay, the two hospitals transhipped everything to the HT *Afric* and sailed for Lemnos, where they arrived on 18 August. All their equipment was moved to Mudros West, and all personnel of No. 1 CSH was in camp by the following day, except for the nursing sisters, under Matron Eleanor Charleson, who arrived shortly afterwards.[34] No. 3 CSH also set up hospital adjacent to No. 1, and both admitted their first patients on 22 August. The arrival of these new hospitals at Mudros West had considerably increased the capacity for accommodating sick and wounded. Each of the Canadian stationary hospitals had accommodation available for 600 cases. The accommodation was provided in 'Hospital Marquees of eastern pattern obtained from Ordnance; size 35' x 17'. These marquees erected in rows of six – ends joined – giving a ward capacity of 100 beds.'[35]

During the course of its service on Lemnos, No. 3 CSH was to lose two of its nursing staff to dysentery: Sister Mary Frances Munro died on 7 September, and Matron Jessie Brown Jaggard died on 25 September. Both are buried in the Portianos Military Cemetery at Mudros West. They were the only nursing sisters of any nation to succumb to the disease during their service on Lemnos.

At the same time as the Canadians were setting up their hospitals, No. 18 BSH arrived to begin work. This hospital had arrived at Mudros on 15 August but remained aboard its transport for three days before being allowed to disembark, at which time the war diary records, 'Site for hospital very rough and dirty'.[36] No. 18 BSH began admitting patients on 23 August. At first, there seems to have been a concept for hospitals specialising in particular types of cases. For instance, at the beginning of its stay, No. 18 BSH seems to have transferred all its enteric cases to

---

33   AWM: AWM41/998: [Nurses Narratives] Sister I G Lovell.
34   Cynthia Toman, *Sister Soldiers of the Great War: The Nurses of the Canadian Army Medical Corps* (Vancouver: UBC Press, 2016), p.186.
35   'War Diary, No. 1 CSH, August 1915', *Canadian Great War Project* <https://canadiangreatwarproject. com/>, (accessed March 2021).
36   TNA: WO 95/4357: War Diary, No. 18 Stationary Hospital, August 1915.

We Had Nothing for Them: Hospitals on Lemnos 175

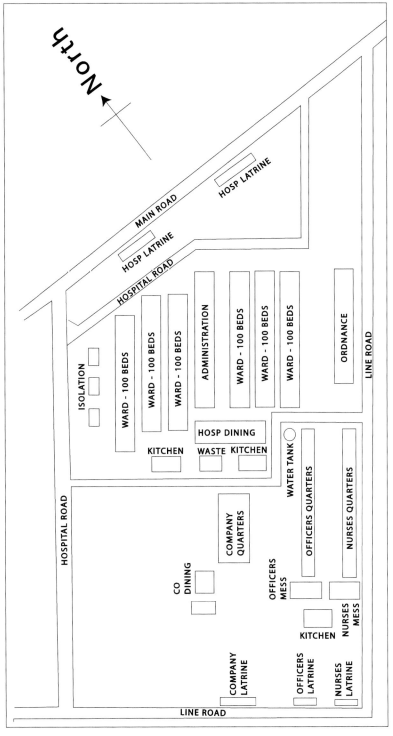

Layout of No. 1 CSH at West Mudros. (Terrence Powell after War Dairy 1 CSH)

No. 3 AGH and its dysentery patients to either No. 1 or No. 3 CSH. It appears that the British hospital concentrated its early efforts on the care of patients with venereal disease, scabies and similar diseases. However, six weeks or so later, the flow of cases seems to have reversed, though infectious diseases such as diphtheria and German measles were still sent to No. 1 CSH, which, at that time, was acting as the infectious disease hospital for Mudros West. Other specialisations, such as ophthalmic and dental cases, were handled solely by No. 3 AGH.[37]

Whilst there was a growing, if sometimes inadequate, accommodation for the sick and wounded, there was also a growing need to consider the convalescence of a patient before being discharged to duty. The call for men to replace those lost through wounds and sickness was, throughout the period of the summer and early autumn, a continual one as units tried to make good their losses through evacuation. COs were always looking for the return of their men as soon as they were considered fit. However, there was a considerable difference between being fit for discharge from hospital and being fit for service in the front line. This had been solved, at least to some extent, by the establishment of a convalescent depot on Mudros East that served the hospitals on that side of the harbour. A similar arrangement was achieved when the 52nd CCS arrived at Mudros West. This unit had embarked at Devonport on the *Marquette* on 9 June, and, like most of the units then leaving the United Kingdom for the Mediterranean, it travelled via Alexandria and, unusually, Port Said before arriving at Mudros East on 2 July. Initially, the 52nd CCS was working at Mudros East, where it established a hospital for the sick and wounded that was capable of accommodating 400 patients.[38] This work on Mudros East continued for a month when the hospital received orders to move to Mudros West to establish a convalescent depot. This move was completed by 10 August when the first patients arrived. This hospital, like some others at Mudros, suffered considerably from the overall supply shortage of basic stores. There were no cooking utensils during the early days, but the hospital was receiving hundreds of patients.[39] There was also difficulty in producing basic sanitation since the hospital could not get any tools to dig latrines. Nevertheless, a week after setting up at Mudros West, the accommodation had grown to 600 beds, and, at this time, it appears that at least some of the patients were not convalescent and that the 52nd CCS continued to serve as both a surgical and medical facility. Gradually, by stages, the capacity at this hospital grew, and, by the end of the month, it was recorded that it held a total of 923 patients.[40]

The final hospital to come into service at Mudros West was No. 27 BGH. This hospital arrived late in the campaign, officially arriving on 30 November, though it is clear that at least some of its personnel had arrived prior to this date and had served in other units.[41] This hospital opened some days later and remained in service until, with the general removal of hospital units from Mudros during January and February, it was embarked and sent to Egypt. By the end of the campaign, the hospitals at Mudros West can be summarised as:

- No. 2 ASH (transferred from Mudros East on 4 August)
- No. 3 AGH

---

37 Butler, *Official History of the Australian Medical Services*, vol. I, p.389.
38 TNA: WO 95/4356: War Diary, 52nd Casualty Clearing Station (Lowland), June–August 1915.
39 TNA: WO 95/4356: War Diary, 52nd Casualty Clearing Station (Lowland), August 1915.
40 TNA: WO 95/4356: War Diary, 52nd Casualty Clearing Station (Lowland), August 1915.
41 Butler, *Official History of the Australian Medical Services*, vol. I, p.393.

- No. 52 CCS (converted to a convalescent depot)
- No. 1 CSH
- No. 3 CSH
- No. 18 BSH
- No. 27 BGH.

The hospitals of Mudros West were supplied through No. 5 Base Depot Medical Stores, which remained on the island as long as the hospitals. Ordnance stores for hospitals both at Mudros East and Mudros West were served by the Army Ordnance Corps (AOC) depot ships in Mudros Harbour. In the early days of the campaign, this was the 3,000-ton SS *Umsinga*, but, as the need grew, the 12,000-ton SS *Minnetonka* took over the duty as the ordnance depot ship. The use of ships for these sort of stores was not without its challenges and difficulties, and the comments in war diaries of hospitals on Lemnos often refer to shortages of one sort or another, such as that of the 52nd CCS noting the complete lack of cooking utensils when it was first opened.[42] The importance of the supply of ordnance stores to hospitals should not be underestimated, and often the quartermaster of a hospital unit would spend days at the store ship in an effort to locate particular items, often without any success.[43] Nevertheless, without the opportunity to set up more permanent ordnance stores, the depot ships made considerable effort to supply the needs of hospitals, and other units, based on Lemnos and the peninsula.

Imbros was also provided with a hospital when the 25th CCS was established there. This hospital also suffered from supply problems during the summer months, and, following his visit there on 15 July, Sir Ian Hamilton was to write in his diary:

> Walked through the different wards talking to some twenty officers and two hundred men, mostly medical cases. Did not think things at all up to the mark. Made special note of the lack of mosquito nets, beds, pyjamas and other comforts … Too bad when so much money is being spent to see men lying on the ground in their thick cord breeches in this sweltering heat, a prey to flies and mosquitos.[44]

The 25th CCS remained at Kephalos on the island until 5 October 1915, when it was transferred to Salonika for duty. Its work on Imbros was taken over by a smaller unit known as the 'Kephalos Hospital', and its purpose was to care for the sick arising from the rest camps on the island. It was enlarged in anticipation of casualties arising from the evacuation of the peninsula, and, when it was taken over by No. 19 BSH on 13 December, it had accommodation for 600 sick or wounded soldiers.[45]

---

42 Major General A. Forbes, *A History of the Army Ordnance Services* (Facsimile of 1929 edition, Uckfield: Naval & Military Press, 2010), p.223; TNA: WO 95/4356: War Diary, 52nd Casualty Clearing Station (Lowland), August 1915.
43 'Diary of Service with No. 15 Stationary Hospital', <https://wellcomecollection.org/works/yfvzvc4a>, accessed April 2021.
44 Hamilton, *Gallipoli Diary*, vol. 2, p.10.
45 Macpherson, *History of the Great War: Medical Services*, vol. 4, p.41.

9

A Night of Bloodshed and Pain

In the three months following the unsuccessful landings, the campaign developed in to trench warfare. Heavy casualties during the fighting following the landing and the fact that the Turks continued to hold the high ground made any advance very difficult and had made trench warfare inevitable. Living conditions deteriorated, with the summer weather bringing very hot winds stirring up clouds of dust. Unburied corpses encouraged a plague of flies and rats to feed off the rapidly decomposing bodies. Poor sanitation control in both the trenches and surrounding ground meant that widespread disease was also inevitable. The troops were not in good health, in sharp contrast to their fitness levels on 25 April.

Lieutenant General Sir William Birdwood proposed a breakout plan at Anzac using only a single division. This plan was enlarged to include a landing at Suvla Bay, and fresh troops of New Army divisions of IX Corps were promised together with a number of territorial divisions. The commander-in-chief, General Sir Ian Hamilton, proposed a major plan to break the deadlock in what was to become known as the 'August Offensive'.

Birdwood's plan was for a broad flanking manoeuvre from the north of Anzac Cove to capture Hill 971, Hill Q and Chunuk Bair, the dominating peaks on the Sari Bair Ridge. From there, the Turks would be pushed back from the surrounding areas of Baby 700, Battleship Hill and 400 Plateau. This would allow the attacking forces to advance towards Mal Tepe and wrest control of the peninsula away from the Turks. To help in this assault, diversionary attacks would be made at Helles and in the Anzac areas including at Lone Pine and the Nek. The objective of these was to keep the Turkish troops in these areas fully occupied and, in doing so, to prevent them from rushing north to defend the main assault on the Sari Bair Ridge.

Following the problems that had arisen as a direct result of the hasty planning for the landings on the peninsula, and the consequent impact on the medical services, there was a considerable responsibility upon the General Staff to make better arrangements for the August operations. The months after the landings had seen some regularisation of the work of the medical services. Field ambulances had been able to establish collecting stations, and a system whereby the wounded were evacuated through CCSs to bases in Egypt or Malta had been put in place. Also, during these months, there had been a considerable development of Lemnos as a forward base to allow the transfer of wounded and sick to hospital care in as short a time as possible. By June, there were four stationary hospitals established on Lemnos around the town of Mudros. Whilst, ideally, these should have been sited nearer the fighting on the peninsula, the overall lack of success of the landings, and the failure to make much progress from the beachheads, particularly at Anzac, had dictated that, for the most part, stationary hospitals were placed on Lemnos, and casualties from the fighting were ferried there.

The early days following the landings had been filled with confusion as far as the evacuation of wounded by hospital ships was concerned. This improved slowly, and, although never ideal, a system using a variety of vessels from the simple hospital barges to trawlers, military transports and hospital ships had been developed in the attempt to remove all the wounded from the beaches, which were frequently under enemy fire. This system was not always a success or satisfactory since it depended on such things as the weather and the uninterrupted supply of vessels to carry wounded. This latter criterion was seldom met, and, at times of stress, during major fighting, the limited supply of vessels all but caused the scheme for evacuation to collapse. Nevertheless, by August, there was a system in place that was, on the face of it, capable of handling casualties from the peninsula. It was a system that had developed out of necessity and had not been strictly planned, as it was adapted to fit the needs of the actions on the peninsula, but was, for all that, a functioning system that worked better sometimes than others. There was, therefore, an important, pressing need for the planners of the August operations to ensure not only that the system continued to function but also, where possible, that improvements were made to ensure that the wounded arising from a major offensive could be handled more efficiently than at the time of the landings.

One aspect of the evacuation of wounded that received considerable criticism after the landings was that of the effectiveness and suitability of hospital ships and transports. This question was revisited during the planning phase for the medical services in readiness for the August operations. On 16 July, three weeks before the offensive began, Surgeon General W. G. Birrell submitted to GHQ his scheme for the seaborne evacuation of wounded, and this is worth reproducing in full:

Proposed Scheme for Evacuation of Wounded. Operations August.

Part B

Hospital Ships
All available Hospital Ships to be off Anzac and Helles. I estimate that only six Hospital Ships will be available and propose stationing 4 off Anzac and 2 of Helles. These when filled will clear direct, under orders of the DMS, to Bases.

Temporary Hospital Ships
I have estimated that our requirements to meet casualties will be 30. Of these 8 will remain behind the boom at Imbros and the rest at Mudros. Of the 8 at Imbros six will fill with cases whose destination is the Base and will proceed direct when filled and will be replaced by others from Mudros called up by telegraph as required. The other two at Imbros will fill up with slightly wounded, and when filled will clear for Mudros, returning to Imbros when empty, and continuing on this duty till themselves required to take cases for clearance to the Base, by which time all stress will be over and their places can be taken by Fleet Sweepers.

Fleet Sweepers
Six Fleet Sweepers will be required; of these three will ply from Anzac to Imbros, one from Gully Beach to Imbros and two from Helles to Imbros, These ships should be the best available.

Tows
The following tows are necessary, at Anzac 4, Gully Beach 2, Helles 2, Mudros 2.

Launches
At Imbros I shall require two launches placed at the disposal of the DMS and Staff so that incoming Fleet Sweepers might be met and proper supervision exercised as to the distribution of the wounded, to ensure that lightly wounded cases go to Mudros and all others to the Bases.[1]

Perhaps one thing that is immediately obvious in Birrell's scheme is that there appears to be no provision for evacuation to hospital ships from the beaches at Suvla. Bearing in mind that there was to be a landing involving initially two divisions in the first 24 hours of the offensive at Suvla Bay, this would seem to be a marked oversight. From the scheme presented, it would appear that, three weeks before action was to take place, Surgeon General Birrell had no idea that a third beachhead was to be opened, unless, of course, Birrell anticipated that all evacuations from Suvla were to take place through Anzac. This would seem to be an unlikely scenario. Thus, it must be assumed that, as at the time of the landings in April, the SMOs responsible for planning the evacuation of wounded were unaware of the scale of operations that were to be undertaken or of their precise location. This should be seen as error in planning at the GHQ level if this were the case. It should also be noted that Birrell's plan allows for sufficient sorting of wounded into slight and serious cases and that there would be three times as many serious cases as slight cases. The latter would seem to be an unlikely, possibly worse case, scenario, but the criterion used by Birrell to define a 'serious' case is unknown.

On the same day as Birrell submitted his proposals to GHQ, Sir Ian Hamilton recorded the text of a cable that he had sent to the War Office some days earlier in his personal diary:

> It seems likely that during the first week of August we may have 80,000 rifles in the firing line striving for a decisive result, and therefore certain that we shall need more medical assistance. Quite impossible to foresee casualties, but suppose, for example, we suffered a loss of 20,000 men; though the figure seems alarming when put down in cold blood, it is not an extravagant proportion when calculated on basis of Dardanelles fighting up to date. If this figure is translated into terms of requirements such a battle would involve conversion of, say 30 transports into temporary hospital ships, and necessitate something like 200 extra medical officers, with Royal Army Medical Corps rank and file and nurses in proportion. If my prognosis is concurred in, these should reach Mudros on or about 1st August. Some would … prove superfluous, and could be sent back at once, and in any case could return as soon as possible after operations, say, 1st September. Medical and surgical equipment, drugs, mattresses in due proportion.[2]

---

1 The National Archives (TNA) WO 95/4275: War Diary, General Headquarters ADMS, July 1915.
2 Hamilton, *Gallipoli Diary*, vol. 2, 16 July.

It is not clear whether Hamilton's cable was influenced by discussions with Surgeon General Birrel or the other way round. Either way, by 16 July, the commander-in-chief and the surgeon general had similar ideas of the numbers of casualties and the numbers of ships that would be needed to evacuate them from the peninsula. Whilst Hamilton made requests of the War Office, it would seem that they were a little late in the planning stage for all to be fulfilled by the start of the operations. Although some new hospitals had been established on Lemnos, some arrived after the fighting had actually begun. For the field ambulances and CCSs on the peninsula, there was little change in personnel in the run-up to the major offensive, with most suffering staff shortages well into it. For instance, it appears that the only reinforcements received by the 1st AFA, working near Dawkins Point during July, was when it was joined by its own tent division on 11 August.[3] The latter had been working on lines of communication up to that date, leaving the ambulance in the field understaffed as the fighting continued.

This field ambulance also complained of the lack of medical supplies on 27 July and commented on the difficulty in treating men parading sick. This can only have been exacerbated by the August fighting. Whilst a similar situation seems to have obtained in other medical units on Anzac, including the CO of the 108th IFA recording a shortfall of MOs in late July, it is perhaps noteworthy that the additional CCSs – such as at the 13th BCCS and the 16th BCCS – were added to the compliment of medical units in the run-up to the offensive. The 13th BCCS had been in Aldershot on 10 July, but, on 8 August, it had landed at Suvla Bay and made its way to the left flank of Anzac to No. 2 Advanced Post. In addition to these, of course, the new divisions that were landing had their field ambulances, which were disembarked as soon as possible behind their respective divisions.

At Anzac, by the start of August, the medical units that were available were mainly those that had arrived at or shortly after the landing in April. That is, there were the three field ambulances of the 1st Australian Division and the field ambulances of the New Zealand and Australian Division. These evacuated wounded through the 1st ACCS, which had arrived on the peninsula shortly after the landings. During August, the number of medical units was increased not only by the arrival of the 13th and 16th BCCSs, which had arrived on 8 August, but also by the 108th IFA, which had arrived at Anzac on 7 August. The latter unit, stationed at Chailak Dere, was sent to support the 29th Indian Brigade during its attack on the Sari Bair Ridge and mainly handled cases from that brigade during its stay in Chailak Dere. In the second half of August, the first units of the 2nd Australian Division began to arrive as reinforcements for Anzac, and these troops were supported by the 5th AFA of that division. These units were essentially the onshore medical units that were to handle all the casualties arising from the fighting around Anzac during August.

Offshore, the situation is more difficult to define. While both Hamilton and Birrell had indicated requirements for ships for evacuation, it is difficult to be certain of the number of ships that were actually employed in the evacuation of sick and wounded during August. It is known from information in the 1st ACCS war diary that the HS *Sicilia* was on station at Anzac on 6 August and was rapidly filled with wounded.[4] The following day, three different hospital ships arrived, one, the *Seang Choon*, specifically for Indian wounded and wounded Turkish POWs.

---

3   AWM: AWM4/26/44/6: War Diary, 1st Australian Field Ambulance, August 1915.
4   AWM: AWM4/26/62/7: War Diary, 1st Australian Casualty Clearing Station, August 1915, Part 1.

These ships also filled up rapidly and left the same day, leaving Anzac without supporting hospital ships for most of 8 August. During that day, the 1st ACCS managed to evacuate a large number of walking wounded using the SS *Redbreast*, which seems to have acted as a ferry to Imbros. Later the same day, the HS *Gascon* arrived on station; it, too, became filled rapidly before leaving early the following day for Mudros. It unloaded the casualties there and returned to Anzac immediately.

Birrell's scheme had suggested that four hospital ships would be needed at Anzac, and it would appear that the war diary records confirm that at least four such ships were in use during the evacuations of wounded from Anzac between 6–9 August, though not all at the same time. It also appears, from records such as personal diaries, that the HS *Assaye* and one other, possibly the HS *Soudan*, were on station at Helles during a similar period, again meeting at least some of Birrell's proposals.[5] However, it is not clear how many temporary hospital ships (hospital carriers) or fleet sweepers were employed. If the numbers evacuated through 1st ACCS during this period are considered, then there must have been a considerable effort to fulfil Birrell's, and indeed Hamilton's, proposals. Between 6–9 August, the 1st ACCS evacuated 4,411 cases.[6] Not all could have gone to the four hospital ships that appear to have been at Anzac in this period. In fact, probably less than half that number could have been accommodated on the available hospital ships. This means that at least four hospital carriers would have been in use at this period. This applies to Anzac alone, and the effort for evacuation would have been more or less repeated at Helles and Suvla, if on a rather smaller scale at the former.

On 31 July, the 11th Battalion Australian Imperial Force (AIF) was involved in a sharp action that was to herald an intense period of heavy fighting at Anzac. The 11th Battalion attacked from Tasmania Post, on the right flank of the Anzac positions, with the aid of mines, and captured a forward position that was to become known as 'Leane's Trench'.[7] According to the battalion's war diary, it suffered the loss of 36 men killed and a further 76 wounded. The latter '… gave the 1st Field Ambulance a considerable amount of work – casualties were heavy and the difficulties of moving these through narrow trenches and steeply sloping tunnels was remarkably great, the shell fire from the enemy onto the ground behind the trenches was particularly heavy and resulted in a number of casualties amongst our bearers'.[8] Private T. J. Richards was serving with the 1st AFA and left details of the night, recorded on 1 August:

> Today follows a night of bloodshed and pain. All the ambulance was called out, after being warned previously, at 10 pm and from that time until 3 am a stream of wounded came down from the 11th Battalion – West Australians mostly – situated some 400 yards from the extreme right flank … The wounded must have had a very rough time getting in as there is a long travelling way leading right through the hill 5 ft below the surface. The height is about 5 ft and the width very little wider than one's shoulder so you can imagine it's a rough passage of perhaps 100 yds of pitch darkness.[9]

---

5   Australian War Memorial (AWM) PR05050, RCDIG0001390: Transcript of Diary of Mary Ann 'Bessie' Pocock, 1914-1918 (Vol. 2).
6   AWM: AWM4/26/62/7: War Diary, 1st Australian Casualty Clearing Station, August 1915, Part 1.
7   Dixon, *Vital Endeavour*, p.182ff.
8   AWM: AWM4/26/44/6: War Diary, 1st Australian Field Ambulance, 1 August 1915.
9   AWM: 2DRL/0786, RCDIG0001478: [Transcript] Diaries of Thomas James Richards, Vol. 2, 1 August 1915.

This was simply the start, and, as the offensive came into full effect, the field ambulances of the 1st Australian Division all became involved in handling casualties. Perhaps the first notification to all that something big was about to happen was the arrival of 'Three large Hospital Ships' that anchored off Anzac on 6 August.[10] This event would not have been wasted on the Turks, and, no doubt, they made as much preparation for an attack that they saw as happening very soon.

At Anzac, two main columns of assault were to march out on the night of 6 August. The Right Assaulting Column (the New Zealand Infantry Brigade) was to attack the Chunuk Bair peak. The Left Assaulting Column (the 4th Australian Brigade and the 29th Indian Brigade) was to attack the two peaks Hill 291 and Hill Q. Each of the columns had a covering force. The Right Covering Force (the New Zealand Mounted Rifles Brigade (NZMRB)) acted as infantry with two infantry companies of the Maori contingent. The Left Covering Force comprised elements of the recently arrived 40th Brigade, 13th Division, namely, the 4th SWB and the 5th Wiltshire Regiment.[11] The task of the covering forces was to advance in front and cover the movement of the main attacking columns when that commenced. The movement of these columns was to be accompanied by a series of diversionary attacks in rapid succession across Anzac, including the attacks at Lone Pine and the Nek. After three months on the peninsula, the troops were not in the same physically healthy condition as on 25 April and were facing an extremely difficult and dangerous task. The Sari Bair range was a tangled mass of gullies, ravines and spurs, making any form of ascent towards the defended Turkish positions very difficult. These columns began their movement soon after dark on the evening of 6 August, by which time the diversionary attacks at Anzac had commenced.

The start of the assault on Lone Pine brought close-quarter fighting with bombs, and, in the evening of 6 August, Private Richards wrote in his diary:

> It is nearly 6 o'clock. We have been working hard from early morning amongst the wounded and such smashed and battered men one never saw. It was purely a bomb fight … The bombs knocked and shattered our men over the whole body. Some cases were swaddled in cotton wool gauze and bandages from the hips right down to the feet. Sad sights they were. Worse even was the congestion down on the beach where the poor fellows, with marvellous fortitude, lay about in dozens …[12]

On 8 August, after two days of fighting, the 1st AFA war diary records:

> On this date the flow of wounded down the Victoria Gully from Brown's Dip and the Lone Pine was considerable – all night long there was one continuous stream of stretcher bearers which all pass through the Divisional Collecting Station formed by the 1st Field Ambulance. The difficulty of handling all these with only thirty-five stretcher squads and no medical officer besides myself was very appreciable, by 48 hours after the beginning of the engagement the number through the station was over

---

10   AWM: AWM4/26/44/6: War Diary, 1st Australian Field Ambulance, August 1915.
11   The 4th SWB had arrived at Anzac in mid-July, but the 5th Wiltshires had arrived on 4 August.
12   AWM: 2DRL/0786, RCDIG0001478: [Transcript] Diaries of Thomas James Richards, Vol. 2, 6 August 1915.

fifteen hundred treated. Our Bearers were already wearied by the attack on Holly Ridge on the same morning of the day in which the Lone Pine attack took place.[13]

The casualties were heavy. The 2nd AFA Bearer Division established a dressing station at the head of Bridge's Road to handle casualties arriving in their sector of the line. From there, the casualties were carried to Brighton Beach, where its tent subdivision was established, and casualties came in steadily.[14] The 3rd AFA, with Major G. P. Dixon acting as CO, were operating from an ADS at Brown's Dip, where, on 6 August, Major Dixon and Captain Goldsmith worked to handle casualties coming along Victoria Gully.[15] C Section of the same ambulance set up another ADS at Fullerton's Post, halfway along Victoria Gully, where Captains Fry and Conrick handled large numbers of casualties. Both these stations were in place and ready for work by 5:00 p.m., that is, only minutes before the main attack at Lone Pine commenced.[16]

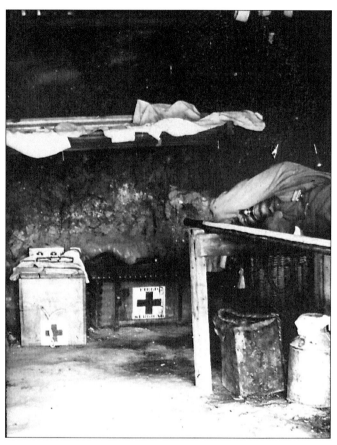

ADS of the 4th AFA at Anzac. Note, in the basic shelter, the use of stretchers and the various medical boxes and panniers. (State Library of South Australia: B45342/57)

The work of the field ambulances was unbroken as the fighting continued, and, in these units, it was the stretcher-bearers who worked hardest. It is no surprise that, on the morning of 7 August, Captain Fry of the 3rd AFA was reporting that his bearers were 'done up' as more cases accumulated, and requests for reinforcements were made immediately. The 2nd ALHFA was sent to their assistance:

---

13   AWM: AWM4/26/44/6: War Diary, 1st Australian Field Ambulance, 8 August.
14   AWM: AWM4/26/45/1: War Diary, 2nd Australian Field Ambulance, 6 August.
15   AWM: AWM4/26/46/1: War Diary, 3rd Australian Field Ambulance, 6 August.
16   AWM: AWM4/26/46/1: War Diary, 3rd Australian Field Ambulance, 6 August.

Joined 3rd Field Ambulance who had two dressing stations … The upper one in Brown's Dip was just behind the trenches from which the attack on Lone Pine had started. There were a great many wounded to be cleared and the bearers started straight away carrying to the 1st F Ambulance at Dawkin's Point. Officers and tent division men assisted in the dressing stations. In the afternoon and evening work slackened considerably. The patients so far dealt with had been those who had fallen at the commencement of the attack. There were known to be a great many in the new position at Lone Pine but they could not be got out yet.[17]

The same day, Private O. H. Gray of C Section 3rd AFA was to write in his diary:

… all went out again, each taking a stretcher, all night long casualties pouring in, up to dark; a lot of shrapnel flying about during night, star shells used which lit up the hills and valley like day … Heavy firing commenced at daybreak. Turks using a great many bombs, caused wounds, and the men bear them without a murmur. Doctors hard at work and some helping others stretcher bearing and helping the wounded.[18]

By the following day (8 August), it was becoming clear that the fighting was beginning to have a considerable effect upon the men:

Some poor fellows suffering from shock, trembling and sobbing like children their nerves all to pieces … A terrible Sunday, terrible sights in many places, pitiful to see the wounded … At daybreak the firing broke out with renewed vigour and Turkish attack repulsed, dozens of bombs thrown in – cruel wounds – men with limbs blown off, covered in blood some dying. It is HELL![19]

The situation at Lone Pine remained difficult as heavy hand-to-hand fighting continued. The 3rd AFA continued to handle the casualties at the Brown's Dip ADS, but the lower ADS at Fullerton's Post was handed over to the 2nd ALHFA. On the evening of 8 August, the situation at Lone Pine allowed for better communication with newly won positions, and it was possible to remove at least some of the casualties to the ADS, where 'in the evening the work became brisk'.[20] Early on 9 August, Private Gray was one of a group of six men ordered to go up to the trenches for duty:

Went through the saps and trenches passing men covered in dust and dirt, some bandaged up, officers calling for reinforcement, for sandbags, bombs. Went through trenches, shrapnel bullets flying overhead, bombs bursting in different places, wounded

---

17   AWM: AWM4/26/40/1: War Diary, 2nd Australian Light Horse Field Ambulance, 7 August.
18   AWM: AWM2018.666.1, AWM2018.785.52: Diary of Oberlin Herbert Gray, August 1915 to March 1916, 7 August. Gray, from Tasmania, later served in France and died of wounds there on 24 August 1918.
19   AWM: AWM2018.666.1, AWM2018.785.52: Diary of Oberlin Herbert Gray, August 1915 to March 1916, 8 August.
20   AWM: AWM4/26/40/1: War Diary, 2nd Australian Light Horse Field Ambulance, 8 August.

186   The Fight for Life

men being carried or crawling to the dressing station. Dressed several and helped two stretchers out. Many dead lying about and near the trenches. Big trenches are being dug for burials.[21]

On the left flank, the New Zealand and Australian Division was to form part of the Right Assaulting Column and was to attack along the gullies, such as Chailak Dere, towards the ridges of high ground, which were the ultimate aim of the August operations:

> The medical units allotted to the force are A and C Sections NZ Field Ambulance and 1st ALH Field Ambulance. C Section will take the Sazli Beit Dere and 1st ALH F Amb Chilak Dere. C Bearer Subdivision under Capt AV Short will follow above force at daylight on Aug 7. OC Bearer Subdivision will send back messages at intervals of 1/4 hour to OC Field Ambulance at Walker's Ridge to inform him of best site for dressing station. On receipt of information C Section with portable equipment on stretcher will proceed to the spot shown getting as near the final destination as possible. The OC will report at 4 hours intervals to OC on Walker's Ridge the progress of events and the number of casualties he has dealt with. A Sections will remain in reserve at Walker's Ridge and if required their services can be obtained by the Senior MO of the Rt Assaulting Column at Divisional Report Centre.
>   C Section Tent Subdivision will, if necessary, take over casualties from 1st ALH Amb to enable latter to push ahead.
>   In case of a shortage of stretcher bearers, messages for reinforcements will be sent to ADMS making clear exactly where they are required.
>   Only absolutely necessary and urgent operations are to be performed and water must be used with the greatest economy.[22]

The remainder of the NZFA, B Section, remained at Walker's Ridge, where it dealt with heavy casualties from Pope's Hill and Quinn's Post.[23] Casualties were evacuated as quickly as possible to Anzac Beach, but the lack of transport from the beach meant that the field ambulances faced great difficulties, as did those they cared for, as they waited in the backlog of casualties that began to build up on the beach.

The Right Assaulting Column's attack on Chunuk Bair began at 9:30 p.m. on 6 August. There were early successes. The Auckland Mounted Rifles seized the Old No. 3 Outpost, the Otago Mounted Rifles and the Canterbury Mounted Rifles took Bauchop Hill, and the Wellington Mounted Rifles stormed Table Top. The fighting took its toll on the men, and, by dawn on 7 August, the advanced parties, in a very wearied state, lay spread over the Apex, some 500yd from the Chunuk Bair crest. The Auckland Battalion mounted an attack on Chunuk Bair at 1:00 a.m. but, for a gain of just 100yd, suffered over 300 casualties. Lieutenant Colonel William Malone

---

21   AWM: AWM2018.666.1, AWM2018.785.52: Diary of Oberlin Herbert Gray, August 1915 to March 1916, 9 August.
22   AWM: AWM4/35/27/5: War Diary, New Zealand Field Ambulance, Part of Summary for Week 1–7 August.
23   AWM: AWM4/35/27/5: War Diary, New Zealand Field Ambulance, Part of Summary for Week 1–7 August.

A Night of Bloodshed and Pain   187

refused an order to attack with his Wellington Battalion, thinking it was an act of suicide. Further attack was delayed until the following day, 8 August. The Wellingtons did manage to occupy the Turkish trench on the Chunuk Bair ridge, but the Turks mounted a fierce counterattack to regain the trench. Men dug trenches on the seaward slopes, heavy fighting continued throughout the days of 9–10 August, and the Turks regained the slopes from the now thoroughly exhausted troops. The attack on Chunuk Bair was over after the bitterest of fighting.[24]

In the sector of the Right Assaulting Column, on 7 August, the field ambulances moved forwards with the assaulting troops and prepared to set up dressing stations. The 3rd ALHFA was in Aghyl Dere with part of the 4th AFA, whilst the NZMFA set up a dressing station at the mouth of Chailak Dere. The 1st ALHFA set up a dressing station about halfway along Chailak Dere, whilst C Section NZFA had set up a collecting post at Sazli Beit Dere and an ADS at No. 2 Outpost. However, it became increasingly difficult to get wounded away along Chailak Dere, as it was becoming heavily congested with men moving to the front and wounded moving in the other direction. Furthermore, when the wounded reached the beach, there was no sea transport:

> The picket boats cannot get into the pier owing to the tidal conditions: we are evacuating into two ships. It is impossible to handle stretcher cases, motor driven lighter the only means … I would suggest that F Ambs hold cases as there is no hope of evacuating those we have at the beach. In all today evacuations at this station 350, principally sitting … If 1st ACCS could clear, we could send along beach parties of bearers from units now around No 3 Post.[25]

By 8:30 p.m. on 9 August, Major O'Neil, CO of A Section Tent Division, had set up a dressing station near the head of Chailak Dere in a valiant attempt to assist the casualties. The Rhododendron Ridge was left covered with wounded. The 16 stretcher-bearers in each battalion had struggled manfully before they were overwhelmed with the number of casualties.

Priority was given to getting men, water and ammunition forwards. The following order was issued:

> No officer, NCO or man is to fall out to assist to the rear a wounded man. To do this is a serious military offence. Stretcher parties will follow all columns and will attend to the wounded. Stretcher parties are not to block or interfere with the forward movement of the troops. They are not to make use of any Communication Trench or Sap till all movement of fighting troops through it has ceased for the night.[26]

Colonel Manders, ADMS New Zealand and Australian Division, did all he could to get the wounded cared for and evacuated, but the narrow ridges defeated his plans. It was left to the

---

24 Christopher Pugsley, *Anzac: The New Zealanders at Gallipoli* (New Zealand: Reed Children's Books, 2000), pp.74–79.
25 Butler, *Official History of the Australian Medical Services*, vol. I, p.307, part of a report from the 4th AFA, 7 August 1915.
26 AWM: AWM4/1/53/5: War Diary, General Staff, Headquarters New Zealand and Australian Division, August 1915, Part 2, Appendix 77: Instructions Issued to Commanders in Accordance with Divisional Order No. 11, 5 August 1915.

troops to assist in any way they could. Trooper H. E. Browne, Wellington Mounted Rifles, commented, 'I had taken two bottles up the hill and did what I could among them. The first lay in a four-inch hollow evidently scooped out by himself … he asked me if there was any hope of stretcher bearers that night, I had to tell him no. Another voice called for help so I left him'.[27] Stretcher-bearer Ormond Burton was busy clearing the wounded from the Apex, saying:

> In the darkness we reached the Regimental Aid Post … heavy and continuous firing went on all night … we took stretchers that were waiting and went down the Dere. For the next few days, we were up and down with little rest. Chailak Dere was a dangerous highway and sometimes desperately crowded. On the high slopes it took six men to get a stretcher down. Four men were needed for the long carry to the Casualty Clearing Station near the beach but only two were available. Snipers were busy at every exposed bend. As we went up there was an unending line of mules laden with water and ammunition going up – and every kind of carrying party.[28]

At Anzac, as the attack developed in darkness on the night of 6 August, Private Richards, 1st AFA, was soon very busy, commenting that, as the wounded men were taken to the beach to wait for transport, '… "Beachy Bill" and a gun from over their middle front showered the men with shrapnel … so many troops were landed this morning and overnight that small launches did not appear to be available to take the wounded aboard the Hospital Ship. The Ambulance men worked wonderfully well this morning and kept the way open splendidly'.[29]

The following day (7 August), for the 3rd AFA, there was no let-up in the numbers of wounded. Again, the ADMS was asked to send reinforcement stretcher-bearers. As a result of the shortage of stretcher-bearers and the inevitable tiredness of the bearers, there was a minor holdup getting the wounded away from the ambulance between 5:00–9:00 p.m. A visit from the ADMS 1st Australian Division to Brown's Dip at 6:00 p.m. relieved the situation when he called for yet more stretcher-bearer reinforcements.[30] Between 5:00 p.m. on 6 August and 6:00 p.m. on 9 August, the 3rd AFA handled a total of 1,151 cases.

On the same day, on the left flank, the 39th Field Ambulance, 13th Division, formed a dressing station under a hill in Aghyl Dere. Whilst there, a shell fell among them and killed two of their men and three of the attached 41st Field Ambulance. Four hundred and fifteen cases passed through the station on 8 August. On 9 August, an ADS was established one-and-a-half miles along the Dere, moving closer to the RAP, but, the following day, it came under heavy machine-gun fire and was forced to withdraw along the Gully. Nevertheless, 601 cases were treated during the day.[31]

The 40th Field Ambulance, 13th Division, arrived at No. 3 Post in the late evening of 7 August, taking over from the NZFA. The unit was immediately put to work tending to casualties,

---

27 Trooper H. E. Browne, Wellington Mounted Regiment, quoted in Christopher Pugsley, *Gallipoli: The New Zealand Story* (Auckland: Hodder & Stoughton, 1984), p.306.
28 Pugsley, *New Zealanders at Gallipoli*, p.308.
29 AWM: 2DRL/0786, RCDIG0001478: [Transcript] Diaries of Thomas James Richards, Vol. 2, 6 August 1915.
30 AWM: AWM4/26/46/4: War Diary, 3rd Australian Field Ambulance, 7 August.
31 The National Archives (TNA) WO 95/4301: War Diary, 39th Field Ambulance, 12 August.

and, in the first 12 hours, about 350 cases were treated and evacuated. Its work continued over the next three days. On 8 August, a party of 30 men led by Lieutenants Weeks and Letchworth established a dressing station at Aghyl Dere, where they made contact with the 39th Brigade and the 39th Field Ambulance to assist with the work of treating casualties. They were to meet the same fate as the 39th Field Ambulance when very heavy machine-gun fire forced them to retire farther down Aghyl Dere. The bearers from these dressing stations often found themselves under rifle fire during their one-and-a-half-mile journey to the beach carrying wounded for evacuation.[32]

The MOs of the field ambulances were occasionally detailed to act as RMO when that officer had been put out of action. Such was the case when Captain Alec Glen, MO with the 40th Field Ambulance, was detailed to replace the fatally wounded MO, Lieutenant John Cattanach, attached to the 6th South Lancashire Regiment on 27 July 1915.[33] This battalion formed part of the force under General Cox during the attack of 8 August. When Glen arrived at Anzac Cove on 5 August, he settled into a small ravine in which the Australians had prepared an aid post in an extra-large dugout. The following day, the attack started. The ravine was subjected to very heavy shelling, and there was a call for stretcher-bearers, who were soon at work carrying casualties to Glen's RAP. An HE shell landed directly in the midst of the casualties at the aid post. Glen was crouching in the corner of the dugout tending to a casualty and was lucky to escape uninjured. The aid post was in a mess, but Captain Glen recovered and tended to the now more seriously wounded. In the midst of this, he was ordered to move out and found himself climbing the steep sides of Chailak Dere. The battalion came under heavy machine-gun fire during this manoeuvre, and it was ordered to cross a plateau and make its way down Aghyl Dere, at the head of which Glen established an aid post in a small ravine. The battalion was spread out, and casualties soon arrived. Stretcher cases were sent down the Dere, accompanied by walking cases. Over the next few days, the bearers dwindled, as they became casualties. On 10 August, Glen found himself alone. All medical supplies were finished, and he had no morphia left. He made his way down the Dere and located the 40th Field Ambulance, where he was given food, drink and medical supplies, and he returned to his battalion. A few days later, he was relieved and rejoined the 40th Field Ambulance.[34] Meantime, in the diversionary fighting on the right, between 8–10 August, the 1st AFA faced a large number of wounded coming along the Victoria Gully from Brown's Dip and Lone Pine. Fortunately, there was no congestion, allowing all the cases to be sent to the divisional collecting station at Dawkins Point. In the same way, the 3rd AFA stretcher-bearers, numbering just 35 squads, were extremely busy, and, in total, over 1,500 casualties passed through the station over the 48-hour time period.

From 8 August to the end of the month, large numbers of sick cases occurred, with B and C Sections reporting many cases of diarrhoea before the end of the battle, and it was found necessary to set up small rest camps for slight cases of diarrhoea. At Monash Gully Dressing Station, there were increasing cases of enteritis, particularly amongst the British troops. This was thought to be because men had been in the trenches for eight days and were very tired and weakened by persistent attacks of diarrhoea. By the time the battle ended, the general health of

---

32   TNA: WO 95/4301: War Diary, 39th Field Ambulance, 10 August.
33   Lieutenant John Cattanach, RAMC, is commemorated on the Helles Memorial.
34   Alec Glen, *In the Front Line: A Doctor's Life in War and Peace* (Edinburgh: Birlinn, 2013), pp.43–49.

the men was considered fair, and there was an increasing number of men reporting with septic sores to hands and legs.

The general health of the troops going into battle continued to be a matter of great concern for COs and MOs alike. On 13 August, the 1st AFA received, and carried out, an order from the ADMS to shift the tent subdivision to a site above Brighton Beach and open up dugout accommodation for 50 slightly wounded or sick cases. This number gradually increased to 100 in order to accommodate a remarkable rise in sick cases. In one battalion, 180 out of a strength of 220 paraded sick on the same day. Despite more accommodation becoming available, with such overwhelming numbers and the seriousness of the sickness cases, unable to benefit from the usual two-day treatment period, as many as 500 cases per day were sent on to the CCS.

The battle had a very marked effect on the health of the men. After the battle, the ADMS 1st Australian Division felt compelled to bring to attention of the GOC the very poor state of health of the division. His report was written as a result of an inspection of 350 paraded sick out of five battalions. He found the vast majority were suffering from repeated attacks of dysenteric diarrhoea with its consequent anaemia. This had produced a very serious change in the cardiovascular system of the men, with many of them suffering from shortness of breath on any exertion and a fast irregular pulse accompanied by listlessness. He warned that there would be a great increase in the numbers being evacuated unless the men were given a long rest and suitable nutrients to get them back to fighting fitness.[35]

The 29th Indian Brigade had been heavily involved in the assault on Chunuk Bair as part of the Left Assaulting Column of the main attack on the high ground of the Sari Bair. At first, their casualties were sent along the lines of evacuation through Chailak Dere and the field ambulances stationed there. However, at 2:00 a.m. on 7 August, the 108th IFA disembarked from a trawler. Their CO, Major Battye, had not been given any specific order as to where his field ambulance should be stationed, and it was not until 11:15 a.m. that morning that he located BHQ, although he had been able to observe the Gurkhas of the brigade going into action on the slopes above the beach. He was then given orders that he was to send a bearer subdivision, under Captain Stocker, forwards to BHQ whilst Major Brassey set up a temporary dressing station and clearing station at the mouth of Chailak Dere:

> Meanwhile the most necessary equipment for a more permanent ambulance station was sent from Reserve Gully to Chailak Dere on kahars shoulders' as not a single mule was available. The distance was over a mile and a half. Major Brassey's temporary station was under fire and two wounded men were hit so the permanent station was made in a cul-de-sac of the hills near the Chailak Dere about 800 yards or more from the beach. The ground was cleared and shelter put up and by evening it was ready. Then all wounded were brought first in here. From here they are being later sent … on to the clearing post in the ravine for evacuation from the jetty. The O's C regiments and the GOC had arrived at Anzac and studied the conditions and the ground five days before the brigade left Imbros. I was not permitted to accompany them. Had I been allowed to go with them and see the conditions myself the muddle and loss of time in getting the bearers and ambulance to work today would never have occurred. The maps are so

---

35   AWM: AWM4/26/18: War Diary, 1st Australian Division ADMS, 18 August.

sketchy and the landmarks on the map proved to be so few that it is almost impossible to work by the map unless the ground has been studied and the map discussed first.[36]

It is clear from Battye's account in the unit war diary that the organisation was not all it should have been. Nevertheless, by the time he had made the entry on 10 August, he was able to report that, in the three days since its arrival, the 108th IFA had handled 542 wounded.

It was during the 1/6th Gurkhas' attack on the Sari Bair that its RMO was to find himself in nominal charge of the battalion. On the night of 8/9 August, the RMO, Captain E. S. Phipson, was in a shallow dugout that was acting as battalion HQ along with Major C. J. L. Allanson, the CO, and Captain A. W. D. Cornish, awaiting the attack that the battalion was about to make. The attack was successful, in so far as it drove the Turks from the crest of the hill, but they were later forced to retire in the face of HE shell fire – some say it was friendly fire – and the crest was never held again. During the fighting, most British officers of the battalion became casualties, and, suffering from a bayonet wound in the leg, Allanson handed over command to Phipson, the last uninjured British officer. Phipson and Subedar Major Gambirsing Pun then commanded the battalion until it was relieved two days later. Phipson recorded:

> My first thought, oddly enough, was I must cease to claim the protection (if any) of the Geneva Convention, and so I removed my Red Cross Brassard, and put it in my haversack. I might, I thought, have to deal with combatant officers of other units and although at that time I held no combatant commission myself I thought it was just as well to look as if I did. I was soon to put it to the test.[37]

Phipson sought support from nearby units such as the SWB and found that mostly they were in a similar state to his Gurkhas. On 10 August, the 1/6th Gurkhas were withdrawn under the precise control of the Subedar Major, as 'he knew the drill from A to Z'. Phipson remarked on the difficulty of bringing out the wounded of the battalion '… down a rocky declivity, intersected by deep narrow gullies, many of them choked with corpses'.[38] However, under the confident guidance of Gambirsing Pun, Phipson was able to get many of the wounded away. According to the war diary of the 108th IFA on this day, '… for two days until their retirement was carried out the Medical Officer, Captain Phipson, was in command in a very precarious position being the only British Officer left. The regiment being now back in reserve I have ordered him here for two days rest and proper food and have sent another MO to relieve him temporarily'.[39] Phipson commented that, in those two days, he was fed '… tinned chicken instead of Bully – a wonderful change, and I was soon back in the line'.[40] Whilst it is perhaps unusual that the RMO took command of the battalion, it serves to demonstrate the close involvement of the RMO with the actions of the battalion: they were often close to the fighting, carrying on their work under fire before passing their wounded comrades back to field ambulances to begin their evacuation from the front.

---

36   TNA: WO 95/4272: War Diary, 108th Indian Field Ambulance, 7 August.
37   Colonel E. S. Phipson, 'With the Gurkhas on Sari Bair', *Gallipolian*, 147 (Autumn 2018), p.38.
38   Phipson, 'With the Gurkhas', p.39.
39   TNA: WO 95/4272: War Diary, 108th Indian Field Ambulance, 10 August 1915.
40   Phipson, 'With the Gurkhas', p.39.

The work of the RMOs and field ambulances depended upon the efficient working of the lines of communication to their rear. The evacuation of wounded at Gallipoli was particularly difficult since it relied on the arrival of hospital ships and transports to remove wounded from the beaches after they had passed through the field ambulances and, usually, a CCS. At Anzac, the 1st ACCS had been established since the day of the landing, and it was through this station that most of the wounded, and sick, were evacuated to waiting transports of various kinds. For the first few days of the August Offensive, it was the 1st ACCS that handled all the wounded coming from the fighting at Lone Pine and right across the Anzac front. On 8 August, the 13th BCCS and the 16th BCCS landed and set up their hospitals on the new left flank of the Anzac beachhead near to No. 2 Outpost. From 6 August, the 1st ACCS was inundated with wounded and evacuated 508 casualties by the end of the day. However, this figure could have been higher if there had been sufficient transport to get wounded away:

> The facilities provided for the conveyance of wounded from the shore to the Hospital Ships are very inadequate. The two cutters and horse boat fitted with awnings which were set aside for use of sick have been taken for use for the landing of troops and are not available. The steam piquet boat to be used solely for evacuating sick which I had had from the Naval Beach Officer was being sent here as a result of my request to Surg. Gen. Babtie has not arrived. Consequently, we have to wait till such time as tows are not being used for troops and stores to get wounded evacuated. The boats used consist of (a) large lighters holding about 50 stretchers and 75 walking cases. Very easy to load and unload but with no awning, (b) horse boats holding 15 stretchers or 70 walking cases and (c) ship's cutters holding six stretchers and 20 walking or 50 walking cases, not very suitable for stretchers. These are towed by Naval piquet boats which are themselves used to carry about 30 walking cases. The Naval bluejackets take over the cases at the jetty and handle the stretchers carefully.
>
> Today we were unable to get any tows off before 12:15 pm. As a result, the shelters we have to keep the wounded in are greatly overcrowded and we were obliged to keep wounded men waiting on the beach which is intermittently shelled each day. I think the Naval officers on the beach do their best to provide towage but the numbers of piquet boats at their disposal is small. The Hospital Ship *Sicilia* which came in today was rapidly filled to overflowing and reported she could take no more cases. No other hospital ship is at present in sight.[41]

The only hospital ship at Anzac on the first day of fighting was the *Sicilia*, and it was filled very quickly and left on the same day. Dawn of the following day saw three hospital ships in the bay, but, whilst this came as some relief to the MOs of the 1st ACCS, one of these ships, the *Seang Choon*, was intended only for Indian wounded and any captured Turks needing treatment. However, the hospital ships that were available allowed for the evacuation of wounded on what had '… been the heaviest day for casualties we have had'.[42] By the end of the day, 1,937 wounded had been evacuated through the 1st ACCS. The fighting continued without break, and, from

---

41   AWM: AWM4/26/62/7: War Diary, 1st Australian Casualty Clearing Station, 6 August 1915.
42   AWM: AWM4/26/62/7: War Diary, 1st Australian Casualty Clearing Station, 7 August.

the point of view of the evacuation of wounded, 8 August proved to be difficult since there was no hospital ship to be found. The two available hospital ships of the previous day had been filled and had left the area; only the *Sean Choon* remained. There were plenty of wounded arriving at the hospital, and the 1st ACCS managed to get walking wounded away to Lemnos on the SS *Redbreast*. The hospital still managed to evacuate 946 cases, and it would appear that most, if not all, had been evacuated to Imbros on any transport that became available.

Meanwhile, the 13th BCCS had landed at Suvla and had been directed to No. 2 Outpost, where the 40th Field Ambulance, 13th Division, was operating a makeshift CCS for evacuation of wounded from the left flank of Anzac. It appears that this ambulance had sent a tow 'consisting of three cutters full of wounded' from the beachhead to a transport, or hospital ship, that had refused to take them. Possibly, the *Seang Choon* was the ship that refused the wounded since it had been designated for Indian wounded. In any event, the tow was returned to Anzac, landing near to the 1st ACCS, where it came under fire from the Turks, who, no doubt, took the tow as reinforcements being landed. These casualties appear to have been cared for by the 1st ACCS, adding to their workload, since there were no other transports available for evacuation apart from the already hard worked fleet sweepers. These latter vessels carried a considerable responsibility during 8 August, as most casualties, the walking wounded, appear to have been evacuated from the fighting in this manner. At 10:00 p.m., the HS *Gascon* arrived on station at Anzac and, throughout most of the following day, took on casualties. Records for the *Gascon* show that, on 9 August, 647 casualties were taken on board from Anzac before the ship sailed for Imbros.[43] Almost 150 casualties were disembarked there before those remaining were taken to hospitals in Malta. The capacity of the *Gascon*, according to the *Official History*, was 401, and it is therefore clear that the ship must have been considerably overcrowded.[44] Furthermore, although the *Gascon* had embarked 647 casualties, the 1st ACCS had evacuated a total of 1,020 cases during that day. The remainder of the casualties can only have been taken by temporary hospital ships and fleet sweepers. Although casualties continued to arrive at the 1st ACCS, 9 August seems to have been the last day for such large numbers to be evacuated. This may have been related to the arrival and establishment of the two BCCSs on the north flank of Anzac, where they began evacuating wounded from the area of Chailak Dere and Sazli Beit Dere.

The newly arrived BCCSs were placed under the overall command of Lieutenant Colonel W. W. Giblin of the 1st ACCS, and the way in which these hospitals worked together shows some difficulties in the first few days of the fighting at Anzac during August. On 13 August, Lieutenant Colonel Giblin recorded that the 16th BCCS had taken over from the 13th BCCS at No. 2 Outpost and that '... the work was proceeding more satisfactorily, that the state of affairs under No 13 CCS had been a hopeless muddle, very little attempt being made to provide shelter and nourishment for the wounded who had to wait a considerable time before being evacuated'.[45] This is, perhaps, an unfair assessment since the war diary for the 13th BCCS gives a rather different story, in which its CO, Lieutenant Colonel J. G. McNaught, was struggling with similar problems to the 1st ACCS and had to, to a large extent, 'hit the ground running' without its full equipment or means of evacuating wounded from the station. On 10 August:

---

43   AWM: AWM41/1053: [Nurses Narratives] Sister E J Tucker.
44   Macpherson, *History of the Great War: Medical Services*, vol. 1, p.366.
45   AWM: AWM4/26/62/7: War Diary, 1st Australian Casualty Clearing Station, 13 August.

194   The Fight for Life

As wounded are coming in to the station in large numbers, I wired to ADMS Communications Anzac at 9.15 am asking for 3 additional medical officers and 20 orderlies. No orderlies were sent as none were available but two medical officers were attached for duty. Two medical officers on embarkation duty were also placed under my orders. I established a feeding and first aid post at the beach under Lt S.K. McKee. The work at the pier head and on the beach is very dangerous as this locality is constantly sniped and there are also many spent bullets falling. The clearing station itself is not safe as spent bullets are constantly falling and wounded men are again hit during the day; no place in the post is free from risk.

Wrote to the CRE [Commander Royal Engineers] 13th Division asking him to have a sandbag shelter put up at the pier had to help protect wounded being evacuated. He promised to do this tomorrow morning. Obtained 50 fatigue men to act as stretcher bearers. Walking cases are evacuated along the sap to Anzac; evacuation by sea from our pier is rather slow owing to insufficient number and small size of boats. Wired ADMS that improvement to sea transport was urgently required. Up to the night of 10th about 2,000 cases had passed through the station. The accumulation of wounded awaiting embarkation at the gully near pier has been cleared off. During the 24 hours to 6 pm 168 stretcher cases and 350 sitting cases had been evacuated by sea, besides those sent along the sap. 431 stretcher cases remain in the clearing station; this is due to the boat service being insufficient. Operating tent and several tarpaulin shelters have been put up to shelter the wounded but many are in the open after all available shelters have been utilized.[46]

Furthermore, on 11 August, under considerable difficulty, McNaught managed to evacuate over 700 casualties. This does not sound like a hopeless muddle, more like a new unit struggling with inexperienced staff and equipment shortages to make the best job it could. However, on 12 August, it was replaced by the 16th BCCS, commanded by Lieutenant Colonel M. P. Corkery, at No. 2 Outpost, and it moved to a new site near Walker's Ridge. A few days later, Lieutenant Colonel McNaught was invalided sick, and the 13th BCCS came under the command of Captain Leslie Way.

On the other hand, Colonel J. L. Beeston, CO of the 4th AFA, also had a rather poor view of the performance of the 13th BCCS:

The miserable part of the affair was that the Casualty Clearing Station on the beach broke down and could not evacuate our wounded. This caused a block, and we had numbers of wounded on our hands. A block of a few hours can be dealt with, but when it is impossible to get cases away for forty hours the condition of the men is very miserable.[47]

Although Beeston was not specific about the CCS involved, it can be no other than the 13th BCCS since, later in his narrative, he commented that '… evacuation was all done from Walker's

46   TNA: WO 95/4356: War Diary, 13th Casualty Clearing Station, 10 August 1915.
47   Joseph L. Beeston, *Five Months at Anzac: A Narrative of Personal Experiences of the Officer Commanding the 4th Field Ambulance, Australian Imperial Force* (Angus & Robertson, 1916, Kindle e-book), location 614.

Ridge about two miles away. The Casualty Clearing Station here (16th) was a totally different proposition from the other one. Colonel Corkery was commanding officer, and knew his job. His command was exceedingly well administered, and there was no further occasion to fear any block in getting our wounded off'.[48] Although McNaught's war diary entries suggest his unit was working hard, it seems that, at least in the eyes of the Australians, it was not working as well as perhaps it could.

The opening days of the August Offensive had tested everyone at Anzac. The medical services had struggled, at times, on shore to accommodate the large numbers of wounded that had arisen from the heavy fighting. They managed largely to overcome deficiencies in staff, equipment and transport, and, whilst the situation could not have been considered ideal by any of the SMOs, the fact that the services had managed to get so many wounded away in a very short time scale suggests that much had been learned since April, though perhaps not all that had been learned could be put in place in time for the major attack.

Although the work at Anzac was fraught with considerable difficulties, these did not end for the medical services when the casualties had been taken off the beaches and away from the CCSs there. Sister Elsie Tucker of the AANS was serving on the *Gascon* at the time of the August Offensive and had left an account of the early days of August, from 7 August, and the work that was involved on the hospital ship on which she served:

> We have our orders to go to Anzac; arrive there about 11 pm. We are soon called upon, scores of wounded are alongside, the guns are so noisy, we cannot hear ourselves speak, we are taking on steadily, by next evening have 600 cases, we transfer half out cases on one transport and the remainder another and return the same evening to Anzac; have not sufficient linen to change the beds and to the best we can to hide the dirtier parts and get the beds made up and get as much dressing as possible cut and sterilized, we are very short of gauze and are having to cut up lint. We reach Anzac in the evening and in the early hours of the morning we are in our wards, receiving wounded again. By evening we are full again [so] go to Imbros. We wait there a whole day expecting a transport to take our wounded. Then the Captain sails for Lemnos. We are working awfully hard to get dressing done by midnight. We wait another whole day in Lemnos, and still no word of who is to take our wounded boys. Then word comes to proceed to Malta. It is a trying trip, we are short of water, the boys are black and so are the beds. Salt water is not at all satisfactory for washing. The patients all look uncomfortable, cannot possibly get time to make their beds, am dressing from morning till late at night, have several bad jaw cases who need constant irrigation. Arrive at Malta on the 16th, we load take on water and provisions and sail again the same day.[49]

It was not only the *Gascon* that was on station at Anzac. The HS *Devanha* arrived late on the evening of 8 August. Sister Mary Ann Brown, QAIMNS, was one of the nurses serving on the hospital ship and wrote in her diary for the day:

---

48   Beeston, *Five Months at Anzac*, location 671.
49   AWM: AWM41/1053: [Nurses Narratives] Sister E J Tucker.

... we got to the place where the Australians first landed, their lights were twinkling on the shore and over the hill was a continual crack, crack of rifle fire, then on our left there was the sound of very fierce fighting right on till midnight. About 10 pm a boat slipped out from the shore with about a hundred wounded to us, so the fighting didn't interest us further, we worked on till after midnight, and when we finished there was a dead silence and black darkness all around us except for the red and green lights of the hospital ships ...[50]

The following day, the work on the *Devanha* became even more intense: 'Up early this morning, began dressing before 7:30. The men are nearly all Australians, they are badly wounded but are very plucky ... Before we got breakfast a boat load of wounded came alongside, and all day the boats were bringing them over. We dressed nearly a thousand and were hard at it all day'.[51] The *Devanha* was filled by the end of 9 August and sailed to Lemnos prior to sailing to Alexandria. According to Sister Brown, there were 23 burials at sea before they reached Lemnos,[52] and, in her opinion, there would be more before the *Devanha* reached Alexandria.[53]

Whilst the medical services nearest the fighting were working hard to manage a very difficult situation, arising as all the components of that service attempted to act as an organised and unified system, it is interesting to note the entry to the war diary of the DMS for 8 August:

Evacuation at Suvla – smooth. Anzac congested, insufficient tows. Arrangements at Kephalos – smooth, No. 25 CCS expanded to 800. Navy changed evac scheme. Ambulance carriers all going to Mudros; DMS had organized for two out of three to go direct to Base. Kephalos cut out of scheme – weather often bad for landing casualties. Hospital ships to run to Mudros and all Ambulance Carriers to stop there. IGC [Inspector General Communications] overruled scheme as saw fit.[54]

It is clear from this terse entry that, although Surgeon General Birrell had sought to put a scheme in place, he was all too often relying on others to play their part. In particular, it was necessary to rely on the navy, and the entry shows that their cooperation could not be guaranteed, in many cases for operational reasons. However, it would seem that ordering all ships to call at Mudros in the first instance may have been causing as many problems as it solved. The call on the best course of action for the wounded should have lain with the medical services, and hence Birrell, but it would appear that he was at least in part overruled by the navy. Furthermore, it

---

50 Diary of Sister Mary Brown for 8 August, quoted in Malcolm Brown, *The Imperial War Museum Book of the First World War: A Great Conflict Recalled in Previously Unpublished Letters, Diaries, Documents, and Memoirs* (London: Guild Publishing, 1991), p.201. (IWM Document 1001).
51 Diary of Sister Mary Brown for 9 August, quoted in Brown, *Imperial War Museum Book*, p.201. (IWM Document 1001).
52 One of those buried at sea has been identified as Private Charles McJarrow of the 14th Battalion, 20 years old and a native of Girvan in Scotland. He had been wounded in the groin on 9 August and died on the *Devanha* the next day.
53 According to Macpherson, *History of the Great War: Medical Services*, vol. 1, p.366, the *Devanha*, at 8,092 tons, was capable of carrying a maximum of 524 cases. Hence, if over 1,000 men had been dressed, the hospital ship was overcrowded in the extreme. This may account for the trip to Lemnos.
54 TNA: WO 95/4267: War Dairy, General Headquarters DMS, 8 August.

appears that the IGC also had input into the running of the medical services, and the scheme devised by Birrell, and may have been overruling the details of the original plan for the evacuation of wounded. This, to some extent, explains why the *Gascon* was sent in the first instance to Imbros and then to Lemnos with delays at both anchorages before ultimately being sent to a base hospital at Malta. If Birrell's original scheme had been followed, the wounded could have arrived at their destination possibly two days sooner.

Although removing the casualty from the beaches to the hospital ships was of prime importance to the medical staff working on the beaches, it was by the no means the end of the evacuation process. As indicated in the account by Sister Elsie Tucker, the ships were simply the next part of the evacuation network. For the wounded who had managed to reach the hospital ships, the next stage in their journey was their arrival at a base hospital. The base hospitals during the August Offensive were, as in April, mainly in Egypt. It is clear from Sister Tucker's account that Malta was soon to come online as a base for seriously wounded carried by the hospital ships. Malta continued to be used as a base for the remainder of the campaign.

The majority of the casualties arising from the fighting of August were taken to Egypt at the start of the fighting. As in April, the wounded were distributed amongst the hospitals in Alexandria, such as No. 15 BGH, and in Cairo, such as No. 1 AGH. Ships arriving in Alexandria immediately disembarked their wounded, many of the most serious cases being rushed to hospital there whilst others were loaded onto hospital trains for the journey to Cairo. According to Sister Janet Buchan, an Australian serving with the QAIMNS, No. 15 BGH was soon filled with seriously wounded from Gallipoli, and the work was then very heavy. She admitted that the hospital was very well equipped for dealing with the influx of wounded at this time.[55]

In Cairo, men began to arrive at No. 1 AGH at Heliopolis and No. 2 AGH at Gezireh. Both hospitals had been working since before the April landings, and there was, by August, some experienced staff to handle the casualties. Nevertheless, there were still problems to be overcome. At No. 1 AGH, established in the Heliopolis Palace Hotel, Sister Anne Kidd-Hart recorded the difficulty of managing wards that were made up of small rooms that had been the bedrooms of the hotel that had been converted to No. 1 AGH. Once again, the sister was at pains to point out that the hospital was well equipped to handle casualties in large numbers.[56] At No. 2 AGH, Sister Adelaide Maud Kellett, a theatre sister, remarked that, when necessary, two operating theatres were kept going day and night to handle the numbers of wounded needing immediate surgery. Additional nurses were always available to provide the necessary cover for operations at night.[57] No. 1 AGH had expanded rapidly immediately following the landings, and the Atelier and Luna Park sites were maintained for the August casualties. Sister Edith Florence Avenell, writing to her mother on 12 August, just as the first rush of casualties arrived from Anzac, reported, 'I am dead tired and cannot write many lines. We are having a rough and jolly busy time receiving patients galore. Our poor old boys they do look awful, such food and dirty, poor beggars.'[58] Later in the same month, Sister Avenell explained to her mother the work

---

55   AWM: AWM41/1072: Kellett Interviews, Sister J. Buchan.
56   AWM: AWM41/1072: Kellett Interviews, Sister A. Kidd-Hart.
57   AWM: AWM41/988: [Nurses Narratives] Matron A Kellett.
58   Pat Richardson and Anne Skinner (eds), *Queenie: Letters from an Australian Army Nurse, 1915–1917* (New South Wales: Gumleaf Press, 2012), p.51.

during the first immediate rush of the wounded, saying that she was working to dress wounded from 8:30 a.m. until after 7:30 p.m. The wounded were all dressed during the day, some men needing to have dressing changed every four hours whilst others were done once in the day: 'One of my patients was hit with shrapnel in five different places, his eye blown out. Left arm blown off and other wounds on the back and body. He is a brave fellow. He says he is not too bad, but thinks he got more than his share.'[59]

For 18 August, the war diary of the DMS records, 'Egypt and Malta full up'. The casualties arising during the fighting of the first half of the month had all but swamped the medical services. There was little in the way of spare capacity, but, at Mudros, the capacity was immediately increased, and the 25th CCS at Imbros was also enlarged to accommodate casualties and offer some assistance to the stretched services elsewhere. By 22 August, the DMS recorded, 'Operations over: casualties to date 34,000'. It is hardly surprising that all spare capacity was all but filled. For the same date, the diary records that 200 cases were evacuated daily from the peninsula as a result of sickness.[60]

Whilst Egypt's base hospitals handled many of the wounded, the development of Lemnos also meant a greater capacity to care for the variety of wounded that were sent directly to the island. The arrival of No. 3 AGH at Mudros West in early August was meant to provide the equivalent of a base hospital nearer to the fighting. The reality was a little different in the first weeks, for the lack of equipment when the hospital arrived meant that it could not be as efficient as was hoped. The MOs, nurses and orderlies struggled to care for the wounded arriving daily: 'The wounds of the men did very well but so many of them contracted dysentery their general condition did not improve.'[61] When Sister Smith recorded this, she was highlighting a major problem that was developing on Lemnos and, indeed, on the peninsula itself. That was the increase in the numbers of men succumbing to disease, particularly dysentery, as the summer months passed. The conditions for medical care on Lemnos were not good. It was a hot, dry island prone to severe storms, and, during the summer months, there was a large number of flies to spread disease. MOs and nurses did all in their powers to improve conditions, to obtain food, medical stores and basic equipment, to improve the lot of the wounded and, later, the sick. However, on an island so generally short of water, it was often difficult to keep the patients clean.[62] Nevertheless, the medical services prevailed, and, if, at first, they struggled to provide an efficient service, as August gave way to autumn, things improved. Lemnos was never ideal, but the work of the hospitals did improve the overall conditions in their continual fight against disease. At times, the hospitals, too, were affected by disease, as their staff became ill with dysentery. The short-handed units maintained their service to the sick and wounded as best they could and continued to save lives in the face of the most difficult conditions.

The medical services met a significant challenge in preparing for the operations of August, especially as it had been criticised for its performance immediately following the landings in April. There can be no doubt that there had been an attempt by Surgeon General Birrell to improve the situation with his plan for a more extensive use of hospital ships and transports to

---

59 Richardson and Skinner (eds), *Queenie*, pp.53, 55.
60 TNA: WO 95/4267: War Dairy, General Headquarters DMS, August.
61 AWM: AWM41/1045: [Nurses Narratives] N F S Smith.
62 AWM: AWM41/1045: [Nurses Narratives] N F S Smith, and AWM41/1013: [Nurses Narratives] Head Sister N C Morrice.

get the wounded evacuated. Also, the increase in the number, and later the capacity, of hospitals on Lemnos was an effort to reduce transport time and assure primary care for at least some of the casualties as quickly as possible. To some extent, it has to be considered that this had worked, for, in spite of the difficulties, Lemnos had been able act as a base for at least some of the time and hospital ships and other transports were directed to Mudros Harbour in the first instance during August. This may have been an attempt to triage the casualties on the various ships. However, given the rather limited capacity of Lemnos, under 9,000 beds at best, it was perhaps wishful thinking to believe that the large number of casualties that occurred could be effectively sorted in the harbour there. Whilst this had not been the original intention of Birrell's evacuation scheme, it was operated during August and resulted in some delays before ships were directed to proceed to Egypt or Malta.

The hospitals in Egypt could not have been less well prepared than they were in April. The British general hospitals in Alexandria were fully staffed by August, whereas, in April, there had been staff shortage. The medical service in Alexandria was dealing with an outbreak of scarlet fever just as the heavy fighting on the peninsula began, but hospitals such as Ras-el-tin were able to call on staff from other hospitals to carry them through the additional problem of the disease. In Cairo, the Australian hospitals were reasonably well established and were functioning effectively. They were still struggling with some problems such as a good food supply and staff accommodation, but their patient care was good, as all the hospitals involved had at least some staff who had experienced the problems of April and knowledge of the ways in which they could be overcome. This generally suggests an overall improvement in medical services compared with that of the start of the campaign.

On the other hand, the problems with seaborne transport had not really been resolved. There were more hospital ships operating in August than in April, but it was still not enough to handle the large number of casualties. The conditions on the hospital carriers (black ships) had improved, and there were more medical personnel to staff them. Nevertheless, it was necessary to use a large number of such vessels to make up for the shortage of hospital ships. This, in itself, almost amounts to an admission of failure on the behalf of the medical services. However, the task of removing wounded was fulfilled more readily than in April. The evacuation of the wounded relied heavily on the efficient work of the field ambulances and CCSs, and, since at Anzac they had been in place from April, they were well acquainted with the necessary process and routine of evacuation. Again, under the stress of battle, this may have not been ideal, but it worked – over 4,000 patients were evacuated through the 1st ACCS in three days during August.

10

An Inferno of Shrapnel: The Suvla Landings

In conjunction with the attempted Anzac breakout, the landing at Suvla Bay was to take place in a weakly defended part of the peninsula. It was planned that the high ground around the bay was to be captured in the first hours of the attack, thus securing the bay. The IX Corps, commanded by Lieutenant General Sir Frederick Stopford, commenced the landing at Suvla Bay early on 6 August. Leading the assault were the 10th and 11th Divisions of the New Army. A few days later, they were joined by the 53rd (Welsh) and the 54th (East Anglian) Territorial Divisions. Each division had its own complement of medical services. Initially, the 14th CCS and the 26th CCS were provided, followed by the 53rd CCS. Against what was considered to be a weak Turkish force, the objective at Suvla Bay was to advance, establish a base and capture the Tekke Tepe high ground, some four miles inland, in an attempt to turn the Turkish flank on the Sari Bair Ridge.

As part of the August Offensive, the Suvla Bay landing is regarded as being very poorly managed and resulted in chaos and confusion that contributed so much to its ultimate failure to achieve its objectives. In particular, the very poor arrangements for medical services transport from the shores of Britain to the Gallipoli Peninsula were to have a long-term damaging effect on the efficiency of the medical services throughout their stay on the peninsula. During embarkation of the forces in England, there had been an unfortunate mix of the personnel, equipment and animals of the field ambulances depending on what ships and medical units were in the port at any particular time. Specific ships were not allocated to specific field ambulances. The ships used were of different capacity and speed, complicated further as some ships were not suitable to carry animals. This meant that the ships arrived at Alexandria at different times with diverse and sometimes unrelated cargoes. The MOs at Alexandria faced the task of searching for their particular unit's equipment amongst the already off-loaded equipment from other units that were spread out on the portside area. This resulted in ambulances finding themselves short of much-needed items of equipment during the critical days of August. In an extreme case, the equipment of the 34th Field Ambulance, 11th Division, was never found, and the RND 2nd Field Ambulance was hurriedly called in as a replacement.

The ADMS of the 10th Division embarked from Liverpool on the SS *Mauritania* on 9 July.[1] He was rather cautious in stating how, to the best of his knowledge, the field ambulances were

---

1   This was the second voyage of the liner as a troopship, see Humfrey Jordan, *Mauretania: Landfalls and Departures of Twenty-five Years* (Wellingborough: Patrick Stephens, 1988), pp.178–200.

A Night of Bloodshed and Pain 201

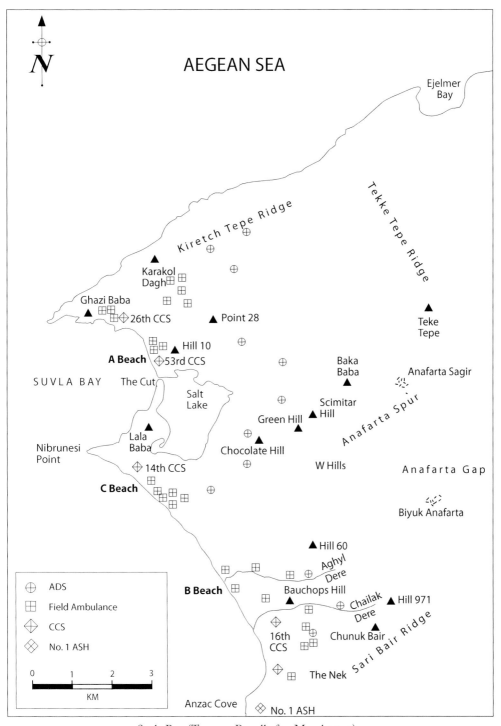

Suvla Bay. (Terrence Powell after Macpherson)

embarked. For the 30th Field Ambulance, the CO, MOs and 100 other ranks were on the SS *Transylvania*; one MO was on the SS *Georgian*; one MO was on the SS *Stetonian*; and one quartermaster and 96 other ranks, with transport, were on the SS *Melville*. The 31st Field Ambulance and the 13th CCS were on the SS *Alvania*.[2] Nevertheless, when the 31st Field Ambulance arrived at Suvla Bay, the ambulance complained that some of its equipment, placed on another ship, had not arrived. The ADMS realised that he may have made a mistake in thinking that the entire ambulance's equipment had boarded the SS *Alvania*. Subsequently, he found that a considerable amount of the equipment had actually been embarked on the SS *Hunsgate* at Devonport around 10 July, and, at the time of the landing, its whereabouts were unknown.[3]

The 10th Division's 30th Field Ambulance Tent Division, of seven officers and 72 other ranks, embarked from Alexandria at 6:30 p.m. on 6 August on the SS *Carron*. Under orders from Alexandria, vehicles were not allowed to be embarked, and only a minimum of equipment, weighing about three tons, would be allowed to be taken by the field ambulance. The medical equipment was complete except for that of B Section Bearer Subdivision, which remained at Lemnos awaiting orders.[4] The 31st Field Ambulance fared no better. It arrived at Mudros on 30 July and found itself in the midst of a diarrhoea epidemic, poor sanitation conditions, swarms of flies and a poor and limited supply of water. Nine officers and 86 men fell sick. As previously reported, they still lacked a considerable amount of equipment known to be on the SS *Hunsgate*. The ADMS then contacted Alexandria in an attempt to locate the ship.[5]

These kinds of problems were experienced by most of the other medical units preparing for the Suvla Bay landing. The 26th CCS lost a lot of its equipment when a lighter, used to offload the equipment, sank in Mudros Harbour.[6] The 1/1st Welsh Field Ambulance (WFA) was embarked on two ships, the *Euripides* and the *Wiltshire*, the latter carrying much of the transport. At Alexandria, the 1/2nd and 1/3rd WFAs were ordered to embark their transport on the *Wiltshire*. While the ambulance's personnel landed at Suvla between 9–11 August, it was 17 August before the transports were landed from the *Wiltshire*, which meant that the offensive was more or less over before these ambulances were fully equipped to carry out their work.

Whilst much is made of the relatively flat ground facing the troops at Suvla Bay as they made their landings, Robert Rhodes James walked the ground in 1962 and commented:

> The plain is scored with deep fissures, washways, unexpected ridges, the ground is coarse, thirsty and difficult. The heat is worse than at Anzac, one finds oneself gasping in the apparently airless atmosphere … it is made for defence, the innocence of the ground luring one into a maze of gullies and a climb only possible by means of winging goat tracks … this was for me was one of the major surprises of my visit.[7]

---

2   TNA: WO 95/4294: War Diary, 10th Division ADMS, 9 July.
3   TNA: WO 95/4294: War Diary, 10th Division ADMS, 7 August.
4   TNA: WO 95/4295: War Diary, 30th Field Ambulance, 6 August.
5   TNA: WO 95/4295: War Diary, 31st Field Ambulance, 30 July.
6   TNA: WO 95/4356: War Diary, 26th Casualty Clearing Station, 2 June.
7   Robert R. James, 'A Visit to Gallipoli, 1962', *Stand-To*, 9:2 (1964), p.5.

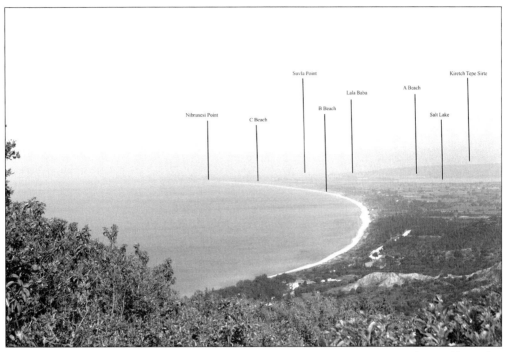

Suvla Bay as seen from Plugge's Plateau to illustrate the main areas of the landing in August. (Author)

The 32nd and 33rd Brigades of the 11th Division landed late in the evening of 6 August at B Beach. Two companies from the 6th Battalion, the Yorkshire Regiment, were able to drive the enemy off Lala Baba after suffering heavy casualties. Only two officers and about one-third of the other ranks escaped being either wounded or killed.

The landing of the 34th Brigade at A Beach was disastrous. Their destroyers anchored about 1,000yd too far south in shallow waters and on the wrong side of the channel draining the Salt Lake into the bay and known as 'The Cut'. Lighters crammed with men ran aground on the reefs and unloaded the men, who had little option but to struggle ashore, heads barely above water. They were met with heavy sniper fire and shelling, causing about 200 casualties.

Progress on 7 August was minimal. Two brigades came ashore later, and, although two hills were taken east of the Salt Lake, the limited gains had come at a cost of 1,700 casualties in the first 24 hours. The GOC IX Corps, Lieutenant General Stopford, perhaps did not make the most of his numerical superiority on 8 August, and, when he called for a pause in operations, Hamilton was unimpressed, insisting that he should push on and capture Tekke Tepe. This did not happen, and an opportunity was lost. Further fighting over the following days was unsuccessful, and, like the attacks at the Sari Bair and Helles, the August Offensive at Suvla had failed when the fighting ended on 13 August.

The field ambulances of the 11th Division landed on 6 August, closely following the infantry of that division. Over the following days, the medical units of the 10th Division and the 53rd Division, together with associated CCSs, landed with the final units arriving on 18 August. These were closely followed by those of the 29th Division, which had been transferred from

Helles on 20 August. Field ambulances were called upon immediately to tend to the wounded. It was a matter of some urgency for the tent divisions to establish themselves at suitable locations immediately and, in such places, as to be as far away as possible and sheltered from artillery and rifle fire. Bearers were sent out at once to search for casualties.

The ADMS 10th Division visited the 32nd Field Ambulance at Suvla Point on 7 August. He found the ground to be so rough, heavy and hilly that he considered it to be all but impossible for stretcher-bearers to carry patients over it in the dark. Messages were sent to the 31st and 32nd Field Ambulances to not send out stretcher-bearers during the night but to wait until daybreak.[8] The 30th Field Ambulance Tent Division landed on Suvla Beach West on 7 August but found itself without bearers and stretchers, so it was only capable of treating walking cases.[9] The CO of the 31st Field Ambulance commented that, on 7 August, there was considerable difficulty in manhandling equipment, weighing over three tons, over the rough ground. This was unfortunate, in so far as the bearers were also needed to search for, and carry in, wounded on the battlefield. The situation that arose could have been avoided since it was a direct result of the lack of wheeled transport, which had not been allowed to land with the ambulances. Despite such conditions, the bearers of this ambulance managed to locate and carry 77 casualties back to the tent division during the day.[10]

The ADMS 11th Division reported on 7 August that all field ambulances had landed on B Beach and had opened their tent divisions in positions as sheltered as possible but still found themselves under heavy shell fire during the whole day. This did not deter all the field ambulances from setting up ADSs. The bearers of the field ambulances were searching out casualties in forward positions because so many of the regimental bearers had been wounded or killed during the opening exchanges of the landing. The 35th Field Ambulance, of this division, landed at 2:30 a.m. on 7 August. At 8:00 a.m., it established a dressing station at Nibrunesi Point. During the greater part of the day, the bearer division and the dressing station were working under shrapnel fire and suffered casualties. Casualties in this area were evacuated to the 14th CCS, a few being evacuated direct by lighter to hospital ship.[11]

The 2nd Field Ambulance of the RND arrived off C Beach on 7 August. The tent division loaded its allocated lighter, which promptly took it to B Beach by mistake, but the unit began disembarking stores immediately. When the error was discovered, the lighter was reloaded and eventually arrived at C Beach, where disembarkation was finally completed. A bearer party remained at B Beach, where a shelter was hurriedly constructed, and casualties of the 33rd Brigade were treated under the direction of Surgeon Foxall of the RND.

The 14th CCS had remained at Imbros until 6 August, when it received orders to embark with only the necessary equipment. All tentage was left behind, but dressings and stretchers were embarked on the HMS *Endymion* and landed at 2:00 a.m. on 7 August at C Beach. The station immediately found itself in an extremely difficult position. Equipment and personnel had barely landed when heavy shell fire swept over the beach and continued all day. Casualties poured in, and soon the CCS was overcrowded. Both the CCS and the main dressing stations of the field ambulances were being very heavily shelled, and wounded on stretchers were being killed whilst waiting to be evacuated. Urgent action was needed to relieve this situation. The

---

8   TNA: WO 95/4294: War Diary, 10th Division ADMS, 7 August.
9   TNA: WO 95/4295: War Diary, 30th Field Ambulance, 7 August.
10   TNA: WO 95/4295: War Diary, 31st Field Ambulance, 7 August.
11   TNA: WO 95/4298: War Diary, 35th Field Ambulance, 7 August.

wounded at the main dressing stations were transferred directly to any available boat, thus saving them from shell fire and suffering from exposure in the chill August nights at Suvla Bay. There was no let up all day, and the non-stop heavy shelling made evacuation onto small boats very difficult. Despite all this, over 500 cases were evacuated. Both the 26th CCS and the 53rd CCS lay idly in the bay, watching the landing whilst awaiting orders, a fact much lamented by the field ambulance officers who were already onshore.

Although 8 August was called a 'Day of Rest' by General Stopford, for the medical services, there was to be no rest. They were keenly aware that there were still many casualties lost amidst the difficult ground between the firing line and the field ambulance and that most were certainly suffering from a lack of water. The stretcher-bearers' search for the wounded continued all day. The CO of the 31st Field Ambulance was able to report that 65 casualties had been brought in but that, as he did not have ambulance wagons, the stretcher-bearers had to carry each casualty for a distance of up to three miles over difficult terrain to the nearest CCS ready for evacuation.

John Hargrave, a bearer in the 32nd Field Ambulance who took part in the landing, described in some detail the difficulty of the search:

> Although our single-file formation allowed us to keep together, and to work methodically, it did not allow us to fan out and search for the wounded who might be lying in out-of-sight gullies or on high rock ledges and who might be too weak to cry for help. This anxiety became more distressing as ever and again in our winding progress towards the firing line we came across casualties that we had missed yesterday in our first frantic and disorganised search: men who had crawled into dells and thickets where their feeble cries of – 'stretcher-bear-e-r-s! stretcher-bear-e-r-s!' could not reach our ears … they had lain there hour after agonising hour in the blazing sun and all through the ague-shuddering dew-soaked night. Some were still alive, their wounds fly-blown. Some needing no attention except a decent burial – or at least burial – which we had no time to give.[12]

The bearers were under great physical strain, but it should be recognised that they were also under great mental strain as they dealt with so much carnage on the battlefield. There was acceptance that they were not able to rescue every single wounded man lost amongst the unforgiving terrain, and this was often difficult for medical units to accept.

The ADMS 11th Division welcomed the arrival of four ambulance wagons and mules at C Beach for the 33rd Field Ambulance on 9 August. Further good news was the improvisation of a pontoon pier erected on A Beach allowing casualties to be transferred directly to the awaiting boats. Thirty-five officers and 920 other ranks were evacuated in this way. Prior to this, it was necessary for the bearers to wade out into the water, up to two-and-a-half feet deep, carrying the casualties on their backs and then lift them onto the boats. The following day (10 August), more horse ambulance wagons and mules arrived, but these were pooled in order to keep a constant supply of wagons going between the main dressing station and the wagon park on the east shore of the Salt Lake.[13]

---

12   John Hargrave, *The Suvla Bay Landing* (London: MacDonald & Co., 1964), p.140.
13   TNA: WO 95/4298: War Diary, 11th Division ADMS, 9 August.

The 1/1st WFA was the only one of the three field ambulances of the 53rd Division that had arrived by 9 August, and it had bivouacked near The Cut in Suvla Bay. It soon placed an ADS near the north-east corner of the Salt Lake, where it came under fire, which caused a number of casualties. Unfortunately, the ambulance was short of six officers and 10 men and greatly deficient in equipment, which had been spread loaded over different ships. The result was that men landed in one place, the equipment at a different place, which inevitably resulted in much confusion and delay. It was of no help that the SS *Wiltshire* had yet to appear, loaded as it was with the 1/1st WFA's remaining personnel, some equipment and wagons, as well as the 1/2nd and the 1/3rd WFAs' equipment. The 53rd Welsh CCS remained aboard the HMT *Huntsgreen* at this time.[14]

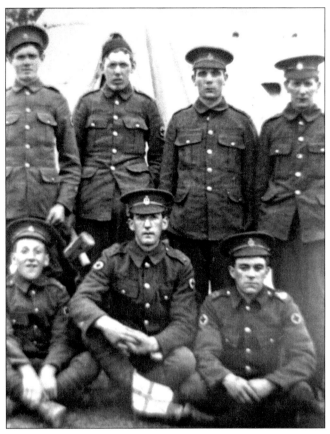

Members of the 1/1st WFA, taken during the last annual camp before the Great War started. Most of these men served in the Gallipoli Campaign. (Author)

The British attacks were resumed, but the battle of the landing at Suvla Bay effectively came to an end as part of the August Offensive, which ended in failure on 13 August.[15] However, the fighting for August was not over since, a week later, a further assault was planned to capture the hills that had been the objective of the first day at Suvla. To assist with this assault, the 29th Division was brought from Helles, and the 2nd Mounted Division arrived in the days preceding the attack from Egypt. Captain Oskar Teichman, RAMC, was the MO of the Worcester Yeomanry, which arrived at Suvla after dark on 17 August. The following day, the unit came under fire, and Captain Teichman set up the first of many dressing stations that he was to use over the next five days:

14   TNA: WO 95/4322: War Diary, 53rd Division ADMS, 9 August.
15   Officially, the Battle Nomenclature Committee refer to the landing as the 'Landing at Suvla' and give the date for the battle honour as between 6–15 August. See Anthony Baker, *Battle Honours of the British and Commonwealth Armies* (London: Ian Allen, 1986), p.305.

I established my dressing station in a little ravine between the first regiment of our Brigade and the Brigade Headquarters. From this spot the wounded were evacuated to the 2nd Mounted Brigade Field Ambulance, and from this unit they were conveyed by Mule ambulance to the beach at the extremity of Suvla Burnu. Here was situate the East Anglian Casualty Clearing Station. A steam launch towing three barges took the wounded from this point to the hospital ships in the Bay.[16]

At least from this account, it would appear that, despite the lack of success of the landing at Suvla, the medical services had been able to establish a method of working and that the lines of communication were functioning properly for the evacuation of the wounded from the battlefield.

The 2nd Mounted Division played an important part in the attack of 21 August when most of its units were engaged and suffered heavily during the crossing of open ground against the Turkish defences. On this day, Teichman reported to the ADMS of the division to be told that he was 'to carry all equipment on stretchers and make my own arrangements with regard to the wounded and that the latter would have to be carried to the beach by hand as the country to the south was too rough for mule transport'.[17] Whilst these instructions would appear to be vague, Teichman and the other MOs of the units that became engaged took their bearer parties and started off behind their regiments when the attack started:

Not a shot was fired until we had gone a quarter of a mile and were well into the plain, when suddenly we seemed to walk into an inferno of shrapnel and HE. Our first casualty was a Worcester yeoman with a spent bullet in his thigh. After that, men seemed to be dropping like flies. Finding an old Turkish trench, we made our first Aid Post, this was soon full of wounded, dressed and labelled and fairly safe, as it was deep.[18]

As the attack moved on, it was the lot of the RMO to move forwards and keep touch with the unit so that wounded could be treated:

Selecting another Aid Post in a slight depression behind a stunted oak tree we were soon busy again bringing in the wounded. It was heartrending work as so many were past hope of recovery; the proportion of killed was very great and many were quite unrecognizable. Three slightly wounded men were killed in our Aid Post as a shell burst over us. The HE caused ghastly effects as men were literally blown to pieces. My bearers worked splendidly and brought the wounded in in a perfect inferno of bursting shells.[19]

As the aid post filled up, Teichman evacuated the casualties to the nearest field ambulance, which, by this time of the attack, was also moving forwards. Once he had made sure his

---

16   Captain O. Teichman, *Diary of a Yeomanry M.O.: Egypt, Gallipoli, Palestine and Italy* (London: T. Fisher Unwin, 1921), p.20, 18 August 1915.
17   Teichman, *Diary of a Yeomanry M.O.*, p.26, 21 August 1915.
18   Teichman, *Diary of a Yeomanry M.O.*, p.27, 21 August 1915.
19   Teichman, *Diary of a Yeomanry M.O.*, p.28, 21 August 1915.

wounded were cared for, he again moved his aid post. In some areas, it was difficult to locate the wounded because of the underbrush and tall reeds: 'About this time the scrub on our right caught fire and burnt furiously. This made the immediate search for wounded very urgent. We could hear those who could not move crying for help as the flames crept up.'[20] Teichman began evacuating wounded through the 1/4th (London) Mounted Brigade Field Ambulance, and the account of the day given in its war diary corroborates the difficulties of the day:

> After marching for about 2 miles found many casualties and opened an ADS about one mile from Chocolate Hill and another East of this place. The Sergt Major and 3 OR were wounded early (all seriously). The gorse on our immediate front was blazing furiously and appeared to be coming towards the Dressing Station. The Dressing Station was therefore moved about 250 yards further back to where the 2nd Mtd Bde FA had left 50 wounded and all our wounded (about 80) were carried by the Bearers. Here many more casualties kept being brought in by our Bearers and by Regimental Stretcher Bearers and so the advance to Chocolate Hill was delayed.[21]

This ambulance alone handled 325 casualties as a result of the fighting, and this would have been similar across the attacking front, as eventually the fighting died away with little to show for it except a long casualty list and men digging in where they were to endure the Turkish shelling. This action had effectively finished the fighting of August at Suvla, and it was the final effort, on any scale, to win ground from the Turks, as the attack petered out to become trench warfare.

20 Teichman, *Diary of a Yeomanry M.O.*, p.29, 21 August 1915.
21 TNA: WO 95/4292: War Diary, 1/4th London Mounted Brigade Field Ambulance, 21 August.

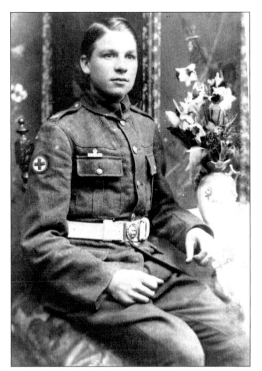

Private William 'Bill' Watkins, 1602, 1/1st WFA, landed at Suvla on 9 August and served there throughout. (Author)

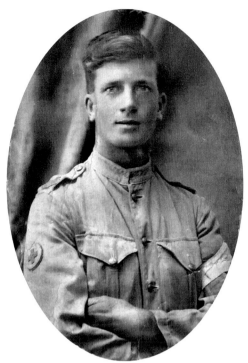

Private Samuel Powell, 1/1st WFA, landed at Suvla on 9 August. This photograph may have been taken while Powell was serving in Palestine after the Gallipoli Campaign. (Author)

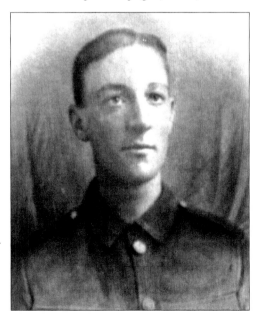

Private Walter Harris, 1700, 1/1st WFA. Harris landed at Suvla on 9 August and was killed in action the same day, becoming the first fatality of the unit. He is commemorated on the Helles Memorial. (Mrs Margaret Blackwell)

11

Only the Dead Remained in the Trenches

In support of both the Anzac breakout and the landing at Suvla Bay, a diversionary attack was planned for Helles. The was intended as an attempt to draw the attention of the Turks away from the attack by the Australians on the Sari Bair. However, the attack that took place became a rather grander scheme than the diversionary attack that had originally been intended. The plan was that an attack was to be made upon on the Krithia Vineyard in the central portion of the British lines. Once this was captured, the idea was to continue the advance and, in so doing, assist the attack made elsewhere on the peninsula. Unfortunately, the attack was an unimaginative head-on attack in much the same manner as the three previous unsuccessful battles in front of Krithia. In outline, the plan was for the 88th Brigade of the 29th Division, with support from the 1/5th Manchester Regiment, to mount an attack on the afternoon of 6 August. The following morning, the 125th and 127th Brigades of the 42nd Division were to mount their follow-up attack on the front from West Krithia Nullah to Kanli Dere. After heavy fighting, resulting in significant casualties, the battle ended in failure for the Allies on 8 August, but, over the next few days, the line around the vineyard was straightened in the face of continued Turkish efforts to prevent any work on the line. The Turkish troops were not kept fully occupied in the area as planned, and some Turkish troops actually made their way from the area to the Sari Bair as early as the second day of the attack, when Liman von Sanders recognised that there was not going to be a significant attack. Not only had the attack failed to capture the ground intended, but it had also failed as a diversionary attack.

As far as the medical services at Helles were concerned, they found themselves committed to dealing with very heavy casualties under battle conditions. The medical services were already under some pressure as a result of the high levels of sickness brought about by the adverse conditions during the months of May–July. Nevertheless, during the preparation for the attack, measures were taken to protect bearers from enemy shelling and rifle fire whilst they tended the wounded. The evacuation lines from the trenches were inspected for their suitability, and those that were considered dangerous were avoided wherever possible. If any given route considered to be dangerous could not be avoided, it was widened and deepened, if possible, to give better access and protection for the stretcher-bearers. The better access for bearers also meant that the casualties being carried out of the line suffered less jolting from hitting the sides of the trenches as the bearers attempted to move them rapidly down the line.

The 29th Division's three field ambulances established dressing stations at the Zig Zag, in Gully Ravine and at Pink Farm to support the division in that part of the line. The 42nd Division's evacuation route for casualties had been established along Kanli Dere by 1 August. However, the route along the Dere was becoming increasingly open to enemy fire, and, for the attack planned for the following week, the route was considered to be unsuitable. Inspections of the route were carried out by the medical services, and suggested were alternative routes that gave good protection from fire and, once widened, would offer a good evacuation route. From the dressing station situated on Sedd-el-Bahr–Krithia Road, the sick and wounded were carried by stretcher to the line of evacuation through Mal Tepe Dere before being transferred to ambulance wagons. On the right of the main assault, the 52nd Division's line of evacuation, from 11 August, was via the Achi Baba Nullah, Mal Tepe Dere and Skew Bridge.[1]

The battle opened at 2:40 p.m. on 6 August. Staff Sergeant Corbridge, 87th Field Ambulance, recorded:

> I counted 11 ships on the horizon, also balloon ships, the observation balloon went up at 2:35 p.m. and at 3.00 p.m. the storm burst. The ships and land artillery started and the noise of the guns and the Turks replying was deafening.
>
> The bombardment was kept up for two hours, then the Essex and Hants were to advance and charge trenches H12 and H13. Poor devils took something on, as before 11:00 pm we had 378 cases in hospital and fearful wounds at that … The moans and cries of the wounded throughout the night and particularly those wounded who had been placed on board the trawler was weird. We were kept busy all night through receiving wounded, redressing them and transferring them to a trawler for designation. The wounds from guns, hand bomb and shrapnel and close rifle fire was very bad. The Essex, Hants and Worcesters suffered very heavily, The Essex suffered 30 officers and 526 men; Hants 12 officers 406 men and the Worcesters 8 officers and 84 men. Never a wink of sleep for any of us. These figures represent up to 6am, 7th inst.[2]

Stretcher-bearers were fully occupied in a seemingly endless search for casualties. Each stretcher case was taken on an arduous and tiring journey to the field ambulance, often suffering much discomfort. The walking wounded were encouraged to make their own way out of the line to the field ambulance. The wounded continued to arrive at the field ambulances in a steady stream all the afternoon of 6 August. The ADMS 29th Division summed up the conditions in his sector:

> The attack failed and heavy casualties received – these men were all in a limited area and occurred in a short time. Walking cases began to come in at about 5pm. Extra Bearers were sent up from both 88th and 89th FA's and evacuation of the large number of casualties then went on well by Zig Zag trench until about 11pm when a bad block occurred owing to the reinforcements being sent up; and to their occupying their trench. Both Brigade HQ's were asked to get this trench clear if possible for the passage of stretchers and about 2am casualties were again got along this trench. About

---

1   TNA: WO 95/4313: War Diary, 42nd Division ADMS, 1–2 August.
2   MMM: PE/1/715/Corb.: Diary of Staff Sergeant Corbridge, 87th Field Ambulance.

212   The Fight for Life

200 cases passed down the other route i.e. by the Eastern Mule Track to the PINK FARM Dressing Station.[3]

At the 87th Field Ambulance, the CO recorded in his war diary later that day:

The wounded continued to flow all day in regular manner, 9 wagons evacuating from ADS number of 87 (2) and 88 (1). Most of the cases are up to now of a minor nature. There are few head wounds, increasingly few wounds of abdomen or chest. The most of the wounds are fairly well dressed when they arrive here but a large proportion of shell wounds which were in a dirty state. Antitetanic Serum was injected.[4]

The timely evacuation of casualties was required, but this was not without problems. The plan to triage cases such that slight cases were sent to minesweepers and serious cases to hospital ships was immediately placed under severe strain. Over 200 cases had built up at the 11th CCS on W Beach before the first trawler arrived late at 9:15 p.m. instead of 6:00 p.m. The sea swell was such that the evacuation of serious cases could not be carried out. The less serious cases, mainly walking wounded, were evacuated as a matter of necessity, and the trawler made its way to an awaiting hospital ship. The second trawler arrived at 11:00 p.m., and, as the sea was much calmer, the more serious stretcher cases were dispatched at 2:45 a.m. onto the hospital ship. The first trawler returned and cleared out all remaining cases. A third trawler arrived and evacuated the late casualty arrivals at 4:15 a.m. About 360 wounded and 50 cases of sickness were evacuated from the CCS during this period. At the end of the day, the hospital ship was full and sailed for Mudros, but it was not replaced immediately.[5] It was significant that, as a result of the shortage of stretchers, Lieutenant Wood, the embarkation officer, was sent off on the second trawler to bring back all the available empty stretchers. Unfortunately, there is no indication as to his success or otherwise.[6]

In the 42nd Division's area, the CO of the 1/1st Lowland Field Ambulance was notified of the part that his ambulance was to play:

Shortly after 0700 message from ADMS instructing me to send 100 Bearers with 25 stretches to report to Dressing Station at PINK FARM. After getting further forward to report to HQ 88th Brigade, all I could muster was 74 Bearers, These were sent off under Capt McInnes and Lt Eadie with 3 Sergeants, 36 stretchers (16 from 3rd LFA) 12 Surgical Haversacks and water bottles and 6 haversacks of Shell Dressings.

… After lunch went in direction of Pink Farm and met Bearer Party returning to Camp after having very little to do. Spoke to officer i/c of Dressing Station there. He told me that my party had turned up on their way forward but that he has had no instructions and did not know what to do with them. He directed them to HQ of 86th Brigade. While I was speaking to him Capt McInnes turned up. He informed me that he had reported to 86th Brigade HQ as directed by me. They knew nothing of

---

3   TNA: WO 95/4307: War Diary, 29th Division ADMS, 6 August.
4   TNA: WO 95/4309: War Diary, 87th Field Ambulance, 6 August.
5   TNA: WO 95/4356: War Diary, 11th Casualty Clearing Station, 6 August.
6   TNA: WO 95/4309: War Diary, 87th Field Ambulance, 6 August.

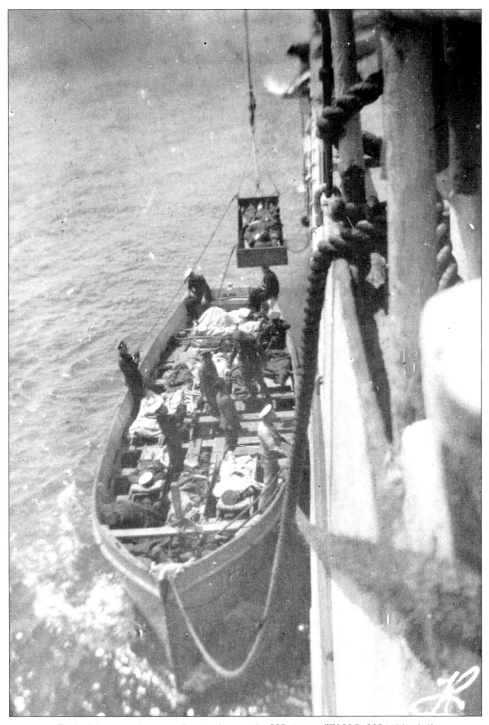

Embarking stretcher cases by winch onto the HS *Sicilia*. (TAHO: NS669/11/18)

214   The Fight for Life

his coming; but the Brigadier ordered him to the trenches to attend to wounded. Capt McInnes told him that he would require informing ADMS as the latter's instructions were not to go further forward with his Bearers to the trenches and having removed the wounded reported again to Bde HQ that only the dead remained in the trenches. The Staff officer with the Brigadier asked him 'did you not bury them?' Capt McInnes told him that was not his duty.[7]

The CO commented further, 'Some combatant officers either fail to understand or contemptuously disregard the organisation of the medical service.' Up to 9:45 p.m. on 6 August, over 214 cases of the 127th Brigade and 92 cases of the 29th Division passed through the 42nd Division's field ambulances. No congestion was reported.[8]

At the Zig Zag dressing station in Gully Ravine, on 7 August, the 89th Field Ambulance stretcher-bearers worked in between relay posts from the RAP at Twelve Tree Copse to the ADS: 'The evacuation is being very well done and in spite of the heat the men are working with tireless energy and courage. The proportion of stretcher cases is very high.'[9]

The bearers stuck to their task often in very difficult and dangerous conditions, although some difficulty was experienced identifying the relay posts in the darkness. Casualties were evacuated down the Zig Zag by horse ambulances to Gully Beach and from there by trawler to available sweeper or hospital ship according to seriousness of wounds. At the Pink Farm dressing station, a total of 211 cases were treated up to 7:00 a.m. on 7 August, and all cases were evacuated to the CCS at W Beach by 8:00 a.m. All this was done under the sole direction of one officer, Captain J. D. Fiddes, dressing every case and overseeing the evacuation process.[10]

There were also men turning up at the field ambulances with self-inflicted wounds. George Davidson, 89th Field Ambulance, 29th Division, recorded the problems of dealing with these. He was at the Zig Zag, three-quarters of a mile up Gully Ravine from Aberdeen Gully:

Today's battle, 6th August, has been a most bloody affair, wounded beginning to drop in at once. As often happens, three out of four first cases were wounds in the left hand – one a bullet through the centre of the palm, another was minus the first phalanx of his fore finger, the third minus another finger. All these were undoubtedly self-inflicted. We are bound to notify all these suspicious cases to their Commanding Officers and until a guard is sent for them we retain them under a guard of our own men. If a hand is found blackened it of course shows that it was done at very close quarters, but to avoid this a glove or bandage is applied before firing.

I was kept very busy and had no time for food during the rest of the day. The wounds were particularly severe, and very few had single wounds, many having four to six.[11]

In the midst of the heavy fighting, it was clearly a distraction to the MOs to be faced with self-inflicted wounds.

7   TNA: WO 95/4319: War Diary, 1st Lowland Field Ambulance, 6 August.
8   TNA: WO 95/4313: War Diary, 42nd Division ADMS, 6 August.
9   TNA: WO 95/4309: War Diary, 89th Field Ambulance, 7 August.
10   TNA: WO 95/4309: War Diary, 89th Field Ambulance, 25 August.
11   Davidson, *The Incomparable 29th*, location 803.

Staff Sergeant Corbridge welcomed the easing of casualties on 7 August, stating:

> Thank God the arrival of wounded is falling off a little. We have had some mental cases, pathetic sights they are with vacant stares and glassy look and partial paralyses.
>
> None of us had any rest for 40 hours but 6 bearers had to remain on duty all night to unload any wagons that may arrive. I asked for volunteers and 22 offered. That's the spirit one sees out here when it is actual duty. I got the 6 men necessary and turned in absolutely knocked up.[12]

On 7 August, the ADMS 29th Division reported that, because most of the regimental stretcher-bearers were ether killed or wounded, there was a huge build-up of wounded in the communication trenches. This, perhaps, is hardly surprising since the attack had caused heavy casualties in the 88th Brigade of the division, where almost 2,000 men had become casualties.[13] Nevertheless, these trenches were vital for the passage of reinforcements and equipment for the front line. However, with the assistance of 74 bearers of the 52nd Division and 50 bearers of the RND, complete with stretchers, the trenches were rapidly cleared. A further trench blockage occurred on the mule track on the Mal Tepe Dere line of evacuation when upcoming mules carrying supplies prevented the stretcher-bearers' clear passage.[14]

In the 29th Division, the ADMS was able to report on 8 August that, by working in conjunction with the ambulances of the 42nd Division, he was able to evacuate 648 casualties through the 87th Field Ambulance from Gully Beach entirely by trawlers. A further 268 cases were evacuated through the CCS at Lancashire Landing and 104 through the dressing stations of the 42nd Division from the extreme right flank of the division.[15]

The shortage of stretchers was a constant problem throughout the months of the campaign. The ADMS 29th Division issued an order that sufficient stretchers must be available at RAPs at the time of a major battle and that stretchers were not to be detained at the CCS, otherwise serious blockages of trenches were inevitable because casualties could not be removed. The officer commanding the CCS pointed out he had to have a sufficient number of stretchers to embark the wounded onto waiting ships. This demonstrates that the real problem was, simply, that there were insufficient stretchers available on the peninsula at any one time to cope with the casualties arising, particularly during a major engagement such as that on 6–7 August.[16]

Hamilton had called a halt to the fighting after hearing of failure of the 42nd Division on 7 August, and, consequently, there was a sharp decline in the number of wounded reaching the field ambulances over the next two days. However, severe shelling by the Turks on 11–13 August resulted in very heavy casualties amongst the forward troops involved in consolidating the positions gained. As a result of this action, the 11th CCS reported heavy firing, particularly on the night of 13 August, and large numbers of bomb wounds were admitted. A total of 38

---

12 MMM: PE/1/715/Corb.: Diary of Staff Sergeant Corbridge, 87th Field Ambulance.
13 Gillon, *Story of the 29th Division*, p.56.
14 TNA: WO 95/4307: War Diary, 29th Division ADMS, 7 August.
15 TNA: WO 95/4307: War Diary, 29th Division ADMS, 8 August.
16 TNA: WO 95/4307: War Diary, 29th Division ADMS, 8 August.

stretcher and 192 walking cases were evacuated to a sweeper sailing to Mudros. Later in the day, 19 stretcher cases and 11 walking cases were transferred to the HS *Galeka*.[17]

The particularly severe and sustained attacks by the Turks over these three days effectively saw the end of the fighting on 13 August. Hamilton was now concerned that the divisions at Helles did not attempt any further assault against the Turks since he wanted to ensure that there was sufficient strength to hold the ground that had already been won. Far from being a so-called 'minor diversion', the battle, however bravely fought by the troops and the sterling work of the medical services, ended in complete failure, and the Turks had not been distracted from the fact that there were more important actions to be fought elsewhere on the peninsula.

---

17   TNA: WO 95/4313: War Diary, 42nd Division ADMS, 11 August.

12

The Physical Condition of the Troops is Very Serious

The so-called 'holding actions' of August had all but taken the last resource of the force at Helles. As might be expected, the conditions affecting the medical services at Helles were much the same as across the rest of the peninsula. During September, the number of men reporting sick grew. There was general concern in the overall deterioration of the men's health largely caused by 'dysenteric diarrhoea' and, as the month passed, an outbreak of 'epidemic jaundice'. By the end of the month, Major A. M. McIntosh, the ADMS of the 52nd Division, was prompted to report:

> Unquestionably the troops are now not in a sufficiently sound condition to stand any severe prolonged strain. During one or two cold nights a marked rise in sickness (chiefly pyrexia) followed. An epidemic of jaundice made its appearance early in the months and has shown a rapid increase until now 15% of sickness is due to this cause. Diarrhoea or dysentery has not increased but shows no abatement as yet and constitutes 45% of sickness.[1]

These were the same issues as faced elsewhere on the peninsula and reported by other MOs, such as Major Battye of the 108th IFA at Anzac and Lieutenant Colonel Shanahan, ADMS 11th Division, at Suvla.

The sickness on the peninsula had a number of root causes. The sanitation was generally poor, and it was difficult to enforce good practices. This caused problems with flies and, in some cases, even pollution of the water supply. Whilst MOs did all they could, including appointing sanitary officers, sanitation and its control remained a significant problem into the autumn on the peninsula. The health of the troops also suffered as a direct result of their diet. At Helles, as at Anzac and Suvla, there were shortages of all kinds of foodstuffs, perhaps most notably, fresh fruit and vegetables. This brought a general deterioration in the health of the men and left them generally more susceptible to other ailments, particularly those of the gastrointestinal type. The quality of bread was often cited by MOs as directly responsible for much of the problems associated with enterica. Whilst there was enough food to keep men alive, it was not suitable to keep

---

1   TNA: WO 95/4318: War Diary, 52nd Division ADMS, 30 September.

218   The Fight for Life

them fit under the extreme conditions of the peninsula, particularly as the weather deteriorated as autumn progressed. Furthermore, when a man reported sick, there was not, in many cases, sufficient medicine or medical equipment for his care:

> From the 4th to the 11th September, we have been instructed to use quinine in all cases of severe diarrhoea. We are finding great difficulty in obtaining it at Advanced Base Medical Stores. We are getting enough to deal with a very small proportion of all cases. We found that there were no syringes for antitetanic serum available at Advanced Base Medical Stores when we indented for them over a month ago. We have daily indent marked urgent in since and we have just got two 10 cc syringes. The proper syringe is 15 cc. We found great difficulty in getting our stores of drugs replenished at first.[2]

The war diary shows that the CO of the 1/3rd Lowland Field Ambulance was feeling the problems of supply very keenly, but this was by no means a unique problem: 'We have been heavily handicapped all this month with an absolute want of chloride of lime which has been found in practise to be most valuable against flies.'[3] In the situation where the health of the troops was in a descending spiral, the inability to obtain the means to combat the problem was frustrating to the MOs. They were faced with the problems daily and could, in some cases, do little more than place a request for the equipment or medicines needed, with little or no belief that they would be sourced or delivered.

Whilst at Anzac much of the water used by the troops was brought in from outside by water tankers, at Helles, there were a number of wells that had done much to support the army in the field. However, increasing sickness during the early autumn, coupled with the knowledge that at least some of the wells were contaminated, led the ADMS of the 52nd Division to conduct a study of the water in some of the wells in his divisional area:

> Started an analysis and classification of all water in area to check and verify weekly reports sent in by MOs of units. Also, in view of reorganising the system of supplying drinking water as there appeared to be leakage in our system which allowed men, in spite of all instructions, to obtain water and not chlorinate or boil it.
>
> In our line new system is to have the best wells set aside for drinking purposes and cooking only. The inferior wells for horses only and the worst for washing only. Each drinking well to have two 400 – 500-gallon tanks so as to allow of one being in use while the other was being chlorinated. Further improved schemes on surface drainage and protection of wells were recommended.[4]

Similarly, in Gully Ravine, the wells were inspected and put under the sanitary officer, and his party, of the 42nd Division to ensure that there was no misuse of the water supply. In spite of the care taken by the MOs and sanitary officers, the ADMS of the 42nd Division asked for samples to be taken from the wells so that they could be tested for purity. However, he was not optimistic and commented, 'It is probable that the analysis of practically all the wells in the peninsula will

2   TNA: WO 95/4319: War Diary, 1/3rd Lowland Field Ambulance, 11 September.
3   TNA: WO 95/4318: War Diary, 52nd Division ADMS, 30 September.
4   TNA: WO 95/4318: War Diary, 52nd Division ADMS, 5 September.

be unsatisfactory.'[5] This officer felt that obtaining good reliable data on the potability of the water had been difficult before bacteriologists had become part of the medical services of the campaign. The effects of poor-quality drinking water had, by the end of September, become clear to just about everybody on the peninsula.

In addition to these issues, it was becoming clear to senior officers across the peninsula that there would need to be significant preparations for a winter campaign. To the MOs, the preparations were all looking to the care of the patients; as early as 8 September, Lieutenant Colonel G. H. Edington, the CO of the 1/1st Lowland Field Ambulance of the 52nd Division, was recording:

> Wrote to the ADMS regarding winter quarters, that any scheme I would suggest implied huts. If present quarters adapted as much wood needed as for huts and quarters damp and insanitary. For patients they would be out of the question. Such talk of makeshifts is futile. I cannot believe that it is impossible to procure material, at least not if the public got to know.[6]

The question of winter quarters was to become something of a major issue, for, although the Royal Engineers were involved in the design of such quarters, at every turn, there was the same supply problems.[7] Two days after the above comments were made, the 1/1st Lowland Field Ambulance was visited by Colonel Yarr, DDMS of VIII Corps, and Surgeon General Birrell, DMS MEF. Whilst both officers expressed satisfaction at the work of the hospital, when the CO raised the issue of huts, he was told that they could not be obtained.[8] No explanation was offered, but such issues were ultimately the responsibility of the home government, and many field officers on the peninsula must have felt that they had been forgotten. As if a demonstration of how much there was a need for good shelter, some days later, the CO of the 1/2nd Lowland Field Ambulance was recording in the war diary:

> A severe thunderstorm accompanied by heavy rain which actually washed us out of our dugouts which were roofless. The whole unit had to get out and seek what shelter could be got. In the dugouts the water stood a foot high. The patients had to be evacuated to the Clearing Station in a drenched conditions which was certain to be prejudicial to them.[9]

Nevertheless, there was little immediate action taken to improve the hospital conditions, and, although the MOs did all they could to care for the number of sick coming from the lines, there was nothing they could do about the inadequate shelters or the lack of supplies. A consequence of bad weather, of course, was that it was often impossible to evacuate the patients from

---

5   TNA: WO 95/4313: War Diary, 42nd Division ADMS, 23 September.
6   TNA: WO 95/4319: War Diary, 1/1st Lowland Field Ambulance, 8 September.
7   Dixon, *Vital Endeavour*, p.325.
8   TNA: WO 95/4319: War Diary, 1/1st Lowland Field Ambulance, 10 September. Note that Colonel M. T. Yarr, formerly ADMS of the 29th Division, had been appointed DDMS of VIII Corps on 4 June.
9   TNA: WO 95/4319: War Diary, 1/2nd Lowland Field Ambulance, 15 September.

hospitals that were essentially unprotected from bad weather. All these issues had a considerable impact on the general health of the men on the peninsula.

Apart from the effects of the weather on the health of the troops, there was a continuing concern on the spread of disease and the appropriate methods to tackle such diseases. A conference of SMOs was convened on 3 September to discuss these issues with Colonel L. S. Dudgeon, who was a member of the Committee for Investigation of Epidemic Diseases. The conference, held at VIII Corps HQ, concerned itself mainly with the chlorination of the drinking water supplied to the troops as a method of dealing with waterborne bacteria. This was considered important since 'The occurrence of diarrhoea and its allied disease conditions is certainly not subsiding. The cause, or causes, of these diarrhoeas etc. cannot be definitely stated without a bacteriological investigation (beyond the possibilities of the present situation) but it may safely be taken that the vast majority of these cases are due to water borne poison.'[10] The report continues with advice on treatment, storage and delivery of water so as to limit the opportunity for contamination at each stage. It also points out that the situation was unlikely to improve with additional autumn rainfall, presumably referring to the increased run-off from the battlefield further contaminating the limited water sources available at Helles. Whilst this was at least in part true, there seems to have been little recognition of the part that flies played as a vector for disease across the peninsula as a whole. This is surprising at this stage of the campaign when many officers had already identified the numbers of flies as a substantial health issue.

Efforts to improve the living conditions for the troops were made by MOs in other areas. Staff Surgeon Edward Leicester Atkinson of the RND conducted a series of experiments in early October on the effects of 'Liquid C' on the control of flies and noxious smells from decaying, unburied corpses of both men and animals in and around the battlefields. No clear indication of the composition of Liquid C is given in the war diary, but it appears to have been volatile and highly flammable, and so it may possibly have been petroleum based. Staff Surgeon Atkinson sprayed the liquid onto corpses near the front line that could not be safely reached for burial and showed that it reduced the smell and had the effect of dehydrating the corpse. The effect of 'mummification' also resulted in reducing the numbers of flies. Atkinson further tested the liquid on flies and found not only that it killed flies but also that surfaces treated with copious amounts of the liquid remained fly free for a number of days. In the effort to show its usefulness against the fly menace, the liquid was also tested on the larval stages of flies found in horse dung, but this proved to be less effective and required additional work to spread the dung thinly first to achieve best results.[11] Whilst Liquid C was thought by Atkinson to be useful in the battle against disease-spreading flies, there is no indication that it was widely adopted for such purposes. This may be partly because, by the time the tests had been completed and reported, autumn was well advanced and the fly problem had abated. There may also have been issues of supply of the liquid, and, since it was highly flammable, perhaps it was not easy to keep in forward trenches, where it would have been needed the most. Nevertheless, the experiment serves to demonstrate the lengths to which MOs were prepared to go to improve the lot not only of patients but also for the troops as a whole.

10   TNA: WO 95/429: War Diary, Royal Naval Division ADMS, report by Surgeon Arthur Gaskell, Appendix for September.
11   TNA: WO 95/429: War Diary, Royal Naval Division ADMS, Report by Staff Surgeon E. L. Atkinson, Appendix 6 for October.

Overall, the conditions did not change greatly throughout October. Weather conditions impacted upon transportation by sea between Y Beach and W Beach and consequently increased the work of already overworked bearer squads. Some supplies of timber started to arrive towards the end of October to provide roofing for winter quarters. This was generally considered to be totally inadequate, with the needs of the infantry taking priority over the support troops. It was also likely to be pilfered by men searching for firewood.

During the autumn, Colonel Yarr raised the issues of mosquitos as a concern at Helles and the cases of malaria that were appearing:

> As the *Anopheles* mosquito is being found in increasing numbers in various parts of the peninsula, please draw the attention of your Sanitary Officers to the necessity of taking the usual precautions as regards treatment of possible breeding places … it should be remembered that many cases diagnosed pyrexia on the peninsula have been found subsequently to be malarial …[12]

It appears that Colonel Yarr's memo to the ADsMS of VIII Corps had been prompted by a letter he received from Surgeon General Bedford reporting a considerable number of malaria cases turning up in the hospitals of Egypt that could only have been contracted on the peninsula. Bedford, whilst accepting that early diagnosis of malaria was difficult, suggested that all cases of fever where there was a suspicion of malaria should receive immediate treatment with quinine.[13] The *Official History of the Medical Services* records that there was a total of 1,473 cases of malaria admitted to hospital from the peninsula.[14]

On a practical note, there were also attempts to improve stretcher transportation to make matters more comfortable for the wounded while easing the work of the stretcher-bearers. A single-wheeled stretcher carriage was trialled in the 42nd Division, and the ADMS, Lieutenant Colonel T. P. Jones, reported:

> I have made a careful trial of the Single Wheeled Stretcher Carriage sent by the AOD [Army Ordnance Department] on the 14th September for trial and report. I am of the opinion that the stretcher carriage is useful for work in long communication trenches or in any road too narrow for the ordinary two-wheeled stretcher carriage. It cannot, of course, be used in a traversed trench. In addition to the saving of road space the single wheel gives it the advantage of being easily steered round stones or obstacles. The pneumatic tyre also prevents the wheel sinking into sand.
>
> It is, however, very unstable and for that reason I consider it unsuitable for a totally helpless patient as he would be likely to fall off. The legs are defective in design and the stretcher can never be allowed to stand without two men to support if. A stretcher squad of three men (as a minimum) is required to work with this carriage.[15]

---

12   TNA: WO 95/429: War Diary, Royal Naval Division ADMS, Appendix 8, 26 October.
13   TNA: WO 95/429: War Diary, Royal Naval Division ADMS, Appendix 9, October.
14   T. J. Mitchell and G. M. Smith, *Official History of the Great War: Medical Services: Casualties and Medical Statistics* (Facsimile edition of 1931 edition, Uckfeld: Naval & Military Press, n.d.), vol. 5, p.207.
15   TNA: WO 95/4313: War Diary, 42nd Division ADMS, Appendix 17, 21 September.

222   The Fight for Life

The ADMS had some concerns about the stretcher carriage but recommended that 18 such carriages should be given to each division for use in the conditions on which he reported.

A week later, the same officer was asked to report on the so-called 'blanket stretcher', 40 of which had been sent out to the 42nd Division. Lieutenant Colonel Jones ordered the 1/1st ELFA to test them in the trenches and prepare a report for him. The ADMS then reported:

> The blanket stretchers may be used by taking out poles and traverses and transporting the wounded men in the blanket until clear of the trench when the poles and traverses can be inserted, but this possesses no advantage beyond carrying in a blanket as usual and subsequent transfer to an ordinary stretcher, The blanket stretcher also has the disadvantage of being no support to keep the patient off the ground if it becomes necessary to lower the stretcher. I hear stretchers are being retained for use in Field Ambulance Tent Divisions where they make excellent beds if supported on trestles.[16]

It can be assumed from his comments that Lieutenant Colonel Jones did not consider the blanket stretchers to be an improvement on those already in use, and it does not appear that he made recommendations for their distribution amongst the forces at Helles. Clearly, moving casualties using blankets was an adopted method in the confines of the trenches, and the blanket stretcher offered little in the way of improvement over the established practices of the stretcher-bearers.

October saw the introduction of the Clayton Disinfectors at Helles. Disinfectors such as the Serbian Barrel Disinfectors and the Thresh Disinfectors had been in use across the area for some time in an effort to keep clothes, blankets and so on free from lice and other vermin. Both had been successful, but, in an effort to increase the volume of fabrics that could be disinfected, the Clayton Disinfector was added. The machine worked by blowing diluted sulphur-polyoxide gas (10–12 percent) over the material to be disinfected, which was contained in an enclosed space such as a small hut or similar. Not only was the gas effective against lice, but it was also reputed to be effective against the germs causing cholera and typhoid. It was a useful addition in the fight against vermin and bacteria, but it is not known how widespread its use was on the Gallipoli Peninsula. Pediculosis remained a problem, and this suggests that, whichever fumigation and disinfection process was used, it was not entirely satisfactory when dealing with tens of thousands of soldiers in the field.

As the autumn weather deteriorated, there were continual calls from the MOs to get improvements to shelters and prepare winter quarters: 'Present site of advanced bearer post at Geoghehan's Bluff is likely to be flooded in rainy season and also does not offer sufficient cover from fire. New site selected adjoining. Ordered to be dug in by the personnel of post.'[17] When Lieutenant Colonel Jones gave this order on 5 November, he could not have known how soon his words would prove to be true for more than just the one advanced bearer post. A little over a week later, there was a violent storm that caused damage to the beach road in front of the 1/3rd ELFA and that continued the following days, making the approach to the field ambulance impassable. The storm caused difficulties for the infantry out of the line since the shelters for them were totally inadequate – winter quarters had not been built by this stage.[18] Within days,

16   TNA: WO 95/4313: War Diary, 42nd Division ADMS, Appendix 18, 30 September.
17   TNA: WO 95/4313: War Diary, 42nd Division ADMS, 5 November.
18   TNA: WO 95/4313: War Diary, 42nd Division ADMS, 16 November.

a supply of corrugated iron for roofing had appeared in the divisional area, but the medical services did not have first call on this material since it was considered to be more important for the infantry in reserve and resting to be comfortable if at all possible. Whilst it was not ideal, at least Jones appreciated the situation. He wrote, 'Many of the men are still in their summer bivouac shelters which are quite inadequate as a protection against the cold and wet.'[19] However, this did not help him nor other MOs prepare their hospitals and dressing stations for the anticipated bad weather.

In the last week of November, a disturbing report was received by the ADMS 42nd Division from the 126th Brigade to the effect that the enemy was pumping noxious gas into the mine workings that were being advanced under their lines. The miners had, by this stage of the campaign, taken the underground war to the Turks and were generally in the ascendancy. As a response to this and to deter further activity, it appears that the Turks had resorted to boring small holes into the mine workings wherever they could, through which they then pumped a noxious gas to prevent work from continuing. Lieutenant Colonel Jones sent the DADMS and the divisional sanitary officer to inspect the workings and, if possible, collect samples of the gas for analysis. The analysis was unsuccessful because sampling had diluted the gas too much for the analytical methods available. The gas was:

> ... of an aromatic nature, irritating to the eyes and causing a certain amount of constriction and pain in the chest. The gas helmets did not protect except in so far as they protected the eyes to some degree. It does not appear to be a gas much to be feared and is obviously only of use in clearing a confined space like a mine gallery. It is comparatively innocuous when diluted with air. Although the expert could not make an analysis of the gas, he considered it to be a halogen derivative of acetic acid.[20]

Miners affected by the gas suffered from headaches and sore eyes, but these symptoms cleared after they had fresh air. The miners took a pragmatic approach and found any possible entrances and boreholes for the gas, blocked them and carried on working. Nevertheless, the threat was taken seriously, and equipment for mine rescue was asked for in case an increase in strength or use created difficulties for the miners.[21]

The work during the autumn at Helles had been hard but not because of fighting such as had gone on in the months before. Now, the force was beginning to fight with the elements as well as the enemy, and, as November neared its close, the Allies could have had no idea just how bad it could become.

19   TNA: WO 95/4313: War Diary, 42nd Division ADMS, 21 November.
20   TNA: WO 95/4313: War Diary, 42nd Division ADMS, 26 November. Note that chloroacetic acids and related halocarbons are considered hazardous substances.
21   Dixon, *Vital Endeavour*, p.354.

13

The Australians and New Zealanders Are Suffering

Following the unsuccessful offensive of August, the troops on Anzac once again fell into the routine of trench warfare, concentrating on holding the ground they had and, wherever possible, preparing for a winter campaign. The 13th BCCS was sited near to Walker's Ridge for most of its time on the peninsula, where it had arrived at the beginning of August as part of the increase in troops for the failed offensive. During much of the autumn, Lieutenant Colonel E. E. Ellery commanded the unit. The war diary kept by this officer records, on a daily basis, the numbers of soldiers evacuated as either sick or wounded. The diary also records the hospital ships to which the CCS was evacuating. From the record kept between 16 August and 14 December, it is possible to see the large disparity between those evacuated sick – a total of 5,344 – and those evacuated wounded – a total of 530 – from the same clearing station. This clearly shows the effects of disease, mostly dysentery and enteric during the early part of the autumn, amongst the troops at this period on the peninsula.[1]

With Ellery's record of the hospital ships, it is also possible to see that, between 6 September and 14 December, there was at least one hospital ship on station at Anzac most days during the autumn, the exceptions being those days when gales were affecting the shipping and hospital ships sought shelter at Lemnos or Imbros. It is also clear that the hospital ships were taking casualties from more than one CCS during their stay at Anzac. The first hospital ship recorded by Ellery was the HS *Maheno*.[2] This was a New Zealand hospital ship staffed by New Zealand MOs and nurses. Its capacity, according to the *Official History of the Medical Services*[3] was a total of 515, with a staff of 10 MOs, six nurses and 61 other ranks.[4] During its stay at Anzac, from 6–9 September, the 13th BCCS evacuated a maximum of 200 cases, suggesting that the *Maheno*, full before its departure, was taking cases from both the 1st ACCS and the 13th BCCS at the same time. However, the 1st ACCS evacuated almost 500 cases from its hospital during this period. This would suggest substantial overcrowding on the *Maheno*, but it should be remembered that a proportion of this number, mainly slightly wounded, would have been evacuated to Mudros by means of smaller vessels and fleet sweepers. The *Maheno* was replaced

---

1   TNA: WO 95/4356: War Diary, 13th Casualty Clearing Station, 16 August to 14 December 1915.
2   TNA: WO 95/4356: War Diary, 13th Casualty Clearing Station, 6 September 1915.
3   Macpherson, *History of the Great War: Medical Services*, vol. 1, p.367.
4   Note that New Zealand sources suggest a staff of only seven MOs and six nurses.

by the HS *Gascon*, staffed by MOs of the IMS and nurses of the AANS, and it remained on station until 12 September. During this period, the 13th BCCS evacuated approximately 180 cases, and the 1st ACCS evacuated a further 230 cases. This suggest that the *Gascon* embarked in excess of 400 casualties from two CCSs before it sailed. This takes no account of those who may have been evacuated from the 16th BCCS during this period. Sister Elsie Tucker, AANS, serving aboard the *Gascon*, recorded that, upon its departure from Anzac at 11:00 p.m. on 12 September, the ship was carrying 465 cases, accounting for a small number evacuated from the 16th BCCS.[5] The *Maheno* was bound for Alexandria and returned to Anzac on 17 September, while the *Gascon* sailed first to Lemnos, where all the Indian patients were disembarked for treatment, probably at the 110th IFA, along with all the diphtheria cases, who were bound for the infectious hospital there. The *Gascon* then departed for Malta, which it reached on 16 September after an 'easy trip'.[6]

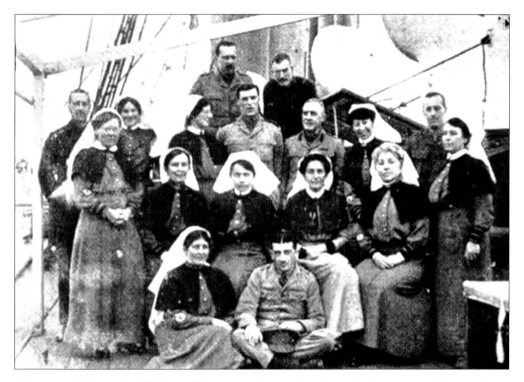

Nurses and MOs on the HS *Gascon*. The photograph was taken during the later stages of the campaign, but the ship had made many trips to collect wounded throughout. Matron Susan Wooler, QAIMNS, is seated in the second row, third from right. The other nurses are all members of the AANS. (*Tasmanian Mail*, 16 March 1916)

5   AWM: AWM41/1053: [Nurses Narratives] Sister E J Tucker.
6   AWM: AWM41/1053: [Nurses Narratives] Sister E J Tucker.

226   The Fight for Life

The arrivals and departures of the hospital ships at Anzac recorded by the 13th BCCS tend to suggest that they were never less than crowded. The HS *Assaye* arrived on station on 1 October, and, by the time it left at 8:00 p.m. on 4 October, it was carrying 650 cases.[7] The accommodation on board was for 488.[8] Like the *Gascon*, the *Assaye* first sailed to Lemnos, where 51 of the patients were disembarked, before it sailed for Malta with the remaining 599 cases. At Malta, the cases were disembarked, but the *Assaye* took on more cases and was ordered to England, where they were to receive extended treatment. This hospital ship did not return to Gallipoli until the last week of November.

In early September, there was an incident that, although not directly affecting the medical services, was recorded by a member of the AAMC who was involved, and it demonstrates the difficulty of keeping the peninsula supplied. Colonel Reginald Jeffrey Millard was a 45-year-old medical practitioner when he embarked for war with the 1st AFA as part of the first contingent in 1914. He served with that unit in Egypt and was aboard the *City of Benares*, which took it to Anzac on 25 April. Millard, then a major, was seconded to the *Derflinger*, a black ship carrying wounded back to Alexandria, and it was not until May that he landed at Anzac.[9] Later, Millard served as MO on the *Seang Bee*, another black ship that he described as very dirty and unsuitable for wounded. On this ship, he completed a trip to Alexandria and then accompanied wounded to Malta, returning to Egypt by the end of July when he was attached briefly to the 5th AFA. However, it was as part of the 5th Australian BHQ Staff that he embarked on the HMT *Southland*, bound for the peninsula on 31 August. Whilst on this voyage, he was engaged in beginning the vaccinations for cholera for the HQ staff of the brigade. This was, in part, in response to the ever-increasing number of men falling sick on the peninsula and to the very genuine fear of the effect of an outbreak of cholera amongst the already weakened men of the force. Two days into the voyage, Millard recorded, 'Definitely cooler, with a fresh head breeze, delightful after Egypt. 9.40 am. Here interrupted by a torpedo striking us on the port side in front of the bridge. A column of water shot up and all was at once excitement. Boats out – men in the water.' He recommenced his account of the events of the day at 3:40 p.m. of the same day on board the HS *Neuralia*, which had come to the aid of the *Southland*:

> There was a considerable explosion which is said to have killed two men and injured others. At once the siren blew and everyone hastened to their appointed collision stations. This meant a good deal of bustle, but no panic the men behaving most admirably. In the lowering of the boats, accidents occurred through bucking of the falls or otherwise and several men were thrown into the water, some being also hurt ... The torpedo was seen distinctly but I do not know of anyone who saw the submarine. However, one of the 4.7 guns at the stern fired at something, and even if it did not hit the submarine, possibly frightened her from giving us another torpedo. As to our steamer, she slowly made water in the forward compartments, but so slowly that there seemed no prospect of the going down suddenly under us so we of the Headquarters (Divisional) Staff having put on our lifebelts awaited developments ... About an hour

---

7   AWM: PR05050, RCDIG0001390: Transcript of Diary of Mary Ann 'Bessie' Pocock, 1914-1918 (Vol. 2), 4 October.
8   Macpherson, *History of the Great War: Medical Services*, vol. 1, p.367.
9   The *Derflinger* was a captured German passenger ship that was later renamed the *Huntsgreen*.

later we saw smoke on the horizon and at 11.40 [a.m.] this hospital ship had come alongside us. By that time another troopship and several destroyers had also hove in sight. Most of our boats that put off early had made in the direction of the island.[10] The other boats and individuals or groups of men were hovering about in the water … Presently all the boats began to gather at the *Neuralia* except the more distant which were rounded up by destroyers.[11]

Of course, there were numbers of men missing because many had entered the water almost immediately when the ship had been struck. Tragically, some died in the water before they could be rescued. According to Millard's account, the *Neuralia* rescued 433 men from the *Southland* whilst others were picked up by the other vessels that had come to its assistance. The *Southland* did not sink, and, with the help of volunteers from the Australians to act as stokers, it was sailed the roughly 30 miles to Lemnos, where it was beached and later repaired. Colonel Richard Linton, brigadier of the 6th Australian Brigade, who had been pulled out of the water, died of heart failure shortly afterwards. Millard summed up by commenting, 'In fact in every way we have cause to be thankful for our preservation'. There was every reason for this sentiment since, from over 1,400 men on board, only 32 died and eight of these were killed by the explosion. No doubt, the casualties could have been higher if ships such as the *Neuralia* had not come to the *Southland*'s assistance.

As a result of the August Offensive, there was an urgent need to make changes to the troops at Anzac. By the beginning of September, the 2nd Australian Division was completing its deployment at Anzac, and with it were three new field ambulances. The fighting to that date had depleted both the 1st Australian Division and the New Zealand and Australian Division, and the addition of fresh troops to Anzac was sorely needed and, indeed, very welcome. With the arrival of the new division, it became possible for commanders to consider the relief of tired, and often sick, troops and to get them away from the peninsula for a rest so that they could become useful to the campaign once more. To this end, Sarpi Rest Camp was set up on Lemnos, not far from Mudros and its hospitals. By the end of August, the first troops from Anzac began to arrive, and, in early September, the 1st and 2nd AFAs also moved to Lemnos, with the 3rd AFA remaining on Anzac to occupy the beach dressing station. A day or so later, the field ambulances of the New Zealand and Australian Division also left for Sarpi along with the troops of that division.

The 5th AFA arrived with its brigade on 19 August and took up position at Walden Point, near Aghyl Dere, on the left of the Anzac position by 22 August, where it set up an operating tent the same day. The unit was soon to be aware of the difficulties of working at Anzac, as its position came under fire regularly, a number of casualties occurring when one of the tents was damaged by shrapnel bullets just days after arrival. The tent was being used to treat wounded at the time, and some were hit again before they could be evacuated.

10 This is a reference to the small island of Strati, which was about six miles distant when the submarine struck.

11 AWM: 1DRL/0499, RCDIG0000181: Typescript Extracts from Diary of Sir Reginald Jeffery Millard, 2 September 1915. The *Southland* had been known as the *Vaderland* until 1915. The submarine was *U-14* which was responsible for sinking the *Royal Edward* two weeks earlier.

The 6th AFA, of the same division, arrived on Anzac on 5 September as the rest of the division arrived and was, at first, bivouacked with the 1st AFA at Brighton Beach, where, after the 1st AFA departed, it took over the hospital camp. Shortly after, the unit began to set up ADSs at Brown's Dip and Scott's Point, together with rest stations on the roads from these to the main 6th AFA. Whilst establishing the ambulance to handle the cases coming in, it was necessary for Lieutenant Colonel Hardy, CO of the 6th AFA, to issue the following instruction relating to information about casualties:

> From official inquiries regarding casualties, and such are increasing in number daily, it is evident that private information of casualties which have not been officially reported or of a contradictory nature to the official reports is furnished to relatives or friends by officers and men of the Army Corps. These unfounded reports, though doubtless made in good faith and with best intention, cause not only a vast amount of unnecessary work in inquiries and replies thereto, but needless pain to the relatives and friends of those falsely so reported.
>
> The army Corps Commander hopes that it will not be again necessary to impress on all ranks that private information of casualties must on no account be communicated until the casualties have been confirmed and officially reported to the AAG 3rd Echelon, and, that the most stringent censorship must be exercised to ensure that any such information is strictly in accordance with the official reports.[12]

The final field ambulance of the division to arrive was the 7th AFA, which reached Anzac on 13 September. The unit was ordered to Walden Point, with one section detailed to Chalk Hill, where it took over from the 4th AFA.

In a similar manner to the units of the 1st Australian Division, the units of the New Zealand and Australian Division were relieved to Sarpi Rest Camp by mid-September. All the units had been in action since the landings, and all had suffered significant losses, some battalions having no more than 300 men to answer the roll call on Lemnos. The medical units were much the same since sickness had hit them every bit as much as the front-line units. Men were tired and drawn from the months of strain of the battlefields, and, whilst Lemnos may not have had much to offer, it was not the peninsula:

> The camp was thrilled when Canadian nurses were discovered on the island. With their wonderful ways … the memory of those nurses working away in that hell-hole of Mudros should never be forgotten … these girls slaved away in Mudros hospitals and saved the lives of many New Zealanders who must have perished had it not been for the devotion of the nurses.[13]

However, for the units remaining on the peninsula, the problems stayed the same, as they fought both the Turks and the prevailing diseases that multiplied rapidly during the late summer and early autumn. The 13th BCCS recorded the number of sick patients through the hospital, and,

---

12 AWM: AWM4/26/49/1: War Diary, 6th Australian Field Ambulance, 16 September 1915.
13 Fred Waite, *The New Zealanders at Gallipoli* (Auckland: Whitcombe and Tombs, 1921), p.263.

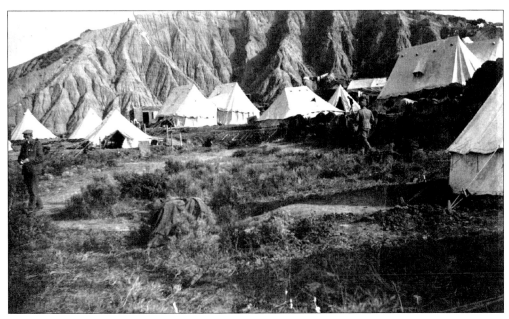
1st ALHFA near Walker's Ridge. (SLSA: B17738/10)

during these months, it was usually that about 90 percent of all cases were those suffering from diseases of one sort of another. Many of the sick were suffering from diarrhoea or dysenteric diarrhoea, which, together with enteric fever and, increasingly, epidemic jaundice, was severely depleting the fighting strength of the force on the peninsula. Private David James White arrived on the peninsula as a replacement for the 20th Battalion AIF on 31 August. Within days, he was taken ill and, on 4 September, was admitted to the HS *Neuralia* and evacuated to Mudros. He had been diagnosed, perhaps incorrectly, with influenza, but, after a brief stay at Mudros, he was once more embarked upon the *Nueralia*, suffering from dysentery, and transferred to Malta, where he died at St Andrew's Hospital on 22 September. This is perhaps an extreme case, but it indicates the problems faced by the medical staff and military commanders in maintaining the health and fitness of the troops on the peninsula. It was undoubtedly clear to the COs that, following the failure of the August Offensive, there was no further likelihood of the engaged force being able to mount another substantial attack on the Turkish lines. There must have been increasing doubt whether such a depleted and sick force could even maintain its line with any prolonged defence should the Turks choose to launch an attack.

The effect of sickness on the fighting force was of especial concern when the men who had been relieved to Sarpi Rest Camp continued to fall ill. These men, it had been hoped, would be able to return to front-line duty after a short rest. The DDMS of ANZAC carried out an examination of the troops at Sarpi at the end of September and reported to Major General H. B. Walker, CO of the 1st Australian Division.[14] The report could not have been very encouraging

---

14   Colonel Neville Howse was appointed DDMS on 11 September.

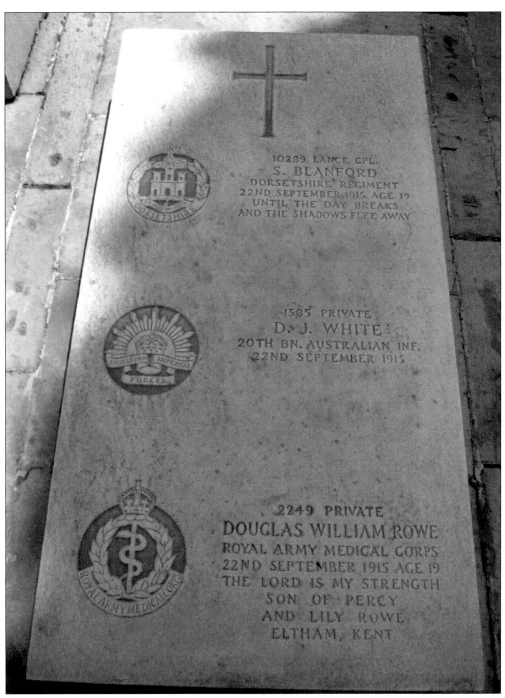

Grave of Private D. J. White at Pieta Military Cemetery, Malta. (Author)

reading for the general: 'The men, on the whole, show definite evidence of improvement in their general condition, but many are still very weak and listless and many also have very bad teeth and would soon become casualties from sickness due to their condition as soon as placed upon a biscuit diet.'[15] Thus, a month after the division had been relieved, the men were still unfit for front-line duty. The DDMS went on:

> With a view to giving some indication of the varying state of the men's health I have classified them under the headings X, Y and Z in the attached list. The X class should be fit to return after a rest of four (4) weeks, the Y class are not likely to be fit with less than eight (8) weeks, while the Z class are likely to be more or less permanently unfit for the front line owing to their suffering from definite pathological lesions. I have included in the Y class many men whose teeth are in a very bad state requiring work which could not be completed in less than eight weeks, if, however, dental attention can be provided at Anzac as well as increased at Mudros, the number of the Y class could be considerably reduced. It is, of course, impossible to predict the state of health of troops even a few weeks ahead and my report has been accordingly guarded.[16]

The DDMS then recorded on a unit-by-unit basis the number of men in each class. The report was based on the examination of 3,263 men of the 1st Australian Division at Sarpi. The DDMS classed 1,609 men as being of X class, ready to return to duty after a further four weeks of rest, 1,604 men as being Y class and 50 as Z class. That is, the best-case scenario was that about 50 percent of the division would be ready for front-line service in four weeks, or after about eight weeks resting on Lemnos since they had been evacuated. It was longer before the Y class men could be considered for front-line duty. At a time when a winter campaign was being considered and some scant preparations were being made, this could not have been considered good news.

Whilst this report tends to give a very bleak picture of those men on Lemnos, two days later (6 October), the DDMS sent a report to the deputy assistant quartermaster general (DAQMG) on the prevailing conditions on Anzac itself:

1. The physical condition of the troops at Anzac is very serious. Many of them who have been here for some months, are extremely feeble, suffering from rapid pulse, shortness of breath on slight exertion, great loss of weight, anaemia and 'dysenteric diarrhoea'.

    Captain Purves-Stewart, who carefully examined many of the men on duty in the trenches, reported very unfavourably on their condition of health …

2. The condition of the troops who have only been at Anzac for a comparatively short period, shows that a very large percentage are suffering from 'dysenteric diarrhoea'. The ADMS of the 54th Division (strength of the division under 6,000) asked for invalid diets for 1,200 men on the 2nd. Of these 350 are being treated under canvas, the remainder are men either off duty or on light duty who are being treated in the lines by RMOs.

---

15   AWM: AWM4/26/14/2: War Diary, DDMS ANZAC Corps, Appendix for October 1915.
16   AWM: AWM4/26/14/2: War Diary, DDMS ANZAC Corps, Appendix for October 1915.

3. In view of the statement made to me by Surgeon General Babtie VC that it is now proved that about 60% of the so called 'dysenteric diarrhoea' are really cases of amoebic dysentery. It is unlikely that many of these cases will be fit for duty under a period of at least two or three months under favourable conditions, and one cannot expect any decrease of this disease with the onset of cold weather. At present efforts are being made to patch up hundreds of men who are being treated by RMO's in the lines. This is possible under the present climatic conditions, but nearly all these cases will have to be evacuated on the onset of bad weather. Another serious difficulty in treating such a number of cases is the supply of medical comforts. I have this day asked for 3,000 invalid diets daily.[17]

This was a further bleak report by the DDMS. The 54th Division had arrived at the beginning of August and, in just two months, had been severely depleted by the fighting and subsequently by the diseases of the peninsula. The other divisions at Anzac, and indeed elsewhere on the peninsula, were not dissimilar. In this report, the DDMS also requested the use of hutting to provide cover for the seriously ill, pointing out the likelihood of bad weather as winter approached. He finished by saying, 'Even under the most favourable conditions, I view, with great apprehension the approaching winter owing to the weak state of the men.'[18] Unfortunately, little was done to prepare the force on the peninsula for the winter, and, consequently, men were forced to endure increasingly difficult conditions.

A common feature of many of the reports and comments made by MOs in war diaries was the shortages of all kinds of stores and supplies for the comfort of the men, not only in hospitals but also those in the line. The ADMS of the 54th Division, Colonel Freeman, was not the only one to ask for medical comforts as sickness increased. Also, MOs were well aware of the generally poor diet of the troops and the effect that it was having on the general health of the force:

> Captain Rennie of this ambulance who has been doing duty with the 5th Gurkhas pending the arrival of another permanent MO has had to come back here for rest and dieting suffering from diarrhoea and vomiting.
>
> Intestinal disturbances of varying degrees are now more common throughout the brigade. The feeding since landing at Anzac on 7th instant had not been so good as it was formerly. Fresh meat has been issued only twice and no green vegetables at all. The Australians and New Zealanders are suffering even worse than we are.[19]

In the 29th Indian Brigade and the Indian Mountain Artillery Brigade, these shortages began to show themselves in the form of scurvy in the troops. The causes of scurvy and its effects upon troops had been well known for a long time before the war. Its prevention was also understood, and so it appearing in troops on the peninsula surprised and troubled the MOs:

> Today I received a telegram from GHQ MEF addressed to me as SMO Indian Brigade stating that 26 cases of scurvy had occurred among the Indian Troops and asking me for recommendations as to diet etc with a view to prophylaxis and treatment.

17 AWM: AWM4/26/14/2: War Diary, DDMS ANZAC Corps, Appendix for October 1915.
18 AWM: AWM4/26/14/2: War Diary, DDMS ANZAC Corps, Appendix for October 1915.
19 TNA: WO 95/4272: War Diary, 108th Indian Field Ambulance, 24 August.

No cases of scurvy from this brigade have come into this ambulance but as cases have occurred in the Indian Mountain Artillery Brigade, I concluded the cases must refer to that force which forms part of the 1st Australian Division and is under the Divisional ADMS.[20]

Although the MO for the 108th IFA was, at first, rather reluctant to admit to the occurrence of scurvy amongst the Indian troops, two days later, he was forced to recognise the fact:

> Today at Captain Evans's invitation I accompanied him unofficially to his hospital and saw three cases of scurvy among the men of the Indian Artillery Brigade. There could be no question as to the diagnosis. He had yesterday received a similar telegram to mine. There is no doubt that there are two main contributing causes in these cases:
>
> 1) a condition of pyorrhoea absolaris;
> 2) a constitutional condition produced by deprivation of fresh vegetables (and fresh meat?).
>
> Lime juice has been given in abundance but with no effect. It appears to have no anti-scorbutic properties. This I think is due to the lime juice issued to us being not the natural product of the lime or lemon but a purely artificial chemical compound probably of citric acid with a little flavouring. If this opinion of mine be correct, I would go further and hazard the opinion that quite possible the lime juice given so freely to the men of the Mountain Artillery has actually aggravated the condition it was meant to prevent or relieve. The citric acid without bases and natural anti-scorbutics or lime had increased the fluid to the blood leading to the intra muscular haemorrhages … I wrote to GHQ recommending an issue of fresh vegetables (which we never get), fresh potatoes (none for a fortnight), 1/2 ounce of vinegar twice a week for every man and dried fruits on alternate days (2 oz).[21]

It is particularly noticeable from Major Battye's record that the use of lime juice had little or no effect on preventing scurvy, possibly even an adverse effect. However, his request for fresh vegetables was by no means exceptional since, across the peninsula, requests of a similar nature were being made by MOs in an attempt to improve the diet and hence the health of the troops. Despite a recognition of the problem, there seems to have been little done about providing the necessary fresh vegetables for the diet, and more cases of scurvy were found amongst the Gurkhas of the brigade later in the month:

> Several cases have recently come in mostly from the 2/10th Gurkhas with swelling, painful … in the muscles of the ham calves and about the knees. They are all unilateral and most of them give a history of some slight strain or blow. These cases are exactly like the haemorrhage of scurvy, but none of the men have spongy gums or even pyorrhoea and they do not appear very ill. Captain Casey Evans tells me that

---

20 TNA: WO 95/4272: War Diary, 108th Indian Field Ambulance, 2 September.
21 TNA: WO 95/4272: War Diary, 108th Indian Field Ambulance, 4 September.

he had considerable experience of scurvy in the Abor expedition and that many cases had theses swellings alone without any gum changes. I cannot yet get fresh vegetables (received only once) or potatoes or vinegar or calcium chloride and the juice (artificial) supplied by the ASC appears to do more harm than good. I am treating these cases or have been doing so with an effervescing mixture of Potassium salts and vinegar, but the mess vinegar has now run out so the cases are being sent away to hospital ship.[22]

The question of vitamin deficiency was not confined to the cases of scurvy occurring in the Indian troops since cases of night blindness, caused by vitamin A deficiency, also started to occur along with a small number of cases of beriberi, a vitamin B1 deficiency disease. These problems were all related to the poor diet that, although frequently plentiful, was monotonous and unbalanced, leading to vitamin deficiency issues and, to some extent, gastrointestinal problems. Whilst the problem may have been recognised, it was a different matter to get anything done about it, and MOs made a point of recording various shortages, such as the CO of the 5th AFA, who made repeated comments on the lack of particular food items throughout the autumn: 'Have reported to ADMS that eggs have not been procurable since Oct 7th, corn flour since 14th and arrowroot since Oct 11th. This is serious as the majority of the sick are suffering from diarrhoea and jaundice.'[23]

In spite of the men falling sick with scurvy amongst the Indian troops, there seems to be no other cases recorded from other units serving on the peninsula. This may reflect the manner in which the records were kept by the MOs at the field ambulances. It may also have been caused by the dietary requirements of these troops or that they were not receiving an equivalent supply of fresh vegetables as the other troops. There is no evidence one way or the other. However, according to Major Battye, and mentioned above, the Indians had not been receiving sufficient good food at Anzac, and the Australians and New Zealanders were in every bit as bad condition as a result of poor diet.[24] This suggests that there was little difference in the rations supplied to the different nationalities serving at Anzac. On this basis, it would have been expected, perhaps, that scurvy would have been found amongst other troops at Anzac. It is also surprising that the *Official History of the Medical Services* records as few as seven cases of scurvy.[25] These can only be those men from the Indian brigade, which appears to have recorded considerably more cases than shown in the statistics in the *Official History*.

The 29th Indian Brigade had arrived on the peninsula with one field ambulance while a further field ambulance was established as a hospital at Mudros. The brigade had not been provided with a CCS of its own and was thus missing a link in the chain of the evacuation of wounded through the lines of communication. Initially, clearing was managed by the 108th IFA, carrying out the normal duties of a field ambulance such as providing stretcher-bearers, setting up dressing stations and so on, as well as clearing wounded that needed to be evacuated to waiting hospital ships. The latter duty obviously added to the workload of the staff of the field ambulance as they sought to care for the wounded and evacuate them to waiting ships. An attempt was made by the DDMS ANZAC in early October to regularise the situation when he gave Battye permission to use one of the CCSs existing at Anzac for clearing Indian

22   TNA: WO 95/4272: War Diary, 108th Indian Field Ambulance, 26 September.
23   AWM: AWM4/26/48/3: War Diary, 5th Australian Field Ambulance, 17 October.
24   TNA: WO 95/4272: War Diary, 108th Indian Field Ambulance, 24 August.
25   Mitchell and Smith, *Casualties and Medical Statistics*, vol. 5, p.206.

casualties.[26] However, it seems that Battye was prepared to carry the burden of the additional work, commenting that the DDMS agreed to take the daily return directly from him, that is, without passing his wounded through a CCS. Battye also pointed out that the evacuation of the Indians from the pier at North Beach was supervised by an MO from his field ambulance.[27] The problems for the IMS were compounded by the fact that there was no provision for the medical care of the Indian Mule Cart Corps, which had been on the peninsula since April:

> With Captain Casey Evans I visited the lines of the Indian Mule Cart Corps, the various units of which are scattered all along our line from Anzac on the South to No 2 Outpost on the north. There are one thousand of these men scattered over this extended area and they have come here without any adequate medical arrangements for their care having been made. There is a Sub A Surgeon attached to them, but no other medical aid provided and no hospital or detention post. Many of them have been here since May at least. Captain Carey Evans, by request, has done his best to look after them though his single section of a field ambulance provided barely adequately for the Indian Mountain Artillery Brigade when fighting was in progress.[28] Further as there has been no Casualty Clearing Station for Indians, Captain Evans has had to clear all his cases through a British Casualty Clearing Station up till now. In the winter when bad weather prevents evacuation, the British Casualty Clearing Stations will not be able to accommodate Indians. It therefore appears to be necessary to open a new temporary hospital for the reception and treatment of Indian Transport Personnel and for the clearing of Captain Evans's cases to the ship. For this purpose, it will be necessary for this hospital to be near the beach pier and central for the transport drivers. For this purpose, I have today, in consultation with Captain Evans selected a site on Walker's Ridge near Walker's Pier and near Mule Gully where our tent subdivision of 108th IFA can be opened under a British MO as an Indian Casualty Clearing Station, if the DDMS can assist with tentage and equipment.[29]

The proposal was approved by the DDMS, and work began on preparing the ground for the new hospital immediately.

As the weather became colder, the COs of the line units responded by issuing orders for an additional ration of rum to be issued to all men. This was not approved by MOs at various levels, with some going as far as suggesting, rightly, that hot drinks and soup should be provided to the troops to fight off the cold rather than an increased ration of rum. The NZFA eventually set up a stall in Chailak Dere to serve hot drinks to men moving up and down the valley, though presumably the men in the firing line still received the additional alcohol.[30] The question of the rum issue was taken to the DDMS ANZAC, and, whilst it is clear that he was in full agreement with the MOs, it does not seem that he was able to prevent the extra issue of rum.

---

26 Colonel Neville Howse was DDMS at this time, and there were three CCSs operating at Anzac, namely, the 13th and 16th BCCSs and the 1st ACCS.
27 TNA: WO 95/4272: War Diary, 108th Indian Field Ambulance, 6 October.
28 Captain Carey Evans was the MO in charge of C Section of the 137th IFA, responsible for the care of the men of the Indian Mountain Artillery Brigade.
29 TNA: WO 95/4272: War Diary, 108th Indian Field Ambulance, 13 October.
30 'Image Number 42871_635001_11844_00099', *Ancestry*, <https://www.ancestry.com/>, accessed Jan. 2021.

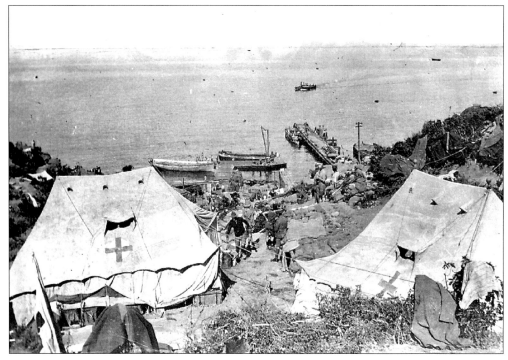
Unidentified field ambulance at Anzac Cove. Note the pier (possibly Watson's) for evacuation of casualties and blankets drying over the bushes. (SLSA: PRG 280/1/12/231)

During early November, Surgeon General Bedford inspected the troops of the 54th Division. His report to the DAG gives some details of the calibre of the soldier engaged with this division at Gallipoli:

> There are a very considerable number of immature lads in the ranks; many of these are of poor physique, and are not robust men, having been recruited from shoemakers, from men working in shops and storehouses. In a draft that joined the 4/Northants on the 8th October there were 36 out of 87 who were under 19 years of age; and one of these (according to the man's own statement) was under 16.[31]

It is hardly surprising that, with such callow youths involved on the peninsula, there were problems with both fighting strength and spread of disease. Bedford noted that there was a need for more variety in the diet but also commented that, by November, fresh meat was issued three times a week with similar issue for bread. There is no mention of the issue of vegetables at all. At this time, the 54th Division was evacuating 'twice the percentage of cases than the Anzac Corps as a whole does'.[32] Bedford gave three reasons for this: the youth of the troops in the division, the

---

31 TNA: WO 95/4324: War Diary, 54th Division ADMS, Appended letter dated 10 November 1915.
32 TNA: WO 95/4324: War Diary, 54th Division ADMS, Appended letter dated 10 November 1915.

poor class of recruit and the high incidence of diarrhoea in the division. Whilst Bedford's report is rather paternalistic, it is no doubt well-meaning, but his suggestion that footballs should be provided to form 'an abstraction and recreation' would probably have increased the casualties since any area to kick a ball was likely to have been under the Turkish guns.

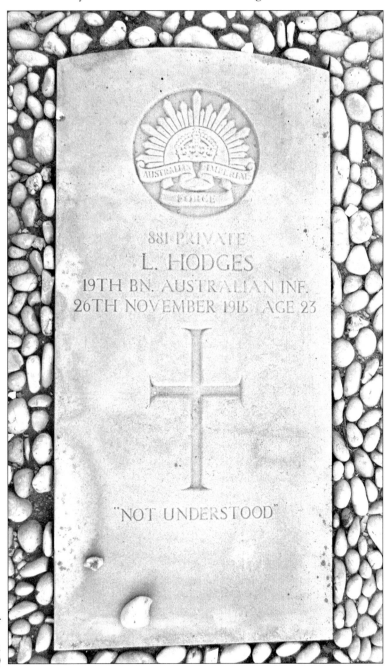

Grave of Lyle Everard Hodges, a 22-year-old blacksmith from Fairfield, New South Wales. He was wounded in action at Gallipoli on 29 October and transferred via the HS *Somali* to Gibraltar, where he died. (Author)

238   The Fight for Life

On 7 November, the ANZAC Medical Association was formed under the direction of DDMS Colonel Howse, in which the MOs of ANZAC could discuss problems and the treatments used at Anzac. The DDMS was president, with a number of SMOs, such as Major Battye, representing the IMS, acting as vice presidents:

> A discussion then took place on 'lice' and their bearing on our work etc. The reading of papers or speaking on the work of other observers and writers was forbidden; only original observations were in order. Capt Phipson MO 1/6th Gurkhas was selected among the IMS officers to speak and he gave quite the best contribution to the discussion of the day and all based entirely on his own observation. Finally, Lt Col Dudgeon, Pathologist to St Thomas's Hospital spoke and said during all his inspections the best and cleanest place was the Suez Canal Area which was run entirely by the IMS and was as near to perfection as it could be. There they are using 'Solar Oil' to combat pediculosis.[33]

The meeting two weeks later dealt with a problem that had emerged on the peninsula during the autumn, namely, epidemic jaundice, otherwise hepatitis A. Major Battye opened the discussion and concluded that the epidemic was different to that experienced by combatants in other wars and that it was not the same as Weil's disease. Whilst on the peninsula, the disease had shown itself during the autumn. The thinking of the day was that epidemic jaundice (*sensu lato*) was essentially Weil's disease and that there was no correlation to weather or season.[34] Thus, the evidence from the peninsula was contrary to the medical research of the day. Later research tended to support the findings of the ANZAC Medical Association.[35] Furthermore, 'When the great outbreak of epidemic jaundice occurred in Gallipoli in World War 1, neither the organism nor any other bacteria was found to explain the disease, and it soon became apparent that Weil's disease or leptospirosis was clinically and bacteriologically different from the predominant form of epidemic jaundice.'[36] The latter research tended to confirm that the epidemic jaundice occurring at Gallipoli in 1915 was viral hepatitis, today known as 'hepatitis A', and was distinct from Weil's disease – the conclusion reached by Battye in November 1915, based upon his observations of the sick on the peninsula.[37]

During the autumn, the staffing levels at the various medical units was to become an issue. In much the same way as illness had affected the front-line troops, it was also affecting all the support troops, including those of the medical services. This was compounded by the fact that men evacuated to Egypt were away for extended periods of time and replaced by reinforcements to the peninsula. As early as 2 October, the DDMS ANZAC was making a lengthy comment to this effect in the war diary:

33   TNA: WO 95/4272: War Diary, 108th Indian Field Ambulance, 7 November. Pediculosis is the infestation with lice.
34   S. Moritz, 'Epidemic Jaundice in War Time', *BMJ*, 2:2860 (1915), p.602.
35   Douglas Symmers, 'Epidemic Jaundice', *Journal of the American Medical Association (JAMA)*, 123:16 (1943), p.1066.
36   Samuel Mirsky, 'Epidemic Jaundice (Viral Hepatitis)', *Canadian Medical Association Journal (CMAJ)*, 70:3 (1954), pp.308–11.
37   Battye's work was a first-rate piece of observational science. It should be remembered that viruses were not identified as vectors for disease for another generation.

Lt Col Newmarch … of No 1 Australian Field Ambulance had been away from his command on sick list for about six weeks when I was informed that he had been appointed 2nd in Command of No 2 AGH Cairo, and later that he had been reported to have him appointed OC No 1 AGH Heliopolis, yet no information had been sent to ADMS of 1st Australian Division and No 1 Australian Field Ambulance had been without its senior officer for many months in fact this officer has not yet landed at Anzac. Another instance is that of Capt Brookman of No 3 Australian Field Ambulance who left Anzac early in May and I am now informed has been given an appointment in Egypt. I also pointed out that AAMC NCO's and men who had been sent from Anzac suffering from slight injury or sickness had on their recovery been detailed for other duties in Egypt. Also, the impossibility of getting MOs for Battalions. I stated that some notice ought to be taken in Egypt of requests for AAMC Reinforcements and also that officers and men might be given written orders when to report … and to return.[38]

There was also a query over the quality of men coming to the peninsula as reinforcements, not only for the AAMC but also for front-line units. In some quarters, whilst it was recognised that the recruits were willing soldiers, their physical condition was such that they were unfit for the hardships of Anzac. Added to this was the issue that, often when men returned from Egypt, they had not regained full fitness and, at least in some cases, had not received the anticipated care:

For some little time past a number of men who had returned here to duty after being in Egypt either wounded or sick have been sent back to this ambulance from their regiments as being unfit for duty. Some of them complain of pain in old wounds, some of them have bullets still in them and have never been X-rayed so they say, some have bullet fragments superficially causing pain and some have other disabilities while some are malingering.[39]

This could have done little to help the MOs on the peninsula, who were then dealing with some men who should not have been returned to active service. This was an issue for the COs of front-line battalions who wanted to see their unit maintained as a fighting force but who could not count on men returning after only slight wounds or on those who did return being suitable to carry out front-line duty:

Many old cripples absolutely unfitted for tough work required by Battalion MO at Anzac, again protested too strongly to DMS MEF upon system of selecting men for the front by Egypt and asked that the young and healthy might be ordered to leave the Flesh Pots of Egypt for Anzac … the extraordinary means adopted by Egypt you would certainly get men whose 'heart was in the right place' but probably not sound enough for hill climbing.[40]

---

38 AWM: AWM4/26/14/2: War Diary, DDMS ANZAC Corps, 2 October.
39 TNA: WO 95/4272: War Diary, 108th Indian Field Ambulance, 19 September.
40 AWM: AWM4/26/14/2: War Diary, DDMS ANZAC Corps, 6 October.

240   The Fight for Life

Anzac was always a difficult area to hold. It was always open to fire from most directions, except from the sea, and the field ambulances looked for every scrap of cover they could in which to place their hospitals and dressing stations. The CO of the 108th IFA was hit by a rifle bullet while in his dugout and was only saved from serious injury because the bullet had been deflected by a bamboo pole supporting the roof of the dugout. The bullet struck him broadside, causing no more than a contusion and grazing on the left shoulder blade.[41] Whilst he escaped serious injury, a number of ward orderlies in the same hospital at Chailak Dere were not so lucky, one being killed by a rifle bullet while working in the operating tent. In the 6th AFA, a similar incident occurred when Captain H. F. Green was killed while assisting in the operation on a wounded man.[42] Perhaps the worst incident of this kind was the shelling of the 16th BCCS on 5 December:

> No 2 Post was badly shelled with 9.2-inch, high explosive shell for about 20 minutes today commencing about noon. A considerable number of shells fell in or about the 16 CCS in which there were 280 patients about 40 of whom were stretcher cases. The first few shells fell outside the gully at No 2 Post. Then two in rapid succession fell immediately above the RAMC officers' dugouts which are placed along the north side of the CCS. Several dugouts and the RAMC officers' mess were totally destroyed. The OC at once gave orders that all wards were to be cleared and the patients directed or carried into the sap the entrance of which is about 20 yards below the west side of the clearing station. The OC had previously published in hospital and company orders instructions in detail as the how the evacuation of patients to places of safety was to be carried out during a bombardment, if such an order was given. While the patients were being removed to safety several HE shells fell into or near the CCS and did consider-able damage. The whole clearing station was full of thick smoke and shell fumes at this time and shells were bursting all round us, the fragments flying in all directions; this made the work of removing the patients to places of safety one of considerable difficulty and danger. One shell exploded in the middle of out surgical ward in which there were about 40 patients mostly stretcher cases who were being removed to safety or awaiting removal. This shell caused a number of casualties and did much damage to hospital equipment.[43]

The difficulties of identifying the casualties where large-calibre shells and HEs were used were demonstrated here since, at first, it was believed that this incident had caused four fatalities. However, the following day, it became clear that there had been a mistake:

> We discovered this afternoon that one of the men killed in the CCS yesterday had been wrongly identified as the man who was supposed to be killed was found to be alive and at the 13th CCS. The mistake arose owing to the remains of the dead man having the tally of the other man entangled in his clothing the body had been literally blown

41   TNA: WO 95/4272: War Diary, 108th Indian Field Ambulance, 28 September.
42   AWM: AWM4/26/49/3, War Diary, 6th Australian Field Ambulance, 29 November. Captain Harry Franklyn Green is commemorated in Lone Pine Cemetery, Gallipoli.
43   TNA: WO 95/4356: War Diary, 16th Casualty Clearing Station, 5 December.

to pieces and was quite unrecognisable. We at once took all possible steps to arrive at a correct conclusion as to the identity of the dead man but were unable to do so. The unidentified man had been a patient in the surgical ward and the ward master had a complete roll of all the patients who were in this ward at the time of the bombardment. A clerk was sent to the various units to which our patients had been transferred to trace all the men who had been in the surgical ward. He was able to account for all but three. All the units to which patients had been transferred had nominal rolls of the cases sent to the with the exception of the 13th CCS. Most of our cases had been received by this CCS and their nominal rolls were incomplete. The space in the 'disposal' column opposite the names of the three men we could not trace was left blank in our A36 Army Form and a note was made with it explaining the circumstances.[44]

Three tents had been blown to pieces, and, when Major Battye of the 108th IFA visited later in the day, he was to comment, there were 'bits of human flesh lying scattered about the vicinity'.[45] It is not clear if this was a deliberate act on behalf of the Turkish artillery, but, on the basis of actions elsewhere and the fact that the hospital was close to Outpost No. 2, it would seem to be very unlikely. The problem at Anzac was that every scrap of space was used for fighting men and non-combatant units. This meant that hospitals were always likely to be exposed to fire, and it is perhaps more remarkable that incidents such as that recorded above did not occur more frequently.

Whilst it has already been mentioned that the hospitals on Lemnos included two Canadian stationary hospitals, it is worth recording that they were not the only Canadian medical units to see service during the campaign. Sister Mabel Lucas was a member of No. 4 Canadian General Hospital (CGH), which had served in France before it was transferred to the Mediterranean theatre of operations. No. 4 CGH was ultimately bound for Salonika but travelled via Alexandria, where it joined the HS *Carisbrooke Castle*, which was to carry it to its final destination. The ship, with the hospital on board, departed Alexandria on 5 November and, two days later, was standing off the beaches of Gallipoli, receiving wounded and sick. Mabel Lucas recorded that the patients were '… dysentery, very sick patients, more than just wounded. We got so many, desperately sick, pitiful, so emaciated patients'.[46] After a few days offshore, the *Carisbrooke Castle* was full and left for Lemnos, where many of the patients were discharged before No. 4 CGH left for Salonika. It was the briefest contribution from No. 4 CGH in the Gallipoli Campaign, but, in taking sick off the peninsula, it had served an important function at a time when the medical services on the peninsula were stretched.

Whilst the medical services, in the normal course of events, dealt with sick and wounded, they were also called upon to give professional advice on perhaps one of the most difficult areas for them, that is, the cases of self-inflicted wounds. The war diary of the 108th IFA records an increasing number of 'self-mutilation' cases throughout the period following the August Offensive and well into the autumn:

---

44   TNA: WO 95/4356: War Diary, 16th Casualty Clearing Station, 6 December.
45   TNA: WO 95/4272: War Diary, 108th Indian Field Ambulance, 5 December.
46   John Gardam, *Seventy Years After 1914–1984* (Sittsville: Canada's Wings, 1983), p.48.

A sick Sepoy of the Burma Military Police attached to the 14th Sikhs was sent here this morning by his CO under guard. He is accused of self-mutilation. The wound certainly favours the theory. A fair number of these cases have occurred in Gallipoli and it seems a great pity that more energetic steps are not taken to put a stop to the practice.[47]

Major Battye made his opinion on the situation very clear by saying that he thought more action was needed. However, some weeks later, it was clear that there were still soldiers prepared to take this extreme action to avoid front-line duty. Yet the major also noted the limitations of the medical evidence:

After the convoy to the pier this morning had been gone some time, I received a note from the OC 1/5th Gurkhas asking me to retain one Bugler Setra Shapa suspected of self-mutilation. The man was caught and brought back from the lighter just in time. The wound on his right index finger was not characteristic and it would have been very difficult to testify definitely that the bullet must have been discharged from close range. On this evidence therefore, although other evidence against the man was very strong the case was dropped. This and other similar cases, I think, show a failure on the part of regimental officers to grasp the scope and value of medical evidence.[48]

Whilst this case was equivocal from the medical point of view, that was not to be the case for:

… a Havildar of the 97th Punjabis, attached to 14th Sikhs, came in with a wound of the right index finger evidently made by the discharge of a rifle at extremely close range and evidently self-inflicted. I reported my opinion to the OC regiment but he declined to take any action. This crime has been very frequent in the 14th Sikhs and hitherto only one man was court martialled for it and he was acquitted. Private information obtained from Sikhs in the regiment leaves no doubt as to the frequency of the crime since landing in Anzac.[49]

Battye was clearly frustrated by these cases since he was asked to provide medical evidence that was then largely ignored. Whilst the question of self-inflicted wounds was a problem for the MOs and regimental officers alike, it was something that was not readily handled, and cases continued to arrive at the hospital:

This evening in the 14th Sikhs trenches I was shown two Sikhs who had self-inflicted wounds of the left hand. One was from a revolver and is being tried for possession of the weapon which he cannot account for. In the other case the professional evidence is clear and I have given my opinion to the OC that the man ought to be court martialled.[50]

---

47   TNA: WO 95/4272: War Diary, 108th Indian Field Ambulance, 12 September.
48   TNA: WO 95/4272: War Diary, 108th Indian Field Ambulance, 10 October.
49   TNA: WO 95/4272: War Diary, 108th Indian Field Ambulance, 7 October.
50   TNA: WO 95/4272: War Diary, 108th Indian Field Ambulance, 11 November.

Perhaps the most unusual case brought to the attention of Major Battye was that brought to him on 22 November:

> Last night a rifleman of the 1/5th Gurkhas came in to hospital having clearly cut off the thumb of his left hand about the middle of the first phalanx with a kukhri while, so he states, cutting some wood with his kukhri in the dark. I made a sketch of the condition and took notes as this method of producing self-mutilation may be adopted in future as being a variation of the rifle bullet and perhaps more easy to account for. There is little doubt the thumb was removed by one clean cut.[51]

The idea of a soldier cutting firewood in the dark with a fearsome weapon such as the kukhri had clearly raised suspicions with the MO, but it again proved to be difficult to show a deliberate act rather than an accident. It did mean one less soldier on the front line. Whilst this was the last self-inflicted wound that Battye recorded, there is nothing to show that it had been stopped completely. The MO of the 108th IFA generally appears to have kept good records, and it is highly likely that such wounds were appearing in other field ambulances throughout the peninsula – they simply went unrecorded. However, Surgeon General Bedford's report of 10 November indicates that there had been 21 cases of self-inflicted injury in the 54th Division in the two months to that date.[52]

Running alongside the problem of self-inflicted wounds was also the occurrence of malingering, which Battye first reported amongst men who had been returned to duty from Egypt.[53] This seems to have been less widespread and more readily dealt with at the regimental level. Again, this problem was unlikely to have been confined to the Indian units. Even so, these were calls on the MOs' time across the peninsula, which could be scarcely afforded when there were such large challenges from the genuinely sick and wounded facing them. Whilst there may have been less fighting during the autumn, there was no reduction in the workload for the medical units on the peninsula.

51   TNA: WO 95/4272: War Diary, 108th Indian Field Ambulance, 22 November.
52   TNA: WO 95/4324: War Diary, 54th Division ADMS, Appended letter dated 10 November 1915.
53   TNA: WO 95/4272: War Diary, 108th Indian Field Ambulance, 19–20 September.

14

Men Who Had Suffered So Much

The lost opportunities of August at Suvla had brought about the trench warfare seen at both Helles and Anzac, and with it came similar problems. By the end of August, the divisions serving there together with their medical services were adapting to the environment, acclimatising to the routines of trench warfare. The medical units established ADSs, aid posts and CCSs. Whilst, by early September, there was a certain amount of organisation and routine, there were occasions that brought the difficulties for the medical services sharply into focus. At the 53rd Welsh CCS, there was an incident that demonstrated the difficulties of working alongside so many troops in an area open to the enemy:

> Morning uneventful. In afternoon two shrapnel shells burst over the Camp, wounding a Private of the 2nd Welsh FA who was at that moment in the Camp. Shells about the same time killed Capt Clark RAMC (TF) and severely wounded a Private in the 1st Welsh FA encamped near us.[1] This shelling appeared to be due to the passing of an Ambulance Wagon loaded with canvas and an ammunition cart along the road behind us. Representations were made at once to Lt Col Kelly, Beach Medical Controller, protesting against the passing of vehicles of this kind so close to the Red Cross Flag and also protesting against the passing of 'formed' parties of Infantry along the Beach just beyond our Camp and in full view of the Enemy, things which had occurred during this afternoon. Many narrow escapes of death and serious wounds occurred (as we thought) owing to carelessness on the part of combatant troops.[2]

The crowded area and the masses of troops also brought other problems, as living conditions deteriorated because of the fighting in August, the flies and bad sanitation:

> In trench warfare, sanitation is the crux of the situation from a medical point of view. Until issues in educating the officers to the value of cleanliness and the comforts resulting therefrom, I despair of success. I see improvements but they are slow in

---

1   Captain John Clark, 1/1st WFA, was killed on 9 September, aged 32, and is commemorated Hill 10 Cemetery, Gallipoli.
2   TNA: WO 95/4356: War Diary, 53rd Casualty Clearing Station (Welsh), 9 September.

formation. Another factor against continuing of policy – or rather the difficulty of carrying it out is from the emergencies of war, the officers and men who are educated in the value of cleanliness today are either killed, wounded or sick next week and a new draft arrives – young officers and soldiers generally – and the whole process must be gone over again. It is a matter of hard pegging along and worrying everybody till the desired result is obtained.

Diarrhoea is the prevailing disease and, in my opinion, this is due to flies and these latter are a pest. They are in their thousands everywhere.[3]

Although this did not bode well, efforts were being made to introduce control, such as the construction of deep latrine pits and the use of quick lime and cresol as disinfectants. By the middle of the month, sanitary squads had set up incinerators for the disposal of waste, and Thresh Disinfectors had been installed by the 1st Field Ambulance of the RND.

However, by early September, there was a firmly established route for the evacuation of sick and wounded from the ADSs through the field ambulances and to the three CCSs located around the bay on either side of The Cut to receive the wounded and sick that arrived more or less continuously. From the CCSs, the wounded were evacuated by sea in the same manner as the other beachheads, and, as at those beachheads, evacuation was dependent upon the availability of hospital ships and small boats and on good weather. Among the hospital ships serving there were the RNHS *Soudan* and the RNHS *Rewa*. Both ships had seen service in the Mediterranean theatre of operations before the landing at Suvla Bay, and their staffs were experienced at handling wounded by the autumn. The MOs of both ships were from the Royal Navy, and the nursing staffs were all members of the QARNNS. Both ships had been intended for use by casualties from the Royal Navy and the RND serving in the campaign. This had not lasted long, and the ships became available in a more general sense to take casualties from the battlefields of the peninsula.

The *Soudan* had accommodation for a total of 302 cases, but, as noted by Fleet Surgeon T. Collingwood, the ship never left its station off the peninsula without being crowded. Indeed, on the last voyage on which Collingwood was in charge, the ship departed Suvla with 472 cases on board, bound for England.[4] At one time, immediately subsequent to the Suvla landing, the ship, and others like it, had acted as a floating CCS, and large numbers of casualties passed through as slightly wounded were treated and then moved on quickly to fleet sweepers bound for Lemnos or Imbros. During the period that the *Soudan* served in the Gallipoli area, between February–December 1915, it handled no less than 12,000 cases and sailed 32,000 miles.[5]

The RNHS *Rewa* was a similar vessel and had similar accommodation for wounded. Fleet Surgeon F. J. A. Dalton, in charge, recorded the way wounded were received from the beaches, which, during the autumn, was Anzac and Suvla:

3   TNA: WO 95/4298: War Diary, 11th Division ADMS, 18 September.
4   Fleet Surgeon T. Collingwood, 'Notes on the Work of the RN Hospital Ship *Soudan* at the Dardanelles', *Journal of the Royal Naval Medical Service*, 1 (1916), p.316.
5   Fleet Surgeon T. Collingwood, 'Notes on the Work of the RN Hospital Ship *Soudan* at the Dardanelles', *Journal of the Royal Naval Medical Service*, 2 (1916), p.203.

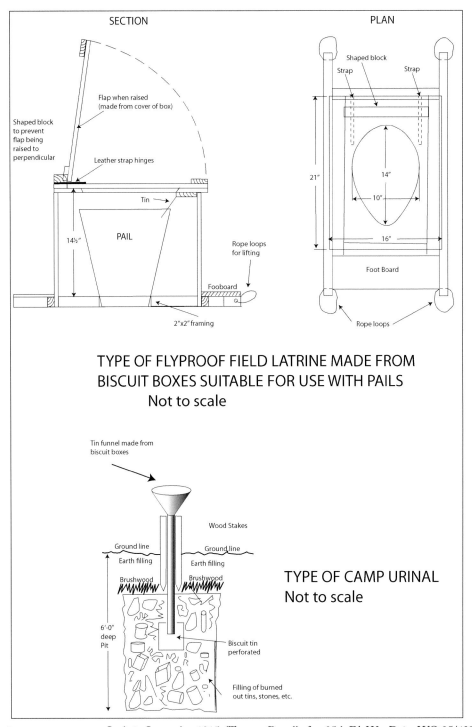

Sanitary arrangements at Suvla in September 1915. (Terence Powell after 35th FA War Dairy WO 95/4298)

… all cases from the Beach come off to the hospital ship serving that beach are sorted on board, and the lighter cases (generally wounded who can walk) are sent to an advanced base by trawlers usually stopping on board for about twelve hours, this allows time to do their dressing, get them clean and fed before passing them on to the advanced base. The more seriously wounded are retained on board the hospital ship and this process of sorting is continued until all available beds are occupied, when the ship is relieved [by] another and takes her load of wounded to one of the Mediterranean bases or home to England. The actual time at the Beach varies very much, if an attack in force is taking place, it is quite possible to have all beds full in under 24 hours, whereas to get the same number on another occasion might take a week or even longer.[6]

The work carried out by this ship was, in all probability, little different to that of any other hospital ship. However, Dalton made some interesting observations during his time in charge. Fleet Surgeon Dalton stressed that, while the MOs had preconceived ideas about certain aspects of treatment, in the end, all the treatment came down to thorough cleansing and efficient irrigating of the wounds. He also remarked that there were differences in the wounded coming off the individual beaches on the peninsula. Those men evacuated from Helles seem to have provided the most septic cases. This was believed to have been the result of the period of time that it was taking to get men evacuated from Helles resulting from the distance of the front-line trenches from the beaches. Dalton stated that evacuation could take 22–24 hours normally and, in the worst cases, as much as three days before some wounded were received on the hospital ships. It appears that wounds were consistently black with flies that soon filled the decks and wards. It was from Helles that the only cases of gas gangrene were recorded on the *Rewa*.[7]

It appears from this account that men evacuated from Anzac were the least likely to have septic wounds. Dalton believed this to have been because of the rapid removal of the wounded from nearby front-line trenches to the beaches and onto hospital ships. At Anzac, the evacuation time could be as little as five hours, and similar wounds received at Anzac did better than those received at Helles. Evacuation from the beaches of Suvla was about 10 hours, and septic wounds from this beach fell between those of Helles and Anzac.[8]

The routine of dealing with cases arriving on the *Rewa* was:

- Every patient was seen by an MO as he was hoisted onto the ship;
- Theatre cases were laid down on the deck outside a theatre to await his turn;
- Walking cases were sent to an onboard dressing station.

The *Rewa* had three operating theatres, and, in rushes, all could be working at the same time for as much as 20 hours without stopping. Temporary Surgeon John Lambert stated that the selection of cases for immediate operation '… is an important problem in the efficient running of

---

6   Fleet Surgeon F. J. A. Dalton, 'Notes on the Work of the RN Hospital Ship *Rewa* at the Dardanelles', *Journal of the Royal Naval Medical Service*, 2 (1916), p.1.
7   Dalton, 'Notes on the work of the RN Hospital Ship *Rewa*', p.2.
8   Dalton, 'Notes on the work of the RN Hospital Ship *Rewa*', p.2.

248   The Fight for Life

a hospital ship'.[9] This was largely down to the fact that batches of wounded arrived, and, as each batch was sorted, it was replaced by another, often leading to a build-up of seriously wounded requiring surgery, which in turn kept the theatres busy for long hours. In particular, compound comminuted fractures of the skull, femur or humerus were considered to need immediate attention.

Nursing Sister Hilda F. Chibnall, QARNNSR, stated that, in time of rushes of wounded, it was important to:

> … remember instead that time is short and an enormous number of men are needing attention and just do the best one can for them under more or less trying circumstances. Our chief difficulties are the endless struggle to get them properly clean and decently clothed, to combat the near collapse, exhaustion and mental shock from which many of them are suffering when they reach us – especially those from Helles Beach who have often been lying out for twenty-four or thirty-six hours without food, exposed to the sun and tormented by flies – and the hopelessness of trying to make comfortable the men who are wounded in so many different places that they can find no easy position in which to rest. They all arrive on board in the clothes they have worn for many weeks or months, these are usually quite stiff with blood and sand, alive with vermin and almost black with flies.[10]

Chibnall's approach was essentially practical. For instance, the staining caused by wounds made it impossible to use drawsheets on cots, but the nurses solved the problem by the use of 'long mackintoshes', which could be easily scrubbed clean with soap and water. This was considered particularly useful for the treatment of cases with diarrhoea. According to Chibnall, however, the most distressing cases to nurse were those with head wounds or abdominal wounds, undoubtedly because recovery rates were commonly very low. Jaw wounds created the most work for the nurses because of the difficulty and time required in feeding such patients. According to Chibnall, the *Rewa* usually departed for base carrying about 300 cot cases and over 400 walking cases. The latter often slept on the deck or in the wards in whatever space they could find. The deck cases seemed to have improved rapidly and enjoyed the fresh air. However, she stated:

> Work in the operation theatres is very different to anything we have seen before. There are two on the salon deck, each with a Sister in charge, and the largest theatre contains two tables. The patients have no previous preparation. They are carried straight to the table, and their dirty, blood-stained clothes have to be cut right off, and skin scrubbed clean before any actual surgery can begin. These duties fell to the share of the theatre attendants and the sister is left to wash and sterilize her own instruments between cases, often to scrub down the table and always do all the odd jobs.[11]

---

9   Temporary Surgeon J. Lambert, 'Two Months' Work in the Royal Navy Hospital Ship *Rewa* at the Gallipoli Beaches: By the Staff of the *Rewa*', *Journal of the Royal Naval Medical Service*, 2 (1916), p.20.
10   Nursing Sister H. F. Chibnall, in Dalton, 'Notes on the work of the RN Hospital Ship *Rewa*', p.27.
11   Chibnall, in Dalton, 'Notes on the work of the RN Hospital Ship *Rewa*', p.28.

The nurses also had to prepare dressings, and this was usually done when the ship had disembarked patients and was on the return trip to the peninsula. A stock of sterilised dressing would then be prepared in readiness for the next load of human suffering. The nurses agreed that they had 'never before nursed men who had suffered so much and complained so little, nor seen patients show so much unselfishness towards each other and gratitude to those who are nursing them'.[12]

Although it may be, as Dalton pointed out, that there were fewer septic wounds arriving from Suvla than Helles, there was little difference in the sick cases being handled by the medical services at Suvla. Diarrhoea was a continual problem, with many of the MOs believing that many of the men reaching the peninsula via Lemnos had picked up the disease in camps on the island. This may or may not be the case. Nevertheless, the field ambulances treated large numbers of cases, and efforts to organise sanitation remained uppermost in the minds of many MOs:

> Survey of area in company with the DADMS 53rd (Welsh) Division re provision of latrine areas. Plan and scheme prepared and submitted showing division of the ground with 8 separate areas together with detailed drawings of various types of fly proof latrines and shelters. Owing to lack of material this scheme has not been carried out with the exception of one Brigade who adopted it when it was found to work in a most satisfactory manner.[13]

While every effort was being made by sanitary officers, it is hardly surprising that there were insufficient materials to complete all the work in the 53rd Division and hence little real chance of preventing the casualties from disease occurring. Similar problems were faced by MOs of all the divisions serving in the area at this time.

There were changes in the Suvla force during September–October. The 10th Division left the peninsula at the beginning of October for service in Salonika, and its three field ambulances accompanied it. In the 29th Division, the 1/5th Royal Scots was withdrawn in September and replaced by the fresh and inexperienced Newfoundland Regiment.[14] Also in that division, the 87th Field Ambulance was returned to Helles for duty. Other units of the division were also reassigned, as the troops at Suvla were reorganised with a view to preparing for a winter campaign. By 3 October, the 10th Division was at Lemnos, where the sanitation required all the attention that had been afforded to that on the peninsula, and the ADMS of the division remarked:

> 3,000 blankets free from vermin were obtained from 18th Sanitary Section and issued to 29th Brigade in exchange for verminous ones. Orders issued that all men's blankets and clothes to be exposed to the sun as much as possible and that crude petroleum was to be obtained and rubbed into the seams of men's underclothing with a blunt pointed stick to kill vermin.[15]

---

12 Chibnall, in Dalton, 'Notes on the work of the RN Hospital Ship *Rewa*', p.29.
13 TNA: WO 95/4322: War Diary, 53rd Division Sanitary Section, 1 October.
14 The 1/5th Royal Scots remained at Mudros until the end of the campaign, sailing for Egypt on 7 January 1916.
15 TNA: WO 95/4294: War Diary, 10th Division ADMS, 3 October.

Four days later, the division left the Gallipoli area for service in Salonika.

The evacuation of the wounded from Suvla was recorded in some detail by Corporal John Gallishaw of the Newfoundland Regiment after he had become a casualty during the second half of October, less than two months after the regiment had landed on the peninsula. John Gallishaw was a student at Harvard University when the war started, and he immediately left to return home to Newfoundland so that he could join the Newfoundland Regiment, then being raised. At this time, Newfoundland was not part of the Federation of Canada, and so the regiment raised did not become part of the Canadian contingent that was sent to Flanders in early 1915. The regiment landed at Suvla Bay on 20 September 1915 and replaced the 1/5th Royal Scots in the 88th Brigade of the 29th Division.

After almost two months at Suvla, Corporal Gallishaw was wounded, shot by a sniper through the left shoulder while working in no man's land:

> I felt a dull thud in my left shoulder blade and a sharp pain in the region of my heart … Until I felt blood trickling down my back like warm water, it did not occur to me I had been hit. Gradually I felt my knees giving way under me, then my head dropped over on my chest, and down I went … I felt everything slipping away from me.[16]

Although he was seriously wounded, he was alert enough to prevent one of the men of his section from applying a dressing out in the open and told him instead to call for B Company stretcher-bearers. These were the regimental stretcher-bearers and not men of the medical services, and, for many of the wounded, they were the first men to respond. When they arrived, 'No women could have been more gentle or tender than those men in carrying me back to the trench … they walked at a snail's pace lest the least hurried movement might jar me and add to my pain'.[17] The bullet had torn across his back from the left shoulder to the right shoulder, but it was not until he was back in the trench and examined properly by the bearers that the extent of the wound was seen. The bearers did the best they could applying a field dressing but were then faced with the problem of getting the casualty out of the front line: 'The stretcher-bearers found that the roughly constructed trench was too narrow to allow the stretcher to turn, so they put me in a blanket and started away.'[18] The two bearers, Privates Hoddinott and Pike,[19] carried him very carefully along the difficult trench, trying not to make contact with the sides and, at the same time, keep their own feet in the muddy and slippery trench so that the journey out of the line could be as good as they could make it. The RMO attended to him in the trench and ordered the bearers to get him to a dressing station as quickly as possible. It was not until the trench widened into a good communication trench that he was transferred to a normal stretcher for the long carry to the nearest dressing station. The end of the first stage of his evacuation was the ADS: 'A great wave of loneliness swept over me when I realized that I was to see the last of the men with whom I had gone through

---

16 John Gallishaw, *Trenching at Gallipoli: The Personal Narrative of a Newfoundlander with the Ill-Fated Dardanelles Expedition* (Location unknown: Alpha Editions, 2020), p.91.
17 Gallishaw, *Trenching at Gallipoli*, p.93.
18 Gallishaw, *Trenching at Gallipoli*, p.94.
19 Private (later Sergeant) Ludwig D. Hoddinott was killed in action at Monchy le Preux on 4 April 1917.

so much. I was almost crying at the thought of leaving them there. Somehow or other it did not seem right for me to go.'[20]

The regimental bearers had been replaced by men of the RAMC to complete the journey to the dressing station, which was described as a rough shelter made of poles across supports made from sandbags. Gallishaw received immediate attention at the station, and, as the doctor worked on him, a bullet dropped from his clothes – it had passed right through his body and out of the right side. During his treatment at the dressing station, he was placed outside at his request, and, while there, he was slightly wounded a second time by the bursting of a shell in the vicinity. These wounds were also tended to at the dressing station. Shortly afterwards, he was marked to proceed to the CCS, and a motor ambulance arrived to remove him: 'Each of the motor ambulances carried four men, two above and two below … we jolted and pitched and swayed … At last, we stopped … We were at West Beach'.

He was at the CCS for only a short time, during which he was given morphine and then loaded onto a lighter to be taken to a hospital ship.[21] The morphine took effect, and, when he awoke, he found himself being hoisted onto a hospital ship. From the deck, he was loaded into a lift that took him to a ward that had been a dining salon on the ship. He was soon attended by a nurse, washed and placed in a clean bed. By that time, he was suffering intense pain and was becoming weaker. Clearly, he was not expected to survive. The nurse screened his bed, and the MO told her to attend his needs and give him anything he wanted: 'She was a woman between thirty and thirty-five, of a type that inspires confidence, every word and movement reflected poise, and there was a calmness and serenity about her that you knew she could have acquired only as a result of having seen and eased much human suffering.'[22]

The ship sailed for Alexandria, and, when the wounded were disembarked, the less seriously wounded went in an ambulance train to Cairo whilst the more seriously wounded, including Gallishaw, were sent to hospitals in Alexandria. He was sent to No. 21 BGH, where he was placed in a ward for the seriously wounded and where he remained for six weeks, slowly regaining his strength. After this time in Alexandria, he was placed on the HS *Rewa*, bound for Lemnos, where he was transhipped onto the *Aquitania*, bound for England. He eventually reached No. 3 London General Hospital at Wandsworth in December. Gallishaw was boarded some weeks later and was found to be unfit for further service, so he was discharged. It was not the end of his war service, however, for he returned to Harvard and, when the United States entered the war, he again volunteered and served with the United States Army 120th Infantry in France, reaching the rank of lieutenant. While there, he was severely gassed and was discharged once more.

For some at Suvla, even the refuge of the hospital ship was not enough after the trauma of the fighting onshore, as one incident on the *Assaye* shows: 'Left Suvla Bay at 5 am. A Pte. McDonald, Scottish Horse, went up on deck in his pyjamas, threw himself overboard. Orderly O'Brian saw him, ship went back, boat lowered, no trace of the poor fellow.'[23] Private Robert McDonald was never seen again. It is not known how he had been wounded at Suvla, but his

---

20   Gallishaw, *Trenching at Gallipoli*, p.96.
21   The CCS was probably the 25th CCS.
22   Gallishaw, *Trenching at Gallipoli*, p.104.
23   AWM: AWM PR05050, RCDIG0001394: Diary of Mary Anne 'Bessie' Pocock, May–December 1915, 22 September 1915.

252 The Fight for Life

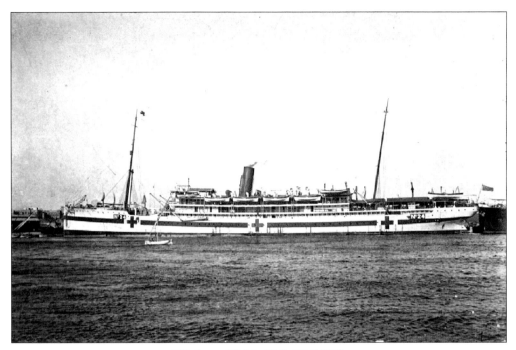

HS *Assaye*. (SLSA: SRG 435/1/282)

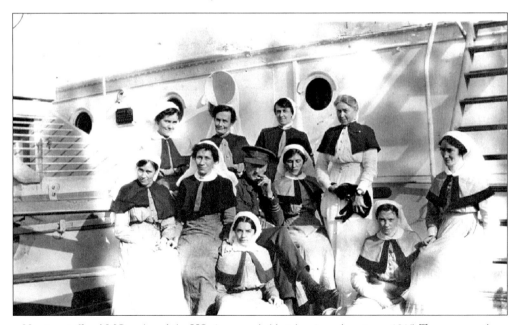

Nursing staff and MO on board the HS *Assaye*, probably taken in early autumn 1915. The nurse on the right of the back row is Matron Bessie Poccock, a veteran of the Boer War, who was in charge of the nursing care on the *Assaye* at this time. Note that the nurses are members of the QAIMNSR and the AANS. (SLSA: SRG 435/1/12)

experience had clearly left him badly traumatised, and, no doubt, he was not the only young man in that position.

The troops at Suvla began to feel the effects of the changes in the weather. There was, as at other beachheads, little or no preparation for the onset of rain and autumn storms, let alone a winter campaign. The 39th Field Ambulance, 13th Division, recorded that rain had created problems for one of its ambulance wagons crossing the Salt Lake since it had begun to soften the salty crust that had formed during the hot, dry summer months. This paled into insignificance with the experience of drivers of the 31st Field Ambulance of the 10th Division:

> Early this morning an Ambulance Wagon of 31FA was returning with 2 lying down and 3 sitting up cases from Chocolate Hill to 31FA. It was in the charge of 35798 Pte T Dickenson, RAMC; 084268 Dr GC Cooper ASC; T/4 071706 Dr W Redwood ASC; 02513 Dr K Baverstock ASC. For about 15 minutes the wagon was shelled, about 20 shells were fired. One mule was wounded and the team was unharnessed and rearranged. After proceeding a short distance more mules were wounded as patients were removed from the wagon and sent in different directions to cover. The above-mentioned men then returned to the wagon, again rearranged the mules and removed the wagon. These men have been sent to GOC, 10th Division for recognition.[24]

As mentioned earlier, there was a never-ending battle with disease and in particular with diarrhoea, which affected most of the men to a greater or lesser degree and to the prevention of which much effort was devoted:

> The main objection is to push along sanitation in the trenches and in the Reserve Areas. Diarrhoea or amoebic dysentery is a prevailing disease and newly arrived drafts are principally affected. Most, if not all, arrive complaining of this complaint. These drafts have been to Mudros for a week or more and it is there they first notice the symptoms of diarrhoea. Latrine trenches in the area occupied by the 11th Division have now been done away with. The bucket system is now everywhere established with boxes and tins but [is] still largely handicapped for the want of latrine buckets … The excreta is disposed of in deep pits. Owing to the nature of the ground these pits have in many places to be blasted through rock. These pits are covered to prevent flies getting in and disinfectants are used freely.[25]

Although a lot had been done in the attempt to improve the general condition of the troops by the improved sanitation, the fly problem persisted well into the autumn. The change in weather, with falling temperatures, tended to reduce the number of flies, but, in early October, rain was interspersed with hot days. Once again, the flies multiplied in almost ideal conditions, leading to general issues of hygiene and the spread of disease as autumn progressed. The problems with diarrhoea amongst the men of the 53rd (Welsh) Division led to an attempt to rationalise the medical services to deal with the number falling sick. The 1/1st WFA was instructed to

---

24   TNA: WO 95/4294: War Diary, 10th Division ADMS, 7 September.
25   TNA: WO 95/4298: War Diary, 11th Division ADMS, 10 October.

treat only diarrhoea cases whilst the 1/2nd WFA took all other sick cases, which, by inference, meant that the 1/3rd WFA took any wounded arising in the division during the second part of October.[26] This perhaps also indicates the impact of the disease on the force as a whole when two field ambulances of a division could be devoted to sick cases whilst only one was needed for wounded. This was further reinforced by the ADMS of the 11th Division reporting that, in spite of all efforts to improve sanitation, he did not '... think the diarrhoea is abating to any considerable extent'.[27] According to one account of the Newfoundland Regiment, recent arrivals on the peninsula, over half the regiment suffered from disease while serving there between 20 September and 8 January, when the regiment finally departed.[28] The effects of sickness were also felt by the medical services, as officers and men of those units succumbed to similar ailments as the men they treated. The CO of the 39th Field Ambulance, 29th Division, was one of the senior officers to be relieved of his duty as a result of sickness on 16 October. However, before handing over his command, he made some interesting comments concerning the service of his field ambulance during the time since it landed at Helles:

> Before handing over command of the Unit to Capt G Davidson, I wish to put on record that this Unit has received no recognition up to now of its heroic work at the Landing on 'W' beach on 25th April and succeeding days – this in spite of a forecast of rewards by the G.O.C. Division on 15th May, and repeated attempts on my part to obtain some recognition for Officers, N.C.Os. and men. This particularly appliers to the Tent Sub Division who in fulfilling their orders, landed on 'W' beach at 6.30am on April 25th, and carried on unaided for at least 24 hours, in what was practically the firing line, and were instrumental in saving many lives by their energetic work. For their magnificent work, the 1st Lancashire Fusiliers have been justly loaded with honours. Are the two Officers and 19 ORs of the Territorial Field Ambulances, who heroically supported them to be denied all recognition? Again, two officers and three N.C.Os. and 108 Bearers of this Unit were on the 'River Clyde' when this ship was beached at 'V' Beach. They did magnificent work at the capture of Sedd-el-Bahr on the 25th and 26th April and on succeeding days – this is acknowledged on all hands – but so far, the only award or recognition has been one officer, Capt. G. Davidson mentioned in despatches.[29]

In general, there would seem to have been a lack of recognition for the work that the medical services had carried out during their stay on the peninsula.

Progress on winter quarters was slow, but preparations were put in place for things such as disinfection of men's clothing, using Thresh Disinfectors, and incineration of camp waste. These methods, coupled with the cooler autumn weather, eventually reduced problems with the spread of disease, which in turn produced a general improvement in men's health, though probably it would be fair to say it still remained below where it should have been for an army in the field. The ADMS of the 11th Division reported on 31 October that the admission rates to

26 TNA: WO 95/4322: War Diary, 1/1st Welsh Field Ambulance, 14 October.
27 TNA: WO 95/4298: War Diary, 11th Division ADMS, 15 October.
28 W. D. Parsons, *Pilgrimage: A Guide to the Royal Newfoundland Regiment in World War One* (St John's: Creative Publishers, 1994), p.23.
29 TNA: WO 95/4309: War Diary, 89th Field Ambulance, 16 October.

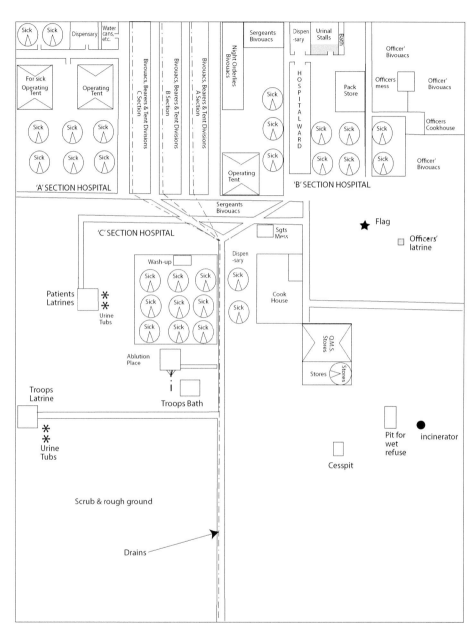

Layout of the 35th Field Ambulance at Suvla. (Terence Powell after War Diary TNA WO95/4298 November 1915)

field ambulances had fallen to between 3–3.5 percent of the division; nevertheless, of these, 85 percent of the cases were from the now familiar bowel-related issues. In conjunction with efforts to improve sanitation and changing weather, there was a big effort to vaccinate men against enteric. Some 98 percent of the men in the 29th Division had been vaccinated by the end of October. Similarly, about 90 percent of the division had been vaccinated against cholera. Whilst disease had been a problem on the peninsula almost from the beginning of the campaign, everything that the medical services could do by way of prevention was being done. Yet, despite the best efforts of the medical services, sickness remained the largest source of casualties throughout the autumn at Suvla:

> There were a great number of diarrhoea and jaundice cases. At one time the latter disease was rampant among the men and was accountable for considerable wastage. The cause of the outbreak was not traceable to any particular condition. There were only a few cases of enteric fever and paratyphoid, all of a mild type. Jaundice cases on an average were about 8 days in Hospital. Of these about 20% were returned to duty and the rest evacuated.[30]

The weather conditions, particularly high wind, became a big problem during November, as evacuation became difficult, if not impossible, on a number of days. On 3 November, the 53rd CCS was 'Unable to evacuate cases owing to adverse winds, the pontoon pier having been blown on to the shore'.[31] However, the same day, the 14th CCS noted:

> Evacuated in 3 clearings. Cleared stretcher cases in 'tea tray'. The difficulty to the Unit lately has been in the serious character of the cases not in true numbers. In order to deal with these properly some strain is thrown on the personnel. This Unit has at times to combine the functions of a CCS with those of a Stationary Hospital. The strain has not reached breaking point but it easily might after a week's non-clearing if there was much sickness combined with military activity.[32]

Other CCSs made similar entries in their war diaries.[33] This added stress to a system that was still attempting to do all possible to reduce sickness and to improve the overall conditions for the sick throughout the area, with continuous work on sanitation:

> The problem of the disposal of faeces and urine is an insistent one. We have adopted the bucket system for faeces removing them to a pit. The soil is very unsuitable for the draining away of water being 3 feet below the surface almost solid rock. Ablution benches are being set up and soakage pits and surface disposal being relied on to get rid of the sullage water.
> The warm weather has caused the appearance of flies which are the great plague of the camp. Cresol and Calcium Chloride are relied on for disinfecting the urinals

---

30 TNA: WO 95/4300: War Diary, 13th Division ADMS, 1–26 November.
31 TNA: WO 95/4356: War Diary, 53rd Casualty Clearing Station (Welsh), 3 November.
32 TNA: WO 95/4356: War Diary, 14th Casualty Clearing Station, 3 November.
33 TNA: WO 95/4356: War Diary, 14th Casualty Clearing Station, 14 November.

and latrines and down the flies to a certain extent. Many cases of jaundice continue to arrive and of late several cases of deafness. Dysentery still continues and we have had some cases of malaria apparently contracted on the Peninsula.[34]

Casualties from fighting were not great, but the Turks persisted to shell the area, and, in the crowded rear areas near the beaches, hospitals suffered as a result:

About 12.30 a British aeroplane fell into the sea near 14 CCS about 50 yards from the shore. The Turks opened fire on it with shrapnel and percussion shell. As our FA was in the line of fire and 8 shells falling short landed in our camp area, one shrapnel shell entered a Hospital Bell Tent and struck No. 1414 Pte WVH Elder of my Unit on the skull fracturing it badly at 13.00.[35] I rendered 1st Aid and removed him to the Scottish Horse FA where Capt Wade operated on him but he died at 19.00 and was buried that night. Pte Elder was one of the best of my nursing orderlies and was a keen active lad, an excellent signaller and had a clean crime sheet. The shell exploded in the sand between the legs of Driver T Fraser HMBFA [Highland Mounted Brigade Field Ambulance] a patient in the tent who escaped with his hair singed. Cpl Davidson also on duty in the tent was gassed with the fumes of the shell and sprained his left ankle. The 24 patients in the tents were removed to shelter in the Officers dugouts. There were no further casualties.[36]

Although there had been a variety of problems to deal with throughout the autumn, no one serving at Suvla could have guessed how bad things could get. Before the end of November, there were to be problems that may have had at least some bearing on the final outcome of the campaign and in which the medical services were totally involved.

34   TNA: WO 95/4301: War Diary, 40th Field Ambulance, 4 November.
35   Private W. V. H. Elder was 18 years old when he died, buried in Lala Baba Cemetery, Gallipoli.
36   TNA: WO 95/4292: War Diary, 1/1st Highland Mounted Brigade Field Ambulance, 6 November.

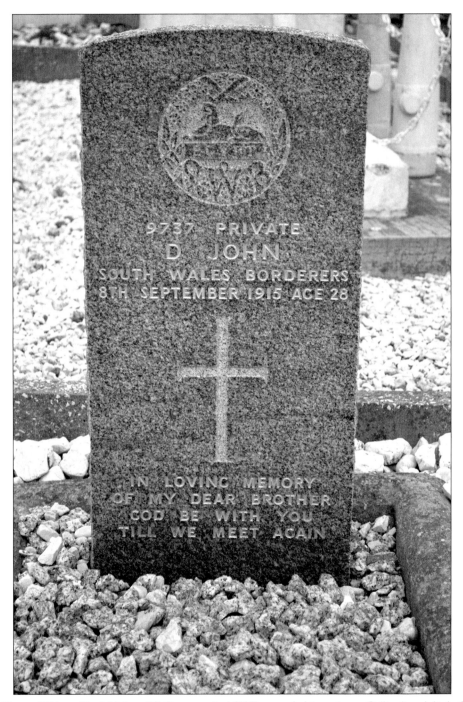

Grave of Private Daniel John of C Company 2nd SWB, wounded in action at Gallipoli and died of wounds at Gibraltar, aged 28. John was a pre-war regular from Aberaman who had joined the regiment in 1907 and had served in Tsingtao with the battalion in 1914. (Author)

15

The MO Died in His Sleep: The Storm

Preparations for a winter campaign on the peninsula commenced during the second half of August as, across the area, the COs and senior engineering officers considered the likely difficulties of surviving through the approaching winter.[1] Whilst this would seem to be a timely consideration of the problems associated with a winter campaign, the implementation of the plans under consideration was impacted by the same problems that had affected the campaign from the beginning, namely, the shortage of everything from manpower to iron sheeting for shelters. The consequence of these shortages was that little progress in providing the basic winter needs, such as shelter, was made. Waterproof, windproof shelters of timber and corrugated iron could not be built in sufficient quantities in readiness for the anticipated bad weather. This affected all parts of the force from the infantryman in the trenches to the MOs manning the CCSs on the beaches. During November, the lack of preparation for winter was to have a severe impact on the Allied forces all around the peninsula. Furthermore, the lack of comprehensive plans for things such as strong piers from which to unload stores and equipment or to evacuate wounded increased the difficulties for everyone, as engineers struggled against the worsening elements to maintain and strengthen wooden and rock-built piers at the beachheads. This was to have a direct bearing on the ability of the medical services to perform efficiently during bad weather since evacuation was frequently interrupted.

The autumn storms that had shown themselves during October continued into November. On 16 November, the peninsula was hit by heavy rain and strong winds, which caused considerable disruption. High winds were always a problem for the medical services since they meant that it was impossible to evacuate from the CCS, which resulted in overcrowding at the station and subsequently at the field ambulances and dressing stations because their casualties could not be moved further down the line of evacuation. Bad weather did not reduce the number of casualties significantly, particularly since there was a tendency for sick cases to rise as men suffered from the effects of exposure to the bad weather. Following this storm, the situation was not immediately eased, as hospital ships did not show up immediately and, even when they did, there was a shortage of small boats to assist with the evacuation of cases built up over several days. The

---

1   Winter quarters were discussed, and a design of a winter dugout was approved as early as 6 September based on discussion that had been started by the CRE, Brigadier General Roper. Dixon, *Vital Endeavour*, pp.322, 325.

108th IFA, for instance, recorded that evacuation 'took place normally' on 23 November, which allowed the ambulance to clear its patients properly for the first time since the storm had hit seven days earlier.[2] It was as well that the hospitals were able to take advantage of the respite to evacuate casualties since it was to be very short. On 26 November, 'In the evening there was a very heavy thunderstorm with torrents of rain from the SW'.[3] This was the beginning of a period of very severe weather that affected everyone on the peninsula: friend and foe alike suffered.

At Suvla, somewhat more exposed than either Anzac or Helles, conditions deteriorated rapidly as trenches quickly became ditches filled with a torrent of water. In the 11th Division, the 6th Lincolns recorded that several men drowned during the storm, as dugouts and trenches filled with water and men were washed out to sea.[4] The 7th South Staffordshires, in the same division, reported their trenches to be four feet deep in water.[5] The wall of water rushing through the trenches towards the Salt Lake and the sea swept all before it; men, animals and equipment were carried away. The men were soon soaked to the skin, and their equipment, blankets and so on were sodden in minutes. There was little in the way of shelter for thousands of men once the dugouts had been filled with water, and many simply left the trenches and drifted back towards the beaches in search of shelter. The conditions were no easier for the Turks, and they, too, left their trenches. There seems to have been very little firing as enemies faced each other in sodden misery.

The 2nd Royal Fusiliers, in the 29th Division at Suvla, recorded:

> November 26th dawned fine and so continued until about 5 pm, when it began to rain … In an hour there was a foot of water in our trenches. From the hills where the Turks lay a tremendous flood of water swept towards the Fusiliers' position … In a few minutes the face of the country had changed. Into the trenches swept a pony, a mule and three dead Turks. Several men were drowned. The communication trenches were a swirl of muddy water … The bulk of the battalion had scrambled out of the trenches and stood about on the spots which remained above water, soaked to the skin, and at least half of them without overcoats or even rifles. The moon lit up these small knots of shivering men on little banks of mud in a waste of water. Not a shot was fired on either side. The common calamity had enforced an efficient truce.[6]

At Helles, the conditions were very similar. The trenches soon became filled with water '… and forced occupants on both sides on to the parapets where they crouched unable to move for fear of falling into the trenches and being swept away by the torrents which poured down them'.[7]

For some, the violent storm was to demonstrate how fragile was their foothold on the peninsula, as the seas crashed against piers built by the Royal Engineers, often under fire, and

2   TNA: WO 95/4272: War Diary, 108th Indian Field Ambulance, 23 November 1915.
3   TNA: WO 95/4272: War Diary, 108th Indian Field Ambulance, 26 November 1915.
4   TNA: WO 95/4299: War Diary, 6th Lincolnshire Regiment, 26 November 1915.
5   TNA: WO 95/4299: War Diary, 7th South Staffordshire Regiment, 26 November 1915.
6   H. C. O'Neill, *The Royal Fusiliers in the Great War* (Facsimile edition, Uckfield: Naval & Military Press, 2002), p.106.
7   F. C. Grimwade, *The War History of the 4th Battalion, The London Regiment (Royal Fusiliers) 1914–1919* (London: HQ of the 4th London Regiment, 1922), p.98.

destroyed them and cast the wreckage of piers and lighters upon the beaches.[8] Again, all transportation by sea stopped.

There was no shelter for most of the troops at Helles, and the scant shelter of tents, tarpaulins and waterproof sheets was soon blown away. The water scoured the battlefield of the detritus of war: 'Stores, timber, equipment, bodies – some fresh some decomposed – pieces of uniform with bones protruding, floated past as the rain and shelling went on without a pause. Men were standing around soaked through, as all available shelter had been swept away.'[9] This was just the start of the storm, and it raged all through the night of 26 November and into the early morning of 27 November: 'With the dawn we were amazed at the devastation around us; it was unbelievable. In the vast quagmire hundreds of men stood stupefied and shivering in the uncanny silence.'[10]

The conditions at both Suvla and Helles were severe, and, whilst the reports from Anzac on the weather at this time are rather few and far between, the conditions there could hardly have been very different. It was perhaps fortunate in this case that the Australians held the steep sided hills of Anzac and that they had spent much of their time securing shelter from fire from more or less all directions so that, at least when the storm hit, there was some semblance of shelter against the weather. The steep slopes also helped with drainage and allowed the water to get away; nevertheless:

> … last night, the 26th, wound up with a terrific westerly gale. Golly it just blew up our gully like one thing. My roof lifted up fully an inch and a half – the whole of it – time after time and whole place fairly rocked about. Great streams of water came tearing down the gully and I thought it was 'good-bye dugout', but they just missed it. Golly, how it blew and blew.[11]

Whilst the rain had increased problems for the medical services in the increased number of men entering both field ambulances and CCSs, there is little mention of it in the Australian records. The 1st ACCS recorded that it was unable to evacuate during this period, but there is no further reference to the rain. Since this appears to be the situation across the Australian medical services, it has to be assumed that there was a different emphasis placed on the way in which their units completed the war diary.

However, whilst the rain had caused difficulty across the peninsula, the weather became much worse over the following days. On the evening of 27 November, the gale-force wind veered to the north-east, bringing with it blizzard conditions for which no one was prepared. With the snow came a rapid drop in temperatures, and soon everything was freezing hard. Once again, the troops at Suvla were hit very hard by the weather. The rain had soaked everything thoroughly, and there had been no chance to get men's clothes dried or replaced by the time the freezing conditions struck. Men stood in wet clothes in waterlogged and flooded trenches as water began to freeze about them. The 5th Dorsets, in the line at Kiretch Tepe Sirte, at Suvla,

---

8 John Ewing, *The Royal Scots 1914–1919* (Edinburgh: Oliver and Boyd, 1925), vol. 1, p.218.
9 Joseph Murray, *Gallipoli 1915* (Bristol: Cerberus, 2004), p.170.
10 Murray, *Gallipoli 1915*, p.170.
11 Sir Ronald East (ed.), *The Gallipoli Diary of Sergeant Lawrence of the Australian Engineers – 1st A.I.F. 1915* (Melbourne: Melbourne University Press, 1981), pp.115–16.

caught the full blast of the northerly blizzard and its freezing conditions: 'The plight of the men could hardly have been worse; drenched to the skin, with their kit sodden, they were completely exposed to the full fury of the blast, most of them being in poor physical condition.'[12] This was echoed by the fate of the 2/3rd London Regiment, attached to 86th Brigade and in the line on the left of the divisional sector and to the right of the line held by the 5th Dorsets. The London's lines were soon flooded completely in the storm, causing many men to be drowned. In the following freeze, the battalion suffered badly since there was no shelter and little in the way of rations. On the night of 27/28 November, the CO recorded, 'We had nothing dry of any kind, no matches, tobacco, paper, clothes. That evening it began to freeze and the night was bitter. The MO died in his sleep and two other men also.'[13] When the battalion was relieved two days later, it came out of the line 45 strong, and many of those men literally crawled away from the line 'on hands and knees'. The battalion had lost over 450 men as a result of the storm, casualties of exposure and frostbite, some drowned by the initial flood and many simply frozen to death where they stood.

The dreadful conditions persisted all night, and, on the morning of 28 November, the ADMS of the 29th Division, at Suvla, wrote:

> Snow and cold wind all last night, at time a hurricane was blowing. At 0730 I received message from General Percival, 86th Brigade, that large number of men who were absolutely dead beat were coming in to 88th and 89th main Dressing Stations. Went personally and saw the CO's of 88th and 89th Field Ambulances and 26th and 54th Casualty Clearing Stations and arranged immediate relief to go out with food, comforts, blankets, braziers etc. Motor and horse transport to go out and bring in bad cases …[14]

The prompt action by the ADMS undoubtedly helped in some cases, but, some hours later, he was becoming fully aware of the situation and the condition of the men: 'Men walking back along Gibraltar Road were hardly able to keep going owing to their utterly exhausted condition. The whole day they have been straggling back along the road in small groups of threes and fours helping one another along.'[15]

In the 53rd Welsh Division, the 1/1st WFA was recording, 'Large numbers of the Herefordshire Regiment [also 53rd Division] were brought in suffering from exposure. Stretcher squads were sent out to fetch in any (cold) casualties to be found and a number were brought into Hospital and treated.'[16]

The medical services were coming under pressure quickly as a result of the blizzard: 'Snow. Rush of cases. Four hundred and twenty-nine (429) admissions. Officers and men were soaked to the waist. Three deaths from exhaustion. 14 Casualty Clearing Station declined to receive any

---

12   Regimental History Committee [C. T. Atkinson], *History of the Dorsetshire Regiment 1914-1919. Part III: The Service Battalions* (Dorchester: Henry Ling, 1932), p.40.
13   C. B. Purdom (ed.), 'Account of Lieutenant Colonel F. W. D. Bendall', in *Everyman at War* (London: Dent & Sons, 1930), pp.290–97. The MO was Captain W. E. Rielly, RAMC. He is commemorated on the Helles Memorial.
14   TNA: WO 95/4307: War Diary, 29th Division ADMS, 28 November 1915.
15   TNA: WO 95/4307: War Diary, 29th Division ADMS, 28 November 1915.
16   TNA: WO 95/4322: War Diary, 1/1st Welsh Field Ambulance, 28 November 1915.

cases, but under great pressure took fifty (50).'[17] This clearly demonstrates the effect of the storm on the manner in which the medical services operated. Without evacuation from the CCS, it was not long before there was a backlog of cases, and, inevitably, these were to be found in the field ambulances and dressing stations – there was nowhere else they could go. The storm had the effect of preventing all movement by sea and hence preventing evacuation whilst creating a large number of men requiring care for the effects of exposure. The CO of the 14th BCCS was to point out that evacuation could be disrupted by a slight south-west breeze since that made it impossible to load the lighters from the piers on the beaches. On the other hand, he pointed out that a strong north-east did not prevent loading from the beaches but did prevent loading the hospital ships safely. This had meant that, during November, there had been 12 occasions when he was unable to evacuate cases at all, and three of these occasions occurred in the days between the evening of 26 November and 30 November. The CO also had some clear opinions on the way his CCS was forced to work at Suvla:

> Character of Unit. This is constantly changing from day to day even hour to hour. At times it is a Stationary Hospital with comparatively few in a tent, patients raised off the ground, well fed and efficiently treated. At other times this unit changes suddenly from a hospital to a dumping ground for the overflow cases from the field ambulances. This happens at times when clearing is impossible. All that we can treat them with is warmth, food and temporary shelter. At other times as in this last rush, clearing is again impossible and becomes the main factor, but owing to the large numbers constantly evacuated from the field ambulances this station is filled up immediately it is emptied, throwing a great strain on all sections (including cooking and clerical) of this unit.[18]

These conditions were exacerbated by the almost normal shortage of small ships able to carry the cases to the hospital ships standing offshore. It is worth noting that, when evacuation was again possible on 30 November, the 14th BCCS evacuated 1,480 cases to hospital ships, and these were mostly those suffering from exposure caused during the storm.[19] The 54th BCCS, also at Suvla, stated that, at 9:00 a.m. on 30 November, there were 1,081 cases in its hospital, pointing out that they were mostly cases of 'exhaustion and frostbite due to exposure'. The hospital had 26 marquees, and 30 cases were packed into each marquee, with the remainder being accommodated in makeshift wooden lean-tos 'made from sections of unbuilt huts', as it called upon all its staff, including all clerical staff and orderlies, to care for the cases coming in.[20] The lack of readiness for the conditions is clearly indicated by the use of sections of wooden huts delivered for use but, at that time, still awaiting the manpower to put them together. In an effort to provide shelter for the many cases of exposure, the cutting for the Decauville railway from West Beach was covered with tarpaulins and braziers installed to heat the makeshift shelter. Elsewhere, packing cases were used to construct shelters to get men out of the weather. Nevertheless, the large number of cases arriving at the beach almost defeated these best attempts:

17   TNA: WO 95/4322: War Diary, 1/2nd Welsh Field Ambulance, 28 November 1915.
18   TNA: WO 95/4356: War Diary, 14th Casualty Clearing Station, November 1915, Appendix III.
19   TNA: WO 95/4356: War Diary, 14th Casualty Clearing Station, 30 November 1915.
20   TNA: WO 95/4356: War Diary, 54th Casualty Clearing Station, 30 November 1915.

Intimation received at 6.30 pm yesterday that a large number of British soldiers were dying of exposure. All British hospitals full. I consented to take 50 of the worst cases. This morning at 7.30 am I received 77 cases none of whom could walk and some of whom were comatose. Hot soup and hot OXO was given to every man at once and their boots and socks and wet clothes removed. Hot chicken curry and rice was then prepared and given to every man. Every available spot in the hospital was packed and we also utilised the Mochi Khana [shoe stores or cobbler's store] to accommodate 36 cases. I don't think at present any cases will die.[21]

Although medical units across the area were doing all they could under very difficult conditions, men still froze to death on their way to the rear, sometimes in each other's arms as they sought warmth. The adverse weather conditions were the last straw for many men already physically reduced by months of trench living, unvaried diet and more or less constant sickness.

Conditions at Helles were no better. On 26 November, the 1/1st ELFA issued winter clothing, but the war diary notes that the supply was inadequate.[22] This undoubtedly had unfortunate consequences on the ambulance. The 1st Lowland Field Ambulance, 52nd Division, reported on 28 November that snow had fallen overnight on 27 November so that the northern faces of the parapets were covered in snow. Icy rain followed, which was then followed by blizzard conditions in the afternoon.[23] Overnight, the conditions deteriorated, and men suffered, although many had been ordered to take extra blankets with them into the trenches. However, with conditions falling to minus four degrees Celsius, an extra blanket was unlikely to provide much comfort for those men who were without any reasonable cover.[24] And there were thousands in the trenches who were in that position. Joseph Murray was to comment on 30 November:

> The walk to the front line has become even more arduous. We have not much strength left and need to rest more often on the way up. Before the deluge we could manage the walk in one stage but not now. Everyone is the same; exhausted men are to be seen all over the place. I fear some will not see out the day.[25]

Although there were many exhausted men suffering from the effects of exposure, the impact upon the troops seems to have been little understood in some quarters. The ADMS of the 52nd Division wrote in his war diary for 30 November:

> Recommended the issue of 3 blankets per man. 16 cases of frostbite, hands and feet, reported from the 1/4th KOSB and 3 from the rest of the division. No deaths from exposure. The general physical condition of the troops has been on the whole fair and they are in good spirits. They stood the cold snap extremely well and the sickness rate showing very slight increase considering the climatic conditions and want of preparation for winter conditions.[26]

---

21   TNA: WO 95/4279: War Diary, 137th Indian Field Ambulance, 28 November 1915.
22   TNA: WO 95/4314, War Diary, 1/1st East Lancashire Field Ambulance, 26 November 1915.
23   TNA: WO 95/4319: War Diary, 1/1st Lowland Field Ambulance, 28 November 1915.
24   TNA: WO 95/4313: War Diary, 42nd Division ADMS, 27–28 November 1915.
25   Murray, *Gallipoli 1915*, p.172.
26   TNA: WO 95/4318: War Diary, 52nd Division ADMS, 30 November 1915.

This would seem to reflect that the ADMS was out of touch with what had happened in the area during the four days of extreme weather, and, although he was able to show only a slight increase in sick admissions in his divisions for the month, he does not seem to have appreciated the full impact of the storm on the admissions at the end of the month and the general state of the men in the division. It is certainly at odds with those conditions reported by Murray in his account. Nevertheless, the medical services at Helles were still under pressure for the same reason as those at Suvla: there was no chance of evacuation for the cases being held in the field ambulances and CCS as a result of the storm. The 11th BCCS at Helles was able to get some light cases away to Mudros on 29 November, but this was on board a sweeper because hospital ships could not be loaded effectively with the more serious cases until the storm had abated on 30 November.[27]

Even at Anzac, the appalling weather conditions did not go unmentioned. Lieutenant F. T. Small, an engineer, experienced a very uncomfortable night although sheltered in a sound dugout:

> During the night I found it impossible to get my feet warm despite the fact that I had three blankets and a pair of bed-socks. I soon saw the reason. The sight was glorious. The whole ground was covered by over three inches of snow while all the trees etc were simply laden with it. To most of us it was a most unique sight, but when you come to examine our trenches and to see the amount of muck and slush in them it would break your heart. I know it breaks the heart of the Engineers, but what of the unfortunate Infantry who spend night and day in them. Already I am mud from head to foot, but not as cold as I expected to be with snow around.[28]

Whilst the snow may have been a novelty to many of the Australians, the men of the Western Australian 10th Light Horse were surprised by the snow but, according to their historian, 'took the snow very well … and carried out their various duties without a murmur'.[29] However, the snow brought with it problems of transporting everything from the beaches up the slopes of Anzac to the front line. This brought about more fatigues for men already in poor shape as a result of the campaign to that date. Perhaps one of the biggest problems at Anzac was the complete loss of water supply, a problem that the front-line troops solved by melting snow until the tanks and pipes in the area could be defrosted. In spite of this, a bathing parade had been scheduled in the 15th Battalion, and this went ahead, with naked men bathing in one quart of water in the almost freezing conditions.[30]

Although the adverse weather lasted no more than four days, it had a significant impact on the medical services at Anzac. With the onset of the gale on 26 November, all evacuation from

---

27 TNA: WO 95/4356: War Diary, 11th Casualty Clearing Station, 30 November 1915.
28 Australian War Memorial (AWM) 2DRL/0778, RCDIG0000252: Diary of Frederick Trouton Small, 1915, November.
29 Lieutenant Colonel A. C. N. Olden, *Westralian Cavalry in the War: The Story of the Tenth Light Horse Regiment, A.I.F., in the Great War 1914–1918* (Facsimile edition of 1921 publication, Uckfield: Naval & Military Press, n.d.), p.68.
30 Lieutenant T. P. Chataway, *History of the 15th Battalion AIF, 1914–1918* (Facsimile edition, Uckfield: Naval & Military Press, n.d.), p.98.

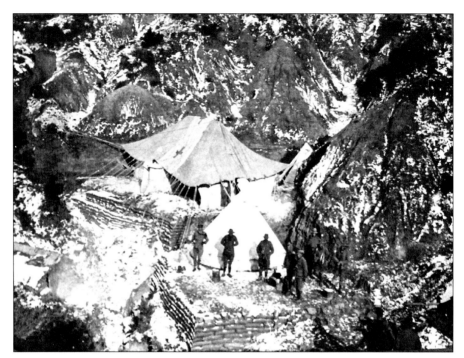

Snow at the 4th AFA (B Section) in Hotchkiss Gully, Anzac, following the blizzard.
(SLSA: PRG 381/22/3)

the beaches had ceased. Hospitals there were full at a time when men were succumbing to exposure and needing treatment.[31] The NZMFA noted that, during and following the bad weather, the regimental sick parade grew and that many of the men required treatment in hospital and even evacuation for rheumatism, cold and some cases of frostbite.[32] The DDMS 1st Australian Corps recorded:

> Bitterly cold day. Wind strong N, in fact blizzard. Snow is falling and has fallen through night. The 54th East Anglian Division struck camp yesterday and were marching to the beach through the cold weather and have suffered much from exposure and frost bite. Arrangements were made for shelter in No 1 Australian Stationary Hospital and structures on the beach but the night bivouac 27/28 was spent in Rest Gully and was very severe on them. All ranks suffered badly from the blizzard and many cases of early frost bite and trench foot are coming in to the Field Ambulances …
> Evacuation of sick and wounded Nil. Rough weather, embarkation impossible …[33]

---

31   AWM: AWM4/26/62/10: War Diary, 1st Australian Casualty Clearing Station, 26–30 November 1915.
32   AWM: AWM4/35/26/5: War Diary, New Zealand Mounted Field Ambulance, November 1915.
33   AWM: AWM4/26/14/3: War Diary, DDMS ANZAC Corps, 28 November 1915.

The MO Died in His Sleep: The Storm   267

At Anzac Cove, the 54th Division was in the process of being relieved when the storm struck and was essentially left without billets once its transport was cancelled as a result of the storm. The 1/1st Eastern Mounted Brigade Field Ambulance (EMBFA) reported:

> … unfortunately, snow fell on the night of the 27th and the following day there was a keen frost, the saps being impossible for stretchers to move along. We had numerous cases of chilled feet and cases of exposure as well as wounded from the whole division to deal with and on the 28th and 29th and today we had a great rush of work. To add to our difficulties the sea was too rough to evacuate any cases to the Hospital Ships and the Beach Hospital reported on morning of 29th that they could not take any more cases.[34]

The 108th IFA had set up its hospital in Chailak Dere on the left flank of the Anzac position. The hospital had been at this site more or less since moving from Helles at the beginning of August and was reasonably well established with tents and dugouts for both staff and patients alike. On 27 November, Major Battye wrote in the unit diary:

> This morning the ground was covered with snow and snow was still falling and fell irregularly nearly all day. There was about an inch on the open ground. A bitter NE wind blew all day. A memo came from Staff Captain asking me to recommend a treble issue of run to be kept in reserve by OC's of against another flood of rain. This I declined and recommended instead a special reserve of cocoa and fuel for supplying hot drinks.[35]

Battye was not the only MO to recommend against the use of rum in the cold of the Gallipoli Peninsula, as he was fully aware of the harm that it could do. It was the following day that Battye was to record the first cases suffering from exposure coming into his hospital when 49 cases from the 2/10th Gurkhas arrived needing treatment.[36] During that day, the hospital admitted 90 cases in total, mostly as a result of the cold. However, things were about to get worse for the unit:

> There was a hard frost last night. Today was bright and clear and no wind. There was a thaw in the sun for part of the day and hard frost again tonight. Yesterday 90 cases and today 92 cases were admitted nearly all suffering from 'trench feet'; 54 of today's cases from 2/10th Gurkhas many of them were in a pitiable condition. Their feet swollen and bleeding, unable to don socks or boots they had walked in from their lines a mile and half or more in bare feet some walking on the ends of their trousers which were too long for them and soaked in mud. On arrival in hospital their feet were washed in tepid water and dried then gently massaged then wrapped in cotton wool and bandages. Dry body clothing was supplied and blankets and hot tea. The men walked from their lines

---

34   TNA: WO 95/4325: War Diary, 1/1st Eastern Mounted Brigade Field Ambulance, 30 November 1915. The beach hospital referred to here is believed to be the 1st ACCS.
35   TNA: WO 95/4272: War Diary, 108th Indian Field Ambulance, 28 November 1915.
36   TNA: WO 95/4272: War Diary, 108th Indian Field Ambulance, 29 November 1915.

as there were not sufficient bearers to carry so many and because the regimental MO considered that in many cases the walk was necessary to maintain circulation.[37]

It will be noticed that Battye used the term 'trench feet' when describing the effect of the cold upon the men in his care. Later, he was asked to separate the cases of trench feet from those of frostbite. He was to comment that he had not made the distinction since all the cases in his hospital were due to the same adverse weather, wet followed by intense cold, and because 'I am not aware that "trench foot" is a properly defined and separate clinical entity'.[38] For his hospital, the cases of frostbite continued to arrive over the next few days, and, gradually, the hospital was overcrowded with suffering men. The capacity of his hospital was nominally 100 cases, but, with one section short, this was reduced to 75, and the weather had meant that well in excess of 200 men were being treated by 2 December. Many of the cases were unable to walk, and, simply to get the men from the firing line, Battye needed to call upon the 1/4th Gurkhas to provide men to act as stretcher-bearers to help his overstretched bearers to bring in the most seriously affected: 'Most of the cases of "trench foot" admitted have been bad cases with commencing gangrene (moist) of toes, half feet and whole feet and others with patches of gangrene, many with haemorrhagic bullae in them and feet and ankles much swollen and oedematous and very tender.'[39] By this time, with his hospital overflowing, Battye was beginning to question why so many men continued to come to his hospital with frostbitten feet even after the general thaw had taken place. He was of the opinion that this had been a result of the lack of regular foot inspection by regimental officers and particularly those in the 2/10th Gurkhas. He wrote to the CO of the regiment to ask that this should be remedied immediately, for, although the weather had improved, he was very keen to ensure that regular foot inspection helped to improve the overall health of the men. In the six days, inclusive, from 28 November to 3 December, the 108th IFA had admitted a total of 443 cases suffering with the effects of the bad weather, and more than half of these, a total of 258, had occurred in the 2/10th Gurkhas.[40] Battye wanted to ensure that this would not be repeated.

The worst storm to hit the peninsula in 40 years had created havoc amongst the forces in the trenches and on the beaches. The medical services had been more or less overwhelmed, and the lack of preparation for winter conditions was at the bottom of the problems faced by all those involved in the campaign. The effects were felt on Lemnos as the stationary and general hospitals there tried to cope with the bad weather. They, too, could not evacuate casualties, and, although they were not receiving casualties from the peninsula, the weather was creating its own problems for hospitals such as No. 15 BSH, which recorded, 'This will be a very bad place for anything but slight surgical cases in the winter. Stoves, heating issued to tents.[41] At the time that the storm started, this hospital had a little over 800 cases in its charge. Following the end of the storm and the evacuation of cases from the peninsula, the number of cases in the hospital

---

37 TNA: WO 95/4272: War Diary, 108th Indian Field Ambulance, 30 November 1915.
38 TNA: WO 95/4272: War Diary, 108th Indian Field Ambulance, 10 December 1915.
39 TNA: WO 95/4272: War Diary, 108th Indian Field Ambulance, 2 December 1915. 'Haemorrhagic bullae' refers to large blood-filled blisters on the feet.
40 TNA: WO 95/4272: War Diary, 108th Indian Field Ambulance, 3 December 1915.
41 TNA: WO 95/4357: War Diary, No. 16 Stationary Hospital, 25 November 1915.

exceeded 1,100 on 3 December. Many of these cases were evacuated the following day on the Cunard liner *Mauretania*.[42]

If there had ever been any question about the viability of a winter campaign in anyone's mind, the storm had done much to swing the balance against such a continued campaign. Whilst figures for the number of casualties arising as a result of the storm vary, there can be no doubt that they were high. The official historian quotes no fewer than 5,000 cases of frostbite for Suvla alone and 200 men drowned by the deluge.[43] The *Official History of the Medical Services* suggests a figure of almost 8,000 for the number of frostbite cases admitted across the peninsula, suggesting that the total figure of hospital admissions for the period of the storm was considerably higher.[44] Nevertheless, the medical services had worked hard under the adverse conditions that the storm had produced and, by their care, had undoubtedly helped to reduce the number of deaths that it caused.

42   TNA: WO 95/4357: War Diary, No. 16 Stationary Hospital, 25 November to 4 December 1915.
43   Aspinall-Oglander, *Military Operations*, vol. 2, p.434.
44   Mitchell and Smith, *Casualties and Medical Statistics*, vol. 5, p.205.

16

Some Were Dying, Some Found Dead

The hospitals on Lemnos had, by the end of August, become reasonably well established. That is not to say they were not suffering from many of the issues that were plaguing the campaign as a whole. There was a shortage of water, generally poor sanitary conditions and a lack of equipment and stores of all sorts. On top of this, the hospitals also had the problems of the thousands of flies that found their way onto all surfaces and the dust that blew into everything.

At first, the hospitals operated without nursing sisters, but, with the arrival of No. 3 AGH, this changed. The nurses of No. 3 AGH, ably lead by Matron Grace Wilson, were not all able to work with their own unit immediately since much of its equipment had not arrived and some were sent to work with No. 2 ASH as early as 8 August. This was partly because No. 2 ASH was itself suffering from the illnesses that were all over the island and peninsula at this time. This meant that the MOs and orderlies were becoming ill and that hospitals were consequently undermanned.[1] The nurses from No. 3 AGH seem to have worked on a daily basis at No. 2 ASH, returning to their unit when their shift was over. This continued throughout the rest of August, with No. 2 ASH using nurses from No. 1 and No. 3 CSHs as they became available. Later, nurses from No. 18 BSH were also called upon to assist.

When 10 of the Canadian sisters were attached to No. 2 ASH, they were met by the CO, who, according to Sister Mabel Clint, did not know what to do with them, seemingly overwhelmed by the situation. If later Australian nurses' accounts of their arrival at No. 2 ASH are to be believed, it would seem more likely that the MOs of the hospital simply did not want the sister there. Nevertheless, as Clint commented:

> We each took a line, and proceeded to do what we could for the worst cases. Some were dying, some found dead. They lay on Egyptian mattresses, about a foot high, almost all had excreta vessels beside them, uncovered except for flies, a cup of water of canned milk here and there had been overturned by a restless sufferer and the delirious were tormented by swarms of insects in a temperature of 100 … Food was the most meagre description and totally unsuited to disease.[2]

1   AWM: AWM4/26/71/1: War Diary, No. 2 Australian Stationary Hospital, August 1915.
2   Mabel B. Clint. *Our Bit: Memories of War Service by a Canadian Nursing-Sister* (Montreal: Barwick, 1934), p.62.

Conditions were far from good in all the hospitals on Lemnos as MOs and sisters did all they could to help those in their care. Shortages hampered their work throughout their stay, and this, too, reflects badly upon the overall lack of organisation of the seaborne invasion of a hostile coast.

Sister Nita Frances Smith, AANS, was one of the nurses detailed from No. 3 AGH for duty at No. 2 ASH:

> There was so much to do and we did not know where to begin – thinking it over now I wish I could have done more, but being quite new to active service then I think I wasted time perhaps – at any rate it was very heart-breaking work, especially when one had to leave No 2 at 6 pm and leave one's patients in the hands of and almost inexperienced man. I can't help thinking if there had been more sisters in those early days a great many more lives would have been saved … We only worked a few days at No 2 Stat, the staff were very good to us and helped us in every way possible to try and make things better for the men … I believe the CO said he would rather have a hospital without sisters, it may sound conceited but somehow, I don't believe many of the patients would have agreed with him.[3]

The presence of sisters in their hospitals was something that the MOs needed to get used to as more arrived on the island. No. 1 and No. 3 CSHs had arrived from Alexandria in the second half of August, both with their full complement of nursing sisters, and started to receive patients on or about 22 August. Sister Mabel Clint commented upon the arrival of the sisters of No. 1 CSH, 'Deposited on the beach, we piled suitcases and started on foot for the hospital camp, a mile or so away. The rough, dry ground, for it had not rained for many months, the sparse scrub, the arid untilled soils, stones, dust and colourless monotony made the walk a long one.'[4] The conditions were harsh, and, as the sisters marched to their camp, they saw groups of sick men 'wandering aimlessly about here and there'. Sister Clint heard one say, 'No place for Sisters'. Over the coming months, the sisters were made fully aware of the conditions behind this sentiment but proved themselves up to the task in the face of all the problems. Mabel Clint described the first weeks on Lemnos as a 'time of acute misery', citing poor sanitary conditions, lack and quality of food, shortage of water and, of course, flies: 'It was difficult to eat or drink without swallowing flies, the tables swarmed with them, every patient's dressing removed required another to stand by fanning vigorously as a cloud of pests prepared to settle. Pus and maggots abounded and wounds would not heal.'[5]

It appears that the conditions and shortages faced by the Canadian hospitals, while not different to those of other nations, were made known in Canada. The government there made immediate contact with London to voice its concern. This seems to have had some effect, in so far as the ADMS Mudros West was instructed to 'redress disabilities'.[6] Whether or not the ADMS was able to make much of a difference is unclear. However, conditions did improve

---

3   AWM: AWM41/1045: [Nurses Narratives] N F S Smith. Sister Smith had embarked from Australia on 15 May 1915 with No. 3 AGH; this was the first active service role for the hospital.
4   Clint, *Our Bit*, p.59.
5   Clint, *Our Bit*, p.60.
6   Clint, *Our Bit*, p.63.

272   The Fight for Life

somewhat throughout the autumn, and, whilst always suffering from various shortages, at least the decrease in the numbers of flies served to help improve the living and working conditions for everyone on the island. Water supplies improved during this period, and this helped in improving sanitation in the hospitals. Canvas huts were also erected for the sisters as winter quarters complete with portable stoves to heat them, which did much to restore the morale and health of the unit as a whole.[7]

The No. 3 CSH war diary notes its arrival and that:

> After strenuous exertion a tent hospital was set up and the first convoy of patients arrived about 10 pm August 23rd. The Army Service Corps and Ordnance Department for Hospitals were totally inadequate at this time. The greatest difficulty was experienced in getting rations for the personnel and hospital comforts for the patients and facilities for cooking were very poor. The heat was intense and prostrating. Conditions at this time left much to be desired. Latrine buckets were practically unprocurable and recourse had to be made to trenches to which innumerable flies had easy access. It was impossible to make [a] proper trench as lava-like rock was found [a] few inches below the surface. Our own personnel were kept more than busy, looking after patients. These unsanitary conditions were particularly hard on our Nursing Sisters. The great proportion of cases treated in hospital at this time were dysenteric.
>
> New wards were opened almost daily to accommodate the influx of patients arriving. Under the strain of work, improper and insufficient food, excessive heat, poor water supply a great many of the staff had to be admitted to hospital.[8]

The war diary also points out that the 'Sanitary conditions at this stage of the campaign were deplorable'.[9] It is perhaps unsurprising that it was not long before the hospital staff were feeling the effects of the living and working conditions on Lemnos. Two nurses, Sister M. F. Munro and Sister E. G. Sunders, were admitted to the hospital with dysentery on 5 September, Sister Munro succumbing to the disease three days later. On 11 September, Matron J. B. Jaggard was admitted to hospital similarly affected, and she, too, died of the disease on 24 September. These two Canadian sisters were the only two members of the nursing staff to die on Lemnos, though many other nurses became ill during their sojourn on the island and, at the time, many more were expected to die.[10] The disease had hit No. 3 CSH particularly hard, for the CO, Lieutenant Colonel Casgrain, was taken seriously ill and was not expected to live. Although he survived, he was evacuated to England by the end of September. Nevertheless, No. 3 CSH was still able to detail two MOs to No. 2 ASH when many of the latter's medical staff were taken ill. Disease was a feature of the work on the island as reflected by the return of No. 3 CSH during its stay and shown in the following table. It is clear from the table that medical cases were by far the largest number treated at No. 3 CSH at Lemnos.

7   Clint, *Our Bit*, p.63.
8   'War Diary, No. 3 CSH, August 1915', *Canadian Great War Project* <https://canadiangreatwarproject. com/> (accessed March 2021).
9   'War Diary, No. 3 CSH, August 1915', *Canadian Great War Project*, <https://canadiangreatwarproject. com/> (accessed March 2021).
10   Clint, *Our Bit*, p.62.

Incidence of Disease at No. 3 CSH, Lemnos, Autumn 1915[11]

	August	September	October	November
Dysentery	73	138	185	212
Diarrhoea	104	132	183	
Jaundice	5	37	150	128
Wounds and Injuries	53	66	33	

In early September, the AANS in Egypt asked for volunteers to work on Lemnos. This probably reflects the level of sickness occurring on the island at this time and the need to maintain good staffing levels in the units already established there. A number of nurses stepped forwards to help their colleagues already on the island, and 25 were embarked upon the HS *Assaye* at Alexandria to work at No. 2 ASH. The *Assaye* sailed at daybreak on 15 September and, after a 'rather rough' crossing, reached Mudros on 17 September.[12] Nevertheless, conditions in Mudros Harbour were too rough to allow the sisters to disembark immediately, and they spent another day aboard the *Assaye* before finally landing at Mudros. Sister Nellie Constance Morrice, AANS, left an account of the conditions she encountered on Lemnos and the type of work in which she and the other newly arrived were involved:

> We disembarked at Mudros where we were met by the Commanding Officer of No 2 Stationary and some of the officers of the unit and taken up to the hospital where we found everything in readiness for us as far as our own personal comfort and convenience to the best of their ability; but being the first Sisters in the unit and not being wanted as we were afterwards told by the officers and orderlies, or some of them, we found our work was uphill to say the least of it.[13] I have known the officers in charge of the ward to come on and fire an order direct to the orderlies, the officer seemed to want the orderly to know that they were quite satisfied with the work the orderlies were doing and that Sisters were quite unnecessary. However, the patients thought otherwise. In the hospital there was equipment with beds for about 250 men. Out of that there was a 'Unit Tent' with beds and everything in the way of equipment that was able to be got. The 'Fighting Man' with dysentery and wounds had to lie on mattresses on the floor of the tents. The first sight that met my gaze was when going over the hospital was some of the dysentery and jaundice patients (both diseases being very prevalent at that time) sitting on commodes outside the tent doors, in the icy wind and sleet with nothing but their pyjamas, doubled up with pain and passing blood and mucus and on going inside the tents found these same patients sleeping on mattresses on the floor which were encased in mud, having had heavy rain the night before. It did not take the sisters long to get patients raised on trestle beds made up on stretchers raised on boxes or anything they could get – kept the sick men in bed and ordered that bed pans should

---

11 'War Diary, No. 3 CSH, November 1915', *Canadian Great War Project*, <https://canadiangreatwarproject.com/> (accessed March 2021).

12 AWM: PR05050, RCDIG0001389: Transcript of Diary of Mary Ann 'Bessie' Pocock, 1914-1918 (Vol. 1), September 1915. Pocock was serving as a member of staff aboard the *Assaye*.

13 The CO was Lieutenant Colonel A. T. White, AAMC.

be given to them. Then again, I noticed the first day I was on duty how dishevelled and dirty the patients looked and there was no need because the Red X supplied plenty of pyjamas, dressing gowns and slippers and razors. The men streamed up to the dressing tent looking more like wild men than anything else, unshaven, long hair and weeks of dirt and vermin on them. In a few days after our arrival the men presented a very different appearance, they had groomed themselves and had a wash and I'm sure were feeling better in consequence. During the first days of Lemnos, I hear the water was very scarce, but when we arrived there in September 1915 there was a good supply and no excuse for neglect of patients. No one will ever realise the personal discomfort the men suffered through vermin, and no change of clothes, except those who actually saw them come in from the peninsula. We used to take their dressing off and find even their wounds crawling with vermin, and even sponging and putting them into clean pyjamas did not always rid them of the vermin. Then when night came, we use to sit on the sides of our bunks and search our own garments one by one till we had found all stray ones. I do not know which worried me the most, those or the big black centipedes that use to crawl from under the tarpaulin on the floor and occasionally find their way into our beds.[14]

It is clear from Sister Morrice's account that things were not good at No. 2 ASH when the sisters first arrived for duty, although there had been some help from other nurses since the arrival of No. 3 AGH. The disconnect between officers of the AAMC and the sisters was not unique to Lemnos. This was partly down to the fact that the AANS was not strictly part of the structure of the Australian Army, and, as such, its nurses had no official place in the chain of command. This had been a problem from the time of the Australians landing in Egypt and had led to the recall of Lady Superintendent Jane Bell of the AANS and Colonel Ramsay Smith of the AAMC, who simply could not work through the issues relating to the role that the nurses were supposed to have in the structure of the hospitals. Senior sisters felt that they could not carry out their work if they had no control over the way in which orderlies worked, whilst many MOs would not allow sisters to give any orders to members of the AAMC.[15] It is sad to say that, given Sister Morrice's account, the issues had not been entirely sorted out satisfactorily even under the near battlefield conditions of the stationary hospitals on Lemnos. The attitude of the orderlies needed to be improved, for, as Sister Morrice went on to say:

> … in the operating tent one day I asked the orderly for a bundle of sterile dressing towels and he handed me some which I happened to know were not sterilized, so I said, 'Those will not do, the surgeon will need sterilized ones,' so the orderly said. 'Never mind Sister, the Captain won't be any the wiser, I never thought of sterilizing the towels for him and he never knows.' Of course, I put this down to ignorance, he little knew the danger he was exposing the patient to.[16]

14 AWM: AWM41/1013: [Nurses Narratives] Head Sister N C Morrice.
15 Dixon, *Army Nurse*, pp.75–77.
16 AWM: AWM41/1013: [Nurses Narratives] Head Sister N C Morrice.

It is, at least in part, because of these kinds of incidents that the sisters of the AANS needed some measure of control and the ability to instruct and correct orderlies, or indeed junior MOs, when they saw error or likely problems for the patients. By this time, the sisters were officially classed as officers but were given little authority at first to go with the rank. It was very different, for instance, in the Canadian hospitals, where the sisters, with the rank of officers, were classed as part of the army and hence were part of the chain of command and fully recognised as such.[17]

Nevertheless, Sister Morrice and the rest of the nurses remained at the hospital throughout the autumn, enduring the difficulties and the oncoming winter. In December, in anticipation of the evacuation of the peninsula, No. 2 ASH was enlarged to accommodate 1,200 beds. There seems to have been no effort to increase the staffing levels in this or, indeed, any of the other hospitals on the island. Typically, the staff would have been expected to carry on through any difficult period, and, at least in this case, they, too, were fortunate that the evacuation did not bring the expected large number of casualties.

It was during the autumn that there were increased efforts made to rotate the men from the peninsula so all could get a period of rest on Lemnos: 'I shall never forget seeing the first lot march, or rather straggle, past – most of them looked haggard and ill – numbers dropped out on the way to be admitted in to the hospitals that day or the next'.[18] Whilst relieving troops from the peninsula was undoubtedly the correct approach, it certainly also added to the work load of the hospitals on Lemnos, as men who had braved the peninsula for months, often simply to stay with their mates, succumbed to the illnesses that should have seen them removed from front-line duty some time earlier.

It is quite clear from accounts of hospital staff that difficulties over shortages in equipment, food and water continued well into the autumn on Lemnos. It is equally clear that the Royal Navy played an important role in trying to ease these difficulties. Sister Smith mentioned men of warships such as the HMS *Cornwallis* and HMS *Agamemnon* who often provided comforts such as cigarettes for the men in hospital and entertainment from the ships' bands. However, perhaps the greatest contribution was the occasional treat of lunch for the nurses on board one of the warships and the provision of bread for the hospitals when, it seems, that the bread provided by the ASC was not considered good for the men's health.[19]

In the midst of the work and the endless numbers of patients arriving on the island, the staff of the hospitals needed some time off duty. Although time off could be irregular for the staff, a popular excursion for all was a trip to Therma, a town about five miles from Mudros where it was possible, at a price, to bathe in the hot spring from which the town had taken its name. There were just two bathrooms at Therma, and there was always a queue to use the luxury, but it appears that most thought the cost was worth it after the arduous conditions of the hospitals. Such was the demand for the baths that the military eventually took over the running of them; however, it was almost too late to have any real effect upon those who had looked upon them as a special treat for months.[20]

---

17 Toman, *Sister Soldiers*, p.30.
18 AWM: AWM41/1045: [Nurses Narratives] N F S Smith.
19 AWM: AWM41/1045: [Nurses Narratives] N F S Smith, and AWM41/937: [Nurses Narratives] Margaret Aitken.
20 AWM: AWM41/1045: [Nurses Narratives] N F S Smith.

The care of Indian soldiers of the 29th Indian Brigade on Lemnos fell to the 110th IFA. This unit had been earmarked to land on the peninsula in support of both the Indian brigade and the 108th IFA. This had not happened at least in part because insufficient land had been captured and held by the Allied invasion force, which limited the amount of space for it to land with the brigade. Thus, while the 108th IFA had established itself first at Helles and then at Anzac, the 110th IFA was left somewhat without a specific role to play in relation to the Indian forces on the peninsula. The unit arrived in Mudros at the beginning of June and was disembarked to form a hospital for lightly wounded arriving from the peninsula. It should be noted that this ambulance, like the 108th IFA, was intended to care for Indian casualties and any wounded POWs. This was in part because the IMS operated on a slightly different structure to the RAMC and because of the cultural differences in the expected care of the Indian troops. After two weeks functioning as a hospital on Lemnos, three sections of the 110th IFA were ordered to report to transports, most notably to the *Seang Choon*, to provide medical care for those Indians needing evacuation to Egypt. A Section of the ambulance remained on shore at Mudros, providing what was effectively a small stationary hospital for Indian casualties.

At the beginning of August, the hospital was taking casualties arising from the heavy fighting on the peninsula. However, it is clear from the war diary of this time that there was concern over the increase in the number of dysentery and fever cases arriving from the front.[21] At first, the diseases were noticed in men of the Indian Mountain Battery and the Indian Mule Corps and not amongst the infantrymen of the 29th Indian Brigade. However, this situation did not continue, as disease gradually affected everyone on the peninsula.[22]

This unit fared no better in its search to obtain sufficient stores than did any hospital on Lemnos, and its work was continually hampered by shortages of one sort or another. It was a story familiar to the medical units on Lemnos: even if the stores were available on the AOC store ship *Minnetonka*, there were never sufficient small boats to the bring the equipment ashore. Nevertheless, by the end of August, the hospital was treating 189 cases. This meant that the hospital was overcrowded since the nominal capacity for one section of an Indian field ambulance was normally considered to be 25 patients.[23] However, these were not normal times, as all the medical services struggled to manage the numbers of patients arising from the fighting and, increasingly, from disease.

Problems of supply continued well into the autumn, and the numbers of patients in the hospital were always high for A Section. In mid-September, D Section of the recently arrived 137th Combined Field Ambulance was attached to the hospital to help with the workload and remained with it until the 110th IFA was reconstituted with the arrival of Major R. H. Price and the rest of the staff at the end of October. In the period from 4 June to 26 October, the small, one-section hospital had treated 2,047 cases, of which 820 were men suffering from wounds, with the other cases all admitted for a variety of diseases, notably dysentery.

At the beginning of October, one man in the hospital died from relapsing fever. This was the first case to be recorded and was considered special enough to warrant a particular mention in the unit war diary.[24] The relevance of this disease was not lost on the MOs of the unit since it is

---

21   TNA: WO 95/4356: War Diary, 110th Indian Field Ambulance, August.
22   Forbes, *History of the Army Ordnance Services*, pp.223–24.
23   TNA: WO 95/4356: War Diary, 110th Indian Field Ambulance, 31 August.
24   TNA: WO 95/4356: War Diary, 110th Indian Field Ambulance, 1 October.

borne by infected lice and ticks. The occurrence of lice in the trenches of the First World War has been well documented, and so it was perhaps not surprising for a louse-borne disease such as relapsing fever to be encountered at Gallipoli. The disease is spread when a louse infected with a bacterium, such as *Borrelia recurrentis*, bites its human host. Scratching of the bite site then allows the pathogen to enter the host's blood stream and for the disease to develop after a period of between five and 15 days. The symptoms displayed are fever, headaches, joint pain and, sometimes, a rash. These last for some days and then disappear.[25] However, the cycle of fever and recovery can be repeated over several weeks and, unless treated, can ultimately lead to death. Today, the disease is readily treated with antibiotics, and recovery is normal. However, at the time of the Gallipoli Campaign, it was more difficult to cure. In soldiers already weakened by months of fighting, poor diet and living conditions, it could prove to be serious. The vector for the infection at the 110th IFA was not discovered, but the CO took no chances and disinfected everything that may have had contact with the infected man, including the tent in which he had been treated.[26] In view of the likely cause being lice brought from the peninsula, it was not an overreaction.

The cultural differences that were present amongst the forces taking part in the Gallipoli Campaign were brought sharply to the fore at the 110th IFA:

> The body of an Egyptian Christian received for burial. A medical officer – Lt Strehil – was asked by me to go to the ADMS and ask for instructions as to its disposal. The ADMS directed Lt Strehil to see the Church of England Chaplain at No 16 and if he could not find him to see the commandant of the Egyptian Labour Corps. The ADMS also telephoned to the adjutant Camp Commandant's office to ask for instructions and to say that if Lt Strehil would call at his office later when he had man arrangements. Lt Strehil did not find the Chaplain and so proceeded to the Commandant Egyptian Labour Corps. After they had made some enquiries, they decided it would be too expensive to have the body buried by the local Greek priest so Lt Strehil and the Commandant Egyptian Labour Corps proceeded to the Camp Commandant's Office. The adjutant there on hearing their report telephoned to Mudros W where there is an Egyptian Hospital and where arrangements for burying Copts exist and told Lt Strehil he would let him know the answer. The adjutant came personally in the afternoon and spoke about the matter to me and asked me to send for a party of Egyptians to have the body carried to Mudros W. The party arrived and waited for some time for final orders which were promised by the Adjutant but he cancelled the order and said to keep the body till further orders. Later a verbal message came from the ADMS by an orderly saying to take the body at once to the Egyptian Pier where all arrangements had been made by the ADMS for its removal to Mudros W. This was done and the body taken down within half an hour of the message by a party of bearers under a Lance Naik.
>
> They met a sentry (British) on the pier who took the note containing the rank, no., and name of the body and directed them to leave the body there. This sentry next day said his name was Pte Cranston, Howe Battalion No KX 309, that two officers had

---

25   'Relapsing Fever', *Wikipedia*, <https://en.wikipedia.org/wiki/Relapsing_fever>, accessed Nov. 2021.
26   TNA: WO 95/4356: War Diary, 110th Indian Field Ambulance, 1 October.

278   The Fight for Life

called 15 – 20 minutes before the arrival of the body and asked if it had arrived and that as he thought they would return he took delivery of body. These officers did not return.[27]

This incident served to remind the officers of the unit of the issues of treating not only the Indian cases, where caste issues and religious tensions were never far away, but also those coming from other units. Often, such issues were handled by transferring the casualty to the relevant unit or hospital, but this was not so easily handled when the casualty was already dead. It is assumed that the Coptic Christian was eventually buried in the appropriate cemetery.[28]

The hospitals on Lemnos had been warned of the August Offensive in time to make some preparation to take in an increased number of casualties. By 16 August, No. 16 BSH, in Mudros East, had 950 patients in hospital, and this level of casualties remained for the rest of the month. With the numbers of patients in hospitals on Lemnos increasing, there were attempts to take measures to prevent hospitals from becoming overwhelmed. No. 15 BSH began having weekly medical boards from the first week of September to examine convalescents with a view to returning men to duty or transferring them to base. Nevertheless, by mid-September, little had changed at No. 16 BSH, which had over 1,000 cases undergoing treatment. Of course, these hospitals were little different to any of the others on Lemnos – all were full to capacity and beyond. For instance, the 24th BCCS, at Mudros East, was recording over 1,600 cases in hospital at the end of September. Whilst evacuation to base in Egypt, or to Malta and England, was helping to clear some of the cases, the hospital ships generally carried no more than 500 cases. Thus, to clear the number of hospitals on Lemnos, all with large numbers of cases, it was necessary for there to be a significant number of hospital ships plying the water of the Mediterranean Sea constantly. One approach to try and solve this issue was to convert large ocean liners to hospital ships, such as the Cunarders RMS *Aquitania* and RMS *Mauretania*. The *Aquitania*, for instance, was staffed by 41 MOs and 102 nursing sisters and was capable of carrying in excess of 4,000 cases swiftly back to England. This large Cunard liner was commissioned as a hospital ship on 4 September 1915.[29] By 15 September, the ship was in Mudros Harbour taking cases from No. 15 and No. 16 BSHs, as well as other hospitals on the island.[30] Whilst these large ocean liners helped, there were too few of them to make a real impact at this stage of the campaign as casualties continued to arrive. Hospitals were struggling under the increasing number of cases caused by sickness, and attempts appear to have been made to rationalise the casualties handled. For instance, No. 18 BSH, at Mudros West, was transferring all enteric cases to No. 3 AGH and all dysentery cases to either No. 1 CSH or No. 3 CSH while it handled many of the other sicknesses including diarrhoea and even venereal disease.[31] This was continued for about two months when No. 18 BSH began

---

27   TNA: WO 95/4356: War Diary, 110th Indian Field Ambulance, 27 November.
28   The Egyptian cemetery at Mudros West was for those of the Muslim faith; hence, it is likely that Christians of the Egyptian Labour Corps were buried in Portianos Military Cemetery, in which there are five burials that are not of the Commonwealth forces.
29   Macpherson, *History of the Great War: Medical Services*, vol. 1, p.367.
30   'Diary of Service with No. 15 Stationary Hospital', <https://wellcomecollection.org/works/yfvzvc4a>, accessed April 2021; TNA: WO 95/4357: War Diary, No. 16 Stationary Hospital, September.
31   TNA: WO 95/4357: War Diary, No. 18 Stationary Hospital, September.

to receive enteric cases as its focus on treatment shifted. These hospitals also relied upon the large hospital ships, and the days that these were in the harbour were filled with work preparing the cases to be evacuated to base and hoping that there would be sufficient ships to ferry the cases over the harbour.

Of course, the British stationary hospitals were afforded no benefits when it came to obtaining stores and suffered from the same shortages as all the others on the island. The CO of No. 18 BSH, Lieutenant Colonel G. S. Crawford, recorded, 'Great difficulty in obtaining hospital supplies ...' on 29 September and, in November, repeatedly recorded, 'No eggs, oatmeal of butter available'.[32] These items would have been considered essential for the diets of the patients, particularly those suffering from gastrointestinal problems.

The hospitals were also suffering from the effects of their service and were consistently undermanned as MOs and orderlies were taken sick and admitted to hospital. In November, both No. 15 and No. 16 BSHs received reinforcements in the form of 31 nursing sisters. These sisters were the nursing staff of No. 27 BGH, which had arrived on Lemnos to set up a large hospital. The hospital was not completed until December, and the nursing staff and MOs were used to assist elsewhere on the island. According to Mabel Clint of No. 1 CSH, the hospital was too late and was never opened.[33] This contradicts the official account, in so far as that indicated No. 27 BGH was operational before the evacuation of the peninsula.[34] However, opening a hospital only days before the evacuation of Suvla and Anzac suggests it was far too late to be very useful. Nevertheless, when Matron F. M. Hodgins and 11 nurses left No. 15 BSH to join No. 27 BGH on 4 December, there can be little doubt that their temporary duty at the hospital had been much appreciated, with some of the nurses later expressing the opinion that they would rather have remained at No. 15 BSH.[35] It is clear that, by 20 December, No. 27 BGH was operational and remained so until its final evacuation in 1916.

The severe storm that hit the area at the end of November did not have as big an impact on the island of Lemnos as on the peninsula. No. 18 BSH was one of the few to make any reference to the storm, the war diary mentioning that a number of tents were damaged by the high winds of 26 November.[36] However, the extreme cold over the following days presented its own problem, for, though the tents offered some shelter, it was difficult to keep them heated and the patients warm. On 30 November, No. 16 BSH recorded the admission of the first cases with frostbite and trench foot coming from the peninsula. The scale of the problem facing the hospitals following the storm is indicated when No. 18 BSH admitted 107 cases of frostbite on 1 December, with more following on subsequent days. The same day, the war diary of No. 1 CSH records no fewer than 800 cases of frostbite admitted.[37] On 10 December, No. 18 BSH recorded a number of deaths where frostbite was considered to have been contributory, including one death from tetanus 'following frostbite'.[38] The CO of the 110th IFA, Major R. H.

---

32   TNA: WO 95/4357: War Diary, No. 18 Stationary Hospital, September and November.
33   Clint, *Our Bit*, p.64.
34   Macpherson, *History of the Great War: Medical Services*, vol. 1, p.367.
35   The matron is believed to be Matron F. M. Hodgins RRC and Bar, MiD.
36   TNA: WO 95/4357: War Diary, No. 18 Stationary Hospital, 26 November.
37   'War Diary, No. 1 CSH, 1 December', *Canadian Great War Project*, <https://canadiangreatwarproject. com/> (accessed March 2021).
38   TNA: WO 95/4357: War Diary, No. 18 Stationary Hospital, 10 December.

Price, submitted a report to the ADMS Mudros East on the treatment for frostbite used at his hospital, which in part reads:

1. The mildest cases without loss of skin, discolouration blebs etc were powdered with Eupad,[39] wrapped in gauze, wool and lightly bandaged. As they improved warm socks were used only, massage with turpentine was liked by the patients. Aspirin was used to ease pain, tingling etc. For severe pain in all cases morphia was given.
2. Severe cases were treated the same way and a line of demarcation waited for. The foot was elevated, blebs opened, dead skin snipped away to allow pent up serum to escape.
3. When a line of demarcation already existed, but edges septic, they were treated as above with Eupad till clean. When local and general conditions did not improve, amputation was done generally above the ankle. When local and general conditions improved with Eupad, for this interference was delayed.
4. When the foot was entirely lost amputation was done above the ankle and straight across if the condition of the patient was bad. Modified circular amputation in the same position with flaps unstitched if condition of the patient favourable.
5. When it was found that other hospitals had cases of tetanus, prophylactic doses of 1,000 to 1,500 were given to several of the cases.[40]

This general approach to the treatment of frostbite seems to have been adopted across the hospitals on the island, but it should be noted that only in extreme cases was amputation used where gangrene was present and immediate intervention called for.

Whilst, at the time of the storm, no one on Lemnos had any clear indication of the evacuation of the peninsula, it is perhaps sad to note that, in war diaries of the hospitals, every effort was being made to improve the hospitals, with No. 16 BSH recording on 13 December that 'stone hutting commenced'.[41] Staff at all the hospitals probably had little idea that, a week later, the beginning of the evacuation of the peninsula would take place as Suvla and Anzac were evacuated. However, in a matter of days, it must have become clear, as the same hospital was making preparations to increase the number of beds because of 'movements on the peninsula'.[42]

The hospitals remained on Lemnos throughout January, and, as the casualties were evacuated along the lines of communication, they began to close. The 24th BCCS packed up and left Lemnos on 21 January 1916, reaching Alexandria two days later. No. 15 BSH remained at Lemnos a little longer, not reaching Alexandria until 9 February 1916.[43] It appears that the last two hospitals remaining on Lemnos were No. 3 CSH and No. 27 BGH; that is, one hospital remained on Mudros West, and one remained on Mudros East until the island was finally free of casualties during the early months of 1916.

---

39 Eupad is an antiseptic powder containing chlorinated lime and boric acid.
40 TNA: WO 95/4356: War Diary, 110th Indian Field Ambulance, Appendix dated 14 December.
41 TNA: WO 95/4357: War Diary, No. 16 Stationary Hospital, 13 December.
42 TNA: WO 95/4357: War Diary, No. 16 Stationary Hospital, 16 December.
43 'Diary of Service with No. 15 Stationary Hospital', <https://wellcomecollection.org/works/yfvzvc4a> (accessed April 2021).

17

Evacuation: Tents Left Standing and Flags Flying

During the autumn, hospital admissions due to sickness continued to exceed 10,000 cases per month. There was recognition amongst the MOs that the depleted troops were not in a good enough condition to mount another sustained attack or, for that matter, to sustain a robust defence in a winter campaign, and the prolonged inactivity did little for the morale of all ranks.

Whilst Hamilton was making urgent calls for huge numbers of reinforcements necessary to mount a major sustained attack, he received a major setback when he received a message from Kitchener on 26 September. The message in part reads:

> On account of the mobilization of the Bulgarian Army, Greece has asked the Allies to send a force to Salonika in order to enable her to support Serbia should the latter be attacked by Bulgaria, as well as by German forces from the North. No doubt you realize that if by such action Bulgaria joins hands with the Central Powers they will have a clear road to Constantinople and Gallipoli, and be able to send large quantities of ammunition or troops, rendering your position very hazardous ... under these circumstances some troops will have to be taken from the Dardanelles to go to Salonika but it must be clearly understood that there is no intention of withdrawing from the Peninsula or giving up the Dardanelles operation until the Turks are defeated ... The troops now at the Dardanelles which are required for Salonika would be two divisions, preferably the Xth and XIth ... The Yeomanry now *en route* to you would also have to be diverted to Salonika ...[1]

Hamilton was, of course, extremely upset to be losing experienced troops rather than receiving reinforcements. Regardless, it was difficult to dismiss the importance of defending Serbia and, indeed, the threat to the Dardanelles operations. This marked a shift in priorities and brought Serbia and the Salonika Campaign firmly to the fore.

The situation did not improve for Hamilton. He received another cable from Kitchener informing him that the Dardanelles Committee felt that he was adopting a purely defensive attitude, yet, confusingly, Kitchener added that he had no reason to imagine that Hamilton had

---

1   Hamilton, *Gallipoli Diary*, vol. 2, 26 September 1915.

any intention of taking the offensive anywhere along the line as he, Kitchener, had been unable to replace the sick and wounded men. Hamilton, already frustrated by complete inaction since the August Offensive, due to a lack of reinforcements and shells, was somewhat confused. He desperately needed the means to mount an offensive but was receiving no encouragement.

The situation for Hamilton worsened when he received a cable from Kitchener informing him that a 'flow of unofficial reports from Gallipoli' was pouring into the War Office.[2] Kitchener was referring, at least in part, to a letter sent by Keith Murdoch, an Australian journalist, to the Australian prime minister in which he exercises full journalistic freedom when severely criticising the British at Gallipoli. He felt the work of the General Staff was deplorable; he also heavily criticised the quality of the British soldiers, remarking they were young and of poor physique without strength to endure or brains to improve their conditions. To cap it all, he stated that an order had been given on the first day at Suvla to shoot without mercy any soldier who lagged behind or loitered in an advance, which, of course, was vehemently denied by Hamilton and his officers. Murdoch's analysis of the situation came from a short visit to Anzac and Suvla and significantly without a visit to the British lines at Helles. Whilst the letter is more of a demonstration of the ignorance of the newspaperman than a true reflection of the situation, it found its way to British Prime Minister Herbert Asquith, who, in his wisdom, decided to forward the letter to the Dardanelles Committee.[3] Hamilton was not given the opportunity to defend himself and his men, and Asquith's action could only have harmed Hamilton's reputation at home.

On 11 October, Kitchener asked Hamilton what was the estimate of the probable losses that would be sustained by the evacuation of the Gallipoli Peninsula if it were to be carried out in the most careful manner. Hamilton was assured that no decision had been made, 'but I felt that I ought to have your views'. Hamilton's reaction was to feel that such an action would turn the Dardanelles 'into the bloodiest tragedy of the world!' Kitchener also asked what was the cause of the sick rate, remarking, 'some accounts from the Dardanelles indicate the men are dispirited'. This only goes to show just how much Kitchener, and indeed the committee, was out of touch with the reality of the appalling conditions that existed on the peninsula.[4]

Hamilton's reply to Kitchener was to give a gloomy yet carefully measured view of the implications of a possible evacuation. He stressed that there were many imponderables, each of which would have a grave effect on the embarkation process. The weather, with winter approaching, could quickly change from absolute calm to the fiercest of storms whipping the sea sufficiently to make evacuation impossible for an indefinite period of time. He questioned whether it would be possible to deceive the Turks whilst evacuating tens of thousands of troops, thousands of horses and mules, all guns big and small and the tons of equipment without their knowledge. He felt that one-quarter of the force would probably get off the peninsula quite easily but then the troubles would begin. His initial thought was of probably 35–45 percent casualties, but he thought it wise to take the General Staff's estimate of 50 percent. The reply was not what the Dardanelles Committee wanted to hear.[5]

2   Hamilton, *Gallipoli Diary*, vol. 2, 4 October 1915.
3   Keith Murdoch, *The Gallipoli Letter* (Crows Nest: Allen and Unwin, 2010).
4   Hamilton, *Gallipoli Diary*, vol. 2, 11 October.
5   Hamilton, *Gallipoli Diary*, vol. 2, 12 October.

Hamilton was awakened on the night of 16 October to be told a 'secret and personal' cable had arrived from Kitchener informing him he was to receive a second cable that Hamilton himself should decipher. Hamilton knew what was to be in the second cable but decided to leave it for the morning of 17 October. Deciphered, the message reads:

> The War Council held last night decided that though the Government fully appreciate your work and the gallant manner in which you personally have struggled to make the enterprise a success in face of the terrible difficulties you have had to contend against, they, all the same, wish to make a change in command which will give them the opportunity of seeing you.[6]

Hamilton was not to take the news kindly, and, despite his protests, his career had effectively come to an end, as he was never given an opportunity to prove himself again in a senior military post elsewhere.

His successor was General Sir Charles Monro, at the time commanding the Third Army on the Western Front. He was a 'shrewd, hard-headed and capable soldier' with the capacity 'for making up his mind and sticking to it, and a most independent will'. He left Britain on 22 October after researching the situation in the Eastern Mediterranean and meeting Kitchener and the Dardanelles Committee on three occasions.[7] Major General Arthur Lynden-Bell, his chief of staff, accompanied him, and they arrived at Imbros on 28 October. They were met by a memorandum prepared by Hamilton's staff that painted the blackest picture of the future requirements needed at the Dardanelles in order to mount a major offensive. If anything, it probably put Monro on the alert of the reality of extending the Gallipoli Offensive. He could not have been impressed with the call for no less than 400,000 reinforcements.

Monro visited Helles, Anzac and Suvla all on the same day (30 October). For any newcomer, it was an unwelcome surprise to be exposed to the very poor condition of the men's health, their living quarters, their frustration and low morale brought about by prolonged inactivity whilst being exposed to Turkish gunfire on open beaches. Monro was appalled at the conditions he saw. However, before he made a firm decision, he met the corps commanders (Lieutenant General Sir William Birdwood, ANZAC; Lieutenant General Sir Julian Byng, IX Corps; and Lieutenant General Sir Francis Davies, VIII Corps) and their staffs. In typically direct manner, he asked the telling question of 'whether the men are capable of mounting a sustained major offensive and to meet any Turkish counter offensive'. The replies were one of hesitancy, in that yes, an offensive was possible but, with the Turks still occupying the heavily defended high ground, receiving supplies of ammunition and reinforcements to maintain a sustained offensive would be very difficult.

Monro's mind was soon made up, and his decision of 31 October recommending the evacuation of the peninsula was inevitable. His report to Kitchener was one stating the facts as he understood them. The Turkish lines were well established and continually being improved. Heavy guns and ammunition were being made available. Even if the Allies' reinforcements were to be made available, the time taken for them to arrive would give the Turks even more

---

6   Hamilton, *Gallipoli Diary*, vol. 2, 17 October.
7   Aspinall-Oglander, *Military Operations*, vol. 2, p.384.

opportunity to strengthen their positions. The troops were not up to mounting a sustained offensive with sickness depleting units of officers and men.[8]

However, on the question of likely casualties in the event of an evacuation, he was more cautious, appreciating the uncertainties of the weather and Turkish reaction to the withdrawal of the Allies. On further consideration, he estimated a casualty rate of 30–40 percent, which must have given Hamilton a certain sense of satisfaction. Corps Commanders Byng and Davies agreed with the decision. On the other hand, Birdwood, whilst appreciating the difficulty of making any significant advance, felt that to give the Turks a total victory by evacuating the peninsula would have a devastating effect on the morale of the troops involved.

General Monro appreciated the difficulties of carrying out the evacuation, but he could quite justifiably have expected his chief, Field Marshal Kitchener, to have supported his decision. However, Kitchener vacillated, trying to keep his options open. Given this hesitancy, Kitchener decided to visit Gallipoli and see for himself the overall conditions before any firm decision would be made at government level. He arrived on 9 November for a three-day stay and was to see at first hand the situation facing the troops. Nowhere were they safe from the incessant Turkish shelling, the living conditions were appalling, and the sickness levels, coupled with the frustration of a prolonged period of inactivity, had greatly weakened the men's resolve to mount a major 'last throw of the dice' offensive to drive the Turks off the peninsula. Kitchener was soon convinced and, on his return, informed the War Committee that he fully supported Monro's decision. Political objections were raised, without any real appreciation of the desperate situation on the peninsula, over the loss of prestige amongst both enemies and friends. However, when all the facts were made available, good sense prevailed, and it was realised that hard decisions needed to be made sooner rather than later.

After consulting the French, who raised no objection to the evacuation but were strictly subject to maintaining their commitment to Salonika, permission was finally given to evacuate on 7 December, 38 days after Monro's decision. Even so, there was still some hesitancy in confirming that the evacuation was to be limited to Anzac and Suvla areas. The plan to evacuate Helles later was considered to be for naval reasons; however, this could be interpreted as an excuse to keep the vociferous anti-evacuation lobby happy whilst plans were made to finalise the arrangements.

Logistically, the prospect of an evacuation was a problem regardless of the weather and risk of Turkish attention. The task to remove tens of thousands of troops, thousands of horses, hundreds of guns and vehicles and over 2,000 tons of baggage and equipment was daunting. Everything and everybody needed to be moved from the front line to the beaches to be evacuated at night with maximum security measures and all done in the utmost quiet. The evacuation plan was the same for all three locations. The wounded and sick were to leave first, the horses would bring the guns to the beach to be evacuated, and the horses, mules, vehicles and all the unnecessary baggage and equipment would follow. Any wagons left behind would have their wheels broken, and horses and mules considered unfit for transport would be shot. With casualty figures estimated up to 50 percent, the men were not initially told of the decision to evacuate for fear of their reaction to these figures. In an effort to confuse and fool the enemy, a variety

---

8   Alexandra Churchill, 'The Decision to Evacuate the Gallipoli Peninsula' in R. Crawley and M. LoCicero (eds.), *Gallipoli: New Perspectives on the Mediterranean Expeditionary Force, 1915–1916* (Warwick: Helion & Company, 2018), p.164.

of ruses were put in place, including tents not being struck, men being encouraged to go about their normal daily activities, rifles being primed to fire by water dripping into a pan attached to triggers, burning candles being used to set off detonators and empty boxes being stacked up at normal storage points.

It remains a controversial topic as to how much the Turks and Germans knew of what was going on at the beachheads. If the element of surprise could help the evacuation at Anzac and Suvla, this could not be the case at Helles, which was under the full attention of the enemy. However, as had happened at Anzac and Suvla, there were minimum casualties at Helles as the force was finally withdrawn.

Two Germans officers, Admiral von Usedom and Colonel Hans Kannengiesser, offered two opinions on the possibility of an Allied withdrawal. On 31 October, the admiral wrote, 'But I do not think it likely that the enemy abandons his positions without a hard attack. In order to be able to throw them out, a very thorough artillery preparation is required first of all, but there is not sufficient ammunition available, nor can it be produced here'. When the supplies did arrive, the Turks faced a long, time-consuming task of using bullock-drawn carts over poor tracks to deliver them to the far-off battlefields of the Gallipoli Peninsula. Kannengiesser echoed these thoughts: 'Rumours and suggestions that the enemy were going to evacuate Gallipoli naturally swarmed round us on Gallipoli. I, personally, did not believe in such a possibility because, taking into account the English character, I considered it out of the question that they would give up such a hostage of their own free will and without a fight.'[9]

When the Turks were made aware that the evacuation was actually taking place, they were ordered to attack but showed an understandable unwillingness to do so. Frontal attacks such as those on 19 May and during the August Offensive had only resulted in very heavy casualties. Now, as with the British, they were suffering from the severe living conditions and high levels of sickness and saw little reason in sacrificing lives unnecessarily if the enemy was actually running away.

Major Siegert, a member of the German *Luftwaffe*, was ordered to inspect conditions on the Gallipoli front lines. He was flown, together with Second Lieutenant Faller, over the front by Major Serno of the Turkish Air Arm on 5 January 1916. He saw enough to convince himself that he was sure the Allies would withdraw in the next two to three days. Reporting his findings on 6 January, he was disappointed that neither Enver Pasha nor Major Feldman, chief of operations, believed him. His report confirms that German and Turkish military leaders knew of an imminent Allied evacuation just two days before the final Allied withdrawal.[10]

Anzac

The final decision to evacuate Anzac along with Suvla was made on 7 December in London. The news was received at Anzac the next day, and this allowed Lieutenant General William Birdwood and his staff to set the evacuation in progress and issue preliminary orders by 10 December for evacuation on 20 December. This left little more than a week to evacuate tens of

---

9   Klaus Wolf, *Victory at Gallipoli 1915: The German–Ottoman Alliance in the First World War* (Barnsley: Pen and Sword Military, 2020), p.208.
10   Wolf, *Victory at Gallipoli*, p.211.

286   The Fight for Life

thousands of men from the lines and thousands of men, sick and wounded, from the hospitals and ambulances on shore. In theory, the evacuation was to be staged over the days following the issue of the preliminary orders so that only those men essential to holding the position remained for the final days. The instructions for the final evacuation of the medical services out of Anzac were issued on 18 December:

1. *Personnel retained for duty*
    a) No 13 CCS – 5 officers, 69 others.
    No 1 ACCS – 7 officers, 71 others.
    b) Divisional units.
    Ten NCO's and men for each 1,000 troops, drawn from the bearer divisions of field
        ambulances, have been detailed to work under the regimental medical officers.
    All other medical units have been withdrawn.

2. *Equipment and Supplies*
    a) Casualty clearing stations have been stocked with 30 days supplies of food, fuel, light, comforts, etc., for 1,200 patients with ample medical and surgical supplies. Each has under guard and red cross flag 6,000 gallons of water, and an additional 70,000 gallons, not earmarked, with water carts and mule, has been left behind.
    b) The camps of field ambulances, dressing stations and aid posts are still standing and have been equipped with stretchers, blankets, food, dressings, etc., for use by personnel from casualty clearing stations or from the bearer divisions. A total equipment for 3,200 patients has been arranged and 30 days supplies for British and 60 for Indian troops provided.

3. *Embarkation*
    a) Patients. Serious cases are to be embarked only by daylight at first; slight cases can embark with their units. On the last night, very serious cases are not to be brought to the CCS's but are to be left in dressing stations or on the spot where wounded, with a view to being subsequently collected. These sites are to be marked on the last night with red cross flags, their sites being marked on a plan furnished to the SMO remaining.
    b) Equipment. All valuable surplus equipment, except tents, and all permanent records etc., were embarked at an early stage. Temporary records are now being kept.
    c) Medical units and personnel. The two CCS's are held ready to embark at a moment's notice on receiving written orders to that effect from the commander of the rear-guard. All arrangements have been made in advance, and the scale and composition of personnel to be left behind have been laid down in accordance with the number of casualties. Stretcher bearers, unless specially retained, will embark with the units to which they have been attached for the occasion.[11]

---

11   Macpherson, *History of the Great War: Medical Services*, vol. 4, p.52.

It had been anticipated that the evacuation would be accompanied by large numbers of casualties, and detailing CCSs to remain was a recognition of this possibility should the Turks become aware of the movement. All medical units were instructed to leave all their tents in position, for this served two purposes: first, it gave the appearance that everything at Anzac was proceeding normally; second, they would provide cover for those casualties that were anticipated. The medical unit camps were protected under the red cross of the Geneva Convention and would provide a relatively safe haven for any wounded arising during the evacuation. Similarly, the convention would also offer some protection for the medical staff and patients should they be left behind and fall into the hands of the enemy.[12] Nevertheless, heavy casualties were expected, and they were to be cared for by the only two CCSs that would remain solely for that purpose. These were the 1st ACCS and the 13th BCCS.

Immediate upon receipt of the instructions from London, and prior to General Birdwood issuing his preliminary orders, the DDMS ANZAC, Colonel N. Howse VC, reviewed the units and personnel for which it was his responsibility to organise evacuation. These units were as shown in the following table. From this table, which excludes the RMOs, it can be seen that the number of men in the medical services to be evacuated was close to that of an entire brigade of front-line troops then at Anzac, and their evacuation was to require a similar attention to detail.[13] Over the days that followed, each of the units received instructions for the part they were to play in the evacuation, which, generally, coincided with those of the infantry movements in the area.

Medical Units at Anzac, 9 December1915[14]

Unit	Officers	Other Ranks	Attached to	Evacuated
3rd AFA	10	142	1st Australian Division	12 December
4th AFA	6	157	New Zealand and Australian Division	13 December
5th AFA	6	137	2nd Australian Division	18 December
6th AFA	5	122	2nd Australian Division	12 December
7th AFA	6	116	2nd Australian Division	12 December
1st ALHFA	4	51	New Zealand and Australian Division	13 December
2nd ALHFA	5	78	1st Australian Division	11 December
3rd ALHFA	2	31	New Zealand and Australian Division	Before 14 December
NZFA	10	173	New Zealand and Australian Division	18 December
NZMFA	6	71	New Zealand and Australian Division	18 December
1/3rd EAFA	6	142	54th Division	12 December

12   Article 6 of the 1907 Geneva Convention details the protection of the mobile medical units, while Article 12 protects the personnel after capture. See Butler, *Official History of the Australian Medical Services*, vol. I, pp.814–20.
13   AWM: AWM4/26/14/4: War Diary, DDMS ANZAC Corps, 9 December.
14   AWM: AWM4/26/14/4: War Diary, DDMS ANZAC Corps, 9 December.

Unit	Officers	Other Ranks	Attached to	Evacuated
EMBFA	4	75	54th Division	Before 14 December
108th IFA	3	134	29th Indian Brigade	14 December
137th IFA (C)	2	42	Indian Mountain Battery	19 December
1st ACCS	9	77		20 December
16th CCS	7	65		13 December
13th CCS	9	75		20 December
No. 1 ASH	8	83		12 December
21st Sanitary Section	0	17		Before 14 December
24th Sanitary Section	1	18		Before 14 December
No. 4 Advanced Depot Medical Stores	1	4		Before 14 December
Total	**110**	**1,810**		

The procedure for evacuation was such that all valuable medical stores and equipment were embarked first to be followed over the following days by the field ambulances until only the two designated CCSs were left on the peninsula. These two units were to remain until as late as possible in case casualties occurred during the final moves of the evacuation. Furthermore, if there were large numbers of casualties that could not be evacuated to the waiting hospital ships or transports, then the CCSs were to remain to ensure the care for the wounded could continue.

The DDMS ANZAC informed Major Battye of the 108th IFA on 11 December that his field ambulance would be leaving the peninsula shortly. As a direct consequence of this, the 108th IFA began to transfer patients to the recently opened Indian CCS so that, by the following day, the hospital of the 108th IFA had been emptied. During the day, the field ambulance continued to pack equipment for an early move. The CO then received orders that he was to detail two British officers and 89 men to remain. One officer and most of the detailed men were to remain at the 108th IFA HQ while the other officer and a small number of bearers were to assist the 1st ACCS with Indian casualties as the evacuation proceeded. This instruction also meant that the Indian CCS would be evacuated early. Captain Stocker, who had been in charge of the CCS, would remain, but he and his staff would assist the 1st ACCS. This rationalisation of the medical resources over the days before the final evacuation was in line with the overall process carried out across Anzac. It also allowed for the CCSs that were to remain to accommodate 1,200 casualties in the event that it should be needed. Major Battye volunteered to stay behind with the Indian contingent, but this was vetoed since Howse had already appointed a captain of the ACCS to be SMO of the remaining medical units at Anzac and hence could not allow a more senior, and more experienced, officer to remain with another unit. Battye appointed Captain Drake, IMS, as the second officer to remain, and the remainder of the 108th IFA embarked on 14 December but not before:

> I omitted to mention above that at my interview with the DDMS I asked him in view of the fact that the Indian Brigade were on the left flank of our line and four miles from the evacuating piers to let me have at least rowing boats to evacuate our wounded

from the beach due west of our lines, between the mouths of the Azmak Dere and Aghyl Dere and so save much time and more than three miles of road transport, or failing that to provide me with a large motor lorry or at least ten or fifteen or more mule carts in which I could rapidly remove wounded up to the last minute. He replied that not a single spare boat of any kind was available; that the motor lorry had already been removed and that all the mule carts were about to be! And that every case must be removed by hand.[15]

It is also clear from the diary that RMOs were to remain with their units and were expected to use their regimental stretcher-bearers until they reached Captain Drake at the old field ambulance HQ site in Chailak Dere. This is perhaps to be expected, in so far as the 108th IFA could not operate fully without its full complement of staff, meaning that bearers to assist the front-line units were also very limited.

For this particular field ambulance, and there is no evidence to suggest anything different for other units, evacuation from the beaches did not mean that the problems were over. In some aspects, the lack of suitable accommodation and transport faced by the 108th IFA is symptomatic of the entire campaign. The problems began before it left Anzac, as the ambulance was asked to wait five hours on the beach during the evening of 13 December before a lighter showed up to ferry the personnel to a waiting transport, the *Abbassiyeh*. Even then, they had to leave all their equipment behind in the hope that it would follow later. By the time the transport sailed, it was early morning of 14 December, and, later the same morning, the unit reached Mudros, where the personnel were then transferred to the HT *Mercian*, of which Battye had little good to say:

It had no facilities for Indian troops and no rations at all for them and the ship's officers had not news of our coming. The troop decks were clean, except that the cooking pots and plates and dishes of the British troops were still unwashed and contained a lot of remnants of food several days old! The rest of the ship however was very dirty and the horse lines were all deep in horse dung and filthy litter.[16]

This suggests that, although the evacuation of the beaches had been very successful, the organisation farther from the beaches and along the lines of communication was not so good, and, on the basis of Battye's experience, it seems to have been particularly poor. The ship was to be used for Indian troops, and there was an urgent need to put it order to receive as many as possible. There was a need for all decks to be cleaned, and, as Battye pointed out, the ship 'Can take 500 troops immediately. Horse decks could take another 750 if cleaned and whitewashed. In present condition impossible. Officer requires at least 4 days and large party to prepare. Indians will not clean horse dung. Latrine accommodation at a pinch for 750 men and cooking accommodation very restricted.'[17]

---

15 TNA: WO 95/4272: War Diary, 108th Indian Field Ambulance, 13 December.
16 TNA: WO 95/4272: War Diary, 108th Indian Field Ambulance, 14 December.
17 TNA: WO 95/4272: War Diary, 108th Indian Field Ambulance, 14 December. Telegram from Major Battye to DAQMG.

Final layout of the 108th IFA as it was left after evacuation. (Terence Powell after War Dairy 108th IFA, WO 95/4272, 14th December 1915)

Despite the efforts made by Major Battye and his sanitary officer to get the ship ready for use, there was still an attempt to overfill the ship as more Indian troops from Lemnos were packed on board. Nevertheless, the fully laden troopship left Mudros on the afternoon of 15 December bound for Alexandria. The 108th IFA's part in the Gallipoli Campaign was finished as the evacuation of troops continued as fast as possible.

By this date, almost all the field ambulances had departed Anzac, leaving little more than a skeleton medical service in place to handle casualties as troops began to leave the area. The 5th AFA received orders that it was to provide a small number of bearers for each of the battalions of the 5th and 6th Australian Brigades still holding the line. In the event, the ambulance provided 56 bearers for the eight battalions and one light horse regiment of the two brigades. This was in line with the requirement set out by the instructions of providing 10 bearers per 1,000 troops. The total number remaining in the two brigades was 5,517. The field ambulance set up dressing stations at a number of locations to ensure some immediate assistance in the event of a Turkish attack. The CO of the ambulance instructed the RMOs remaining:

> That on final night no seriously wounded case is to be transported to a clearing station and is to be dressed in the spot and left at one of the dressing stations or made comfortable at the place where he was wounded. These wounded will be subsequently collected. Red Cross flags at each dressing station and Regimental Aid Posts are to be erected on last evening. No fresh flags are to be put up till then. I also sent a map of the position of my bearers and dressing stations to the DDMS.[18]

The 5th AFA was then evacuated from the peninsula and disembarked to No. 2 Camp Mudros West on 18 December.

This sort of arrangement was made by other field ambulances at Anzac. For instance, the NZFA detailed 14 men to the New Zealand Brigade, and the New Zealand Mounted Brigade Field Ambulance (NZMBFA) a further seven men to the New Zealand Mounted Brigade. These field ambulances began evacuation of their own staff on 13 December, but the detailed men remained until the unit to which they were attached evacuated on 19 December. As elsewhere, the units left their tents standing to assist the appearance of normality.[19]

The plan was that, by the final night, only two CCSs would remain with such support as could be offered by RMOs and bearer details still remaining at that time. As the medical units evacuated, it was necessary for all their patients to be evacuated. For instance, the 16th BCCS was evacuated to Mudros on 13 December at the same time as No. 1 ASH and the 1/3rd East Anglian Field Ambulance (EAFA), together with 900 sick and wounded.[20] According to Butler, approximately 20,000 sick and wounded were evacuated from the peninsula between 11–20 December, though a proportion of these were from Suvla. On the evening of 19 December, the 13th BCCS received orders to evacuate at 11:10 p.m. This reflected that there had been no casualties as the infantry units began to come away from the line, and this in turn meant that the hospital was no longer needed on the peninsula. A little over three hours later, the first part of the 1st ACCS was embarked on the HS *Dongola*, which set sail for Mudros. The evacuation had

---

18   AWM: AWM4/26/48/5: War Diary, 5th Australian Field Ambulance, 16 December.
19   Carberry, *New Zealand Medical Service in the Great War*, p.133.
20   Carberry, *New Zealand Medical Service in the Great War*, p.133.

292   The Fight for Life

been a success. There had been no casualties and, consequently, no need to leave any wounded or medical staff behind.

During the evacuation phase, a little over 31,000 troops were removed from the Anzac beaches over a period of 10 days, with over half this number remaining until 19 December when the final evacuation commenced. Whilst the medical services were also run down over the same period, the two remaining CCSs needed to provide cover for in excess of 16,000 troops remaining for the last phase of the operation. The fact that the manoeuvre was not challenged by the Turks is no doubt fortunate, but, nevertheless, all pieces of the evacuation worked well to avoid any unnecessary casualties. For the medical units, their work was not over since, when they reached Lemnos, most were retained to handle the sickness that remained. Eventually, all were reassigned as, for them, the war moved into other theatres.

Suvla

The plan for the evacuation of Suvla was similar, in that it, too, gradually reduced the military presence over a 10-day period from 8–17 December. On 11 December, the 89th Field Ambulance of the 29th Division received orders to the effect that an officer was to be selected to report to the marine landing officer at West Beach that evening to prepare for the rest of the ambulance to embark that night. The entry in the war diary for the following day gives some details of the departure:

> Camp was cleaned up, tents left standing and flags flying, a few tents with candles lit. All baggage was carried down to a dump on the road and thence removed by mule carts to West Beach. Advanced dressing station and advanced aid post handed over to A Section of 88th Field Ambulance. Ambulance moved off from camp at 7.15 preceded at 6.30 by Lt Murray as advance officer. Embarked 2100 on HMS *Redbreast*. Embarkation strength seven officers and 152 other ranks.[21]

The unit landed at Mudros, where the 87th Field Ambulance had already arrived, and remained there separated from its division until it, too, was evacuated in early January. The 88th Field Ambulance remained at Suvla for some days longer, and its departure was spread over a number of days. It was to remain split until it rejoined the division in January.

The final two days (18–19 December) saw the evacuation of the remaining troops. The troops were to be thinned out on the night of 18 December, but the firing line would be manned right up to the final moment in the early hours of the next day. On both nights, the troops were to find their way to designated collecting posts. Here, a careful check of numbers was made of incoming troops to ensure there were no stragglers. Only when this condition was satisfied were the troops be allowed to move on down the line to the beaches. There, small boats were waiting to be ready to take them to awaiting ships. As at Anzac, there was the ever-present fear that the Turks would be alerted at any time and turn the entire operation into catastrophe. Added to this was the fear that poor weather conditions would make it impossible to evacuate men off the

---

21   TNA: WO 95/4309: War Diary, 89th Field Ambulance, 12 December.

beaches. In the event, the weather remained calm on the first night, but strengthening winds and a rough sea in the early hours of 19 December caused much concern but did not prevent the eventual successful evacuation of all troops.

Once the decision to evacuate had been made, the medical services were immediately faced with the task of coping with the expected casualties and the prevailing high levels of sickness during this entire period. It was essential to maintain the correct balance of available medical services ready to handle any wounded and sick that may occur at any one time. This required sufficient personnel, animals, wagons, equipment, rations, water supply and so on to allow the units to function. In order for this to happen, it was essential that all MOs had a thorough understanding of the evacuation plans.

A scheme of medical personnel, equipment and transport requirements was made. It was based initially on the assessment by the DDMS IX Corps of the likely number of casualties that would require a 50-bed hospital for one month and a 500-bed for 10 days. The scheme, which was put in place immediately, had to be drastically upgraded when the DDMS asked for an increased provision for 1,000 casualties.[22]

Throughout the preparation, the Turks maintained fire on the area, and there were casualties. Sickness levels stayed high and required continued medical care whilst the evacuation process continued to be organised. The ADMS 2nd Mounted Division included in his December report total admissions of those sick for the week ending 11 December to be 14 officers and 329 other ranks, including cases of diarrhoea, jaundice, trench foot, rheumatism and pyrexia. This gave a total percentage of those sick in the division as 10.9 percent.[23]

During the storm and blizzard in late November, Captain A. Glen of the 40th Field Ambulance decided to take an ambulance wagon across the Salt Lake, by that time frozen hard, and many men were brought back to the safety of the dressing stations. However, on the third day of using this route, the wagon broke through the hard crust of the Salt Lake. The Turks started shelling the wagon. One mule was hurt, and, in the process of freeing the animals, an MO was wounded in the chest. The wagon had to be abandoned. Stretcher cases were collected by bearers, and the walking wounded found their own way back to the field ambulance. Glen came in for some good-natured teasing about his mishap and the highly visible 'Monument on the Lake'. Whilst the wagon could have been abandoned, General Maude, OC 13th Division, ordered it to be recovered from the lake as a means of indicating that everything was continuing normally at Suvla. This was done at night by a section of pioneers.[24]

Surplus equipment including kits, blankets, ground sheets, waterproofs, tents and medical and surgical panniers were sent to the ordnance depot. Unwanted ambulance wagons, drivers and mules were returned to IX Corps Transport. The 26th CCS was able to send about six tons of equipment to the ordnance depot for embarkation before the night of the final evacuation. In the first instance, all men considered too weak and unfit to resume duties within two days were evacuated. As plans for the final days of evacuation were revealed, the manning require-ments became clear for the medical services. This allowed the evacuation of all personnel who would not be required. Field ambulances were instructed to clear their hospitals by sending their casualties to a CCS. It became possible to close the 33rd Field Ambulance, 11th Division,

22   TNA: WO 95/4356: War Diary, 26th Casualty Clearing Station.
23   TNA: WO 95/4292: War Diary, 2nd Mounted Division ADMS, 11 December.
24   Glen, *In the Front Line*, p.53.

294   The Fight for Life

and the 1/2nd South Western Mounted Brigade Field Ambulance (SWMBFA), 13th Division, while the 35th Field Ambulance was detailed to take all divisional casualties but to pass them to the CCS as quickly as possible. The process continued until only those required for the final days remained. The 11th Division evacuated a total 890 'weakly' men and, by 13 December, had reduced its personnel to just 10 officers and 214 men.[25] The 13th Division reduced its numbers on 11 December when it made the following arrangements for each of the three field ambulances (39th, 40th and 41st Field Ambulances):

- A bearer division was formed consisting of three officers, six NCOs and 90 men (18 stretcher squads of five men each) and equipped with surgical haversacks, water bottles, shell dressing haversacks and 22 stretchers.
- A tent subdivision consisted of two officers and 25 other ranks with dressings, medical comforts, cooking utensils and so on.
- Two officers were detailed to replace casualties if required.

A total of 13 officers and 313 other ranks was to be available for duty during the final stage of the evacuation and detailed to form a dressing station at South Pier. Equipment and medical comforts necessary for 300 patients for one week was to be retained, the remainder handed in to the ordnance depot at West Beach and left under guard ready to be evacuated. The remainder consisting of five officers and 165 other ranks with the equipment and baggage of the three field ambulances embarked from C Beach at 6:00 p.m. on 11 December.[26]

On 9 December, the ADMS 29th Division visited the dressing stations of 88th and 89th Field Ambulances and made arrangements for the handling of surplus equipment. The 89th Field Ambulance embarked on 11 December after it had handed over its ADS and advanced aid post to a section of the 88th Field Ambulance. Orders were given for the 1/1st HMBFA, 2nd Mounted Division, to embark on 16 December, but Major L. M. V. Mitchell and 38 other ranks remained to act as stretcher-bearers for the Highland Mounted Brigade.

On 13 December, the 53rd CCS left one NCO and 15 men behind to 'keep the Camp fires and lights burning' before embarking on the *Rowan* and leaving the peninsula in the early hours of the following day. Those remaining left Suvla on 20 December. The 14th CCS embarked on 15 December, and the 26th CCS on 17 December, but both were detailed to leave a detachment behind for the final days. The 14th CCS party to be left behind consisted of three officers and about 20 NCOs and men with sufficient equipment and stores for a month. The 26th CCS left a party of two officers, two NCOs and 10 men.

The plan was to remove the remaining troops over the final two nights. General Maude was concerned over not only the necessity to hold the front line but also the need to avoid the sudden mass movement of troops away from the front lines. There was much concern that such movements carried out at night, when troops could unavoidably make more noise than during daylight, and that the sound made, which could easily carry, would sufficiently alert the Turks that 'something was taking place'.

General Maude on the final day (19 December) wrote in his diary:

25   TNA: WO 95/4298: War Diary, 11th Division ADMS, 13 December.
26   TNA: WO 95/4300: War Diary, 13th Division ADMS, 11 December.

From about 11.30am onwards, our front line of trenches was held by 200 men, till 1.30am, when they finally withdrew. From 11.30am onwards the Salt Lake lines were only held by 100 men and three machine guns., the Lala Baba defences being held by 250 men and six machine guns, we closed the gaps in the wire and withdrew everyone except the Lala Baba garrison, and embarked them, and finally we embarked the Lala Baba garrison and the six machine guns.[27]

Whilst the troops' primary concern was the evacuation process, it is worthwhile pointing out that the medical teams' primary concern was to attend to the expected casualties whilst keeping in mind their eventual evacuation. They were under the strictest orders not to retire until the main body of troops had passed. This placed them under great mental pressure to maintain their composure as up to 1,000 troops passed by and made their way to safety before they could follow.

The medical teams were well spread out along the firing line. The 11th Division's field ambulances were located to the north of the Salt Lake. There were ADSs at Piccadilly Circus, Karakol Gap and Lone Tree Gully and a dressing station in the Reserve Area. This meant that there were no fewer than eight officers and 226 medical personnel from the firing line to the point of evacuation. In addition, there were 10 ambulance wagons manned and available if required. It was planned that wounded were to be sent to West Beach or Little West Beach, where they would be evacuated under the supervision of the embarkation MO.[28]

The men at the Piccadilly Circus ADS retired to the 2nd Line, followed the vacating troops of the 32nd Brigade and prepared to embark. The men at Karakol Gap ADS followed the same routine but fell back to the 3rd Line before proceeding to the 29th Division HQ, where they prepared to embark in the company of the 32nd Infantry Brigade. At Lone Tree Gully ADS, the men retired along the Chanak Road and took up position at the Chanak Chesme Well. This unit was to move through the 2nd and 3rd Lines and join up with the troops arriving from the front line to prepare to embark. The dressing station in the Reserve Area was kept open until the last to accommodate any casualties occurring on the beach. All personnel were finally evacuated on 20 December, taking equipment with them.

The 13th Division field ambulances were located in the mid and south areas of Suvla. Here, the plan was that the wounded were brought to the dressing station at South Pier, Lala Baba, from the front trenches. On 18 December, the 39th Field Ambulance was detailed to send one officer and two NCOs, complete with surgical haversacks and 16 stretcher-bearers with four stretchers, to Well 82 on the old Chocolate Hill Road. They were to wait until approximately two battalions returning from the firing line had all passed before leaving. One officer and one NCO proceeded along the road towards Chocolate Hill to get in touch with the RMOs. If there were any casualties, they were to be sent direct to the 14th CCS for evacuation. On the final day (19 December), the medical personnel of the 13th Division were a total of eight officers and 102 other ranks. The 39th Field Ambulance was split up into two parties. The first party was under the command of Captain Minns. He was ordered to report to GOC 38th Brigade at the dressing station on Chocolate Hill. The party marched via Lala Baba direct to the dump

---

27   Churchill, 'Decision to Evacuate', p.179.
28   TNA: WO 95/4298: War Diary, 11th Division ADMS, 18 December.

at the western foot of Chocolate Hill and waited there to take any casualties that might occur. His instructions were that only stretcher cases were to be taken. Walking cases were to make their own way down with their own battalions and embark with them. Stretcher cases, if they occurred during the early part of the evening, were to be evacuated to the 14th CCS at C Beach. If casualties occurred later in the evening, after 11:00 p.m., they were to be carried straight down to South Pier at Lala Baba and to retire with the troops from that position. No casualties occurred, and the party embarked at 1:15 a.m. on 20 December.

The second party, under Captain I. J. Williams, had orders to report at HQ at 6:45 p.m. to take any casualties that might occur at Lala Baba. They were to be taken straight down to the dressing station at South Pier. As there was only one walking case, the party at Chocolate Hill was able to march down with the party of the 39th Brigade, leaving Chocolate Hill at 11:30 p.m. following in rear of the BHQ. They marched to Lala Baba without incident and embarked at 1:30 a.m. on the HMT *Rowan*. Both parties were instructed to preserve the normal appearance of the camp as far as possible. Any equipment that could not possibly be carried away was destroyed.

A third, small group of 12 men drawn from the 39th Field Ambulance, 40th Field Ambulance and 41st Field Ambulance, under the command of Lieutenant Williams, formed an aid post at the place of assembly near divisional HQ, where the troops formed up prior to embarkation. At the 40th Field Ambulance, Captain Burke, Lieutenant King and 32 men were detailed to report to GOC 39th Brigade at Asmak Dere Bridge at 8:00 p.m., where they came under the orders of the ADMS 11th Division. When the party arrived at Asmak Dere Bridge at 6:00 p.m., Lieutenant King and three squads were sent to the 39th Brigade Dump. They left there with the second-last party to leave the trenches and embarked with them at 1:00 am on 20 December. Captain Burke and the remainder stayed at Azmak Bridge until 2:00 a.m., when the last snipers arrived from the trenches. There was only one wounded man in the brigade, and he was only slightly hurt. The party came behind the infantry and were the last through the wire before the gap was closed. They collected three stragglers who had to be assisted along. The party finally embarked at 4:00 a.m. on 20 December.

Captain Lovell and Lieutenant Burton at the 41st Field Ambulance, with one NCO and 24 men, were ordered to report to GOC 40th Brigade at 8:00 p.m. on 19 December. This party was stationed at Well 82 in order to keep a check on the movements of the stretcher squads to ensure that all were within the defences when the time came to close the gaps in the barbed-wire entanglements in front of the line of trenches. The party retired with the rearguard and embarked on the last lighter leaving South Pier at 3:45 a.m. Lieutenant O'Brian, Lieutenant Murphy and six men from the 41st Field Ambulance formed a collecting post and dressing station in a sandbag redoubt at the entrance to the pier.

On the night of 18/19 December, one NCO and 19 men of the 1/1st HMBFA originally intended to act as stretcher-bearers for the South Western Mounted Brigade were ordered to proceed to the point of rendezvous at Lala Baba and embarked for Imbros on the night of 19/20 December. Major L. M. V. Mitchell, CO of the 1/1st HMBFA, one NCO and 16 men forming four stretcher squads of four men each with eight stretchers remained and were sent to the gap in the Salt Lake defences at Anzac Road, where they arrived at 6:00 p.m. and reported to the divisional staff officer posted there. They were detailed to stay at the firing lines in the Anafarta plain until the line was evacuated. The group accompanied departing troops and reached the gap in the defence line at about 2:20 a.m. on 20 December. This group was the last of the division to arrive at the rendezvous at Lala Baba Beach:

There were no casualties known to us and everything went like clockwork – we embarked on a lighter at 0030 thence to a ship and so off to Imbros. Mention is worthy of the good spirit with which the men of the detachment of this unit waited those 7 hours at the gap in the defences – hours which were made all the more trying owing to their inactivity and the necessary strict silence and no smoking.[29]

The CCS had made the rigorous plans to cater for the possibility of anything up to 1,000 casualties. In the event, there were no casualties of note, and it was allowed to embark on 20 December.

Helles

Any thoughts of retaining troops at Helles were dashed on 23 December by General Sir William Robertson, chief of the Imperial General Staff. He wrote that there was no sound reason to maintain an Allied presence at Gallipoli. He dismissed the argument for keeping the Turks occupied as irrelevant given the total defeat of the Allies and the extreme impossibility of ever mounting another worthwhile offensive. In any case, he pointed out that the Allied forces were already fighting the Turks in the Caucasus, Persia and Mesopotamia. He felt to maintain up to 50,000 men at Helles would provide more problems of supply for the navy rather than the relatively simple task of maintaining a blockade. Coming from such a senior and highly respected officer, the General Staff now called for the peninsula to be totally evacuated.[30]

The evacuation of Helles differed in two significant ways from that of Anzac and Suvla. First, the Turks and Germans were unlikely to be caught unawares and would be on alert guarding against any attempted withdrawal at Helles; that is, the element of surprise had been lost. Second, at Helles, the distance from the firing line to the beaches at some 6,000yd was greater than at Anzac or Suvla. This posed problems for the timing of troop withdrawal from the front lines. It would take time to get these troops away from under the Turks' guns, but to leave the front line unmanned for any lengthy period of time could have alerted the Turks of an Allied withdrawal. To some extent, the French had rather pre-empted the decision since they had removed a portion of their force from Helles as early as October, leaving just 7,600 troops to evacuate as the campaign was finally ended.[31] These were evacuated some days before the British forces, but much of their artillery remained to maintain the necessary fire power in the event of an attack by the Turks.[32]

As a result of these additional problems associated with evacuation at Helles and an estimate of a high percentage of casualties, the medical services were placed in a very difficult position. They had to ensure that, on the days of troop withdrawal and particularly on the final day and night, there would be sufficient medical cover at suitable locations capable of attending to casualties anywhere along the planned routes of evacuation. This included a medical team to accompany everyone to the beach from the first to the last party making its way to the beach.

29   TNA: WO 95/4292: War Diary, 1/1st Highland Mounted Brigade Field Ambulance, 20 December.
30   Churchill, 'Decision to Evacuate', p.181.
31   Aspinall-Oglander, *Military Operations*, vol. 2, p.391.
32   Aspinall-Oglander, *Military Operations*, vol. 2, p.470.

298 The Fight for Life

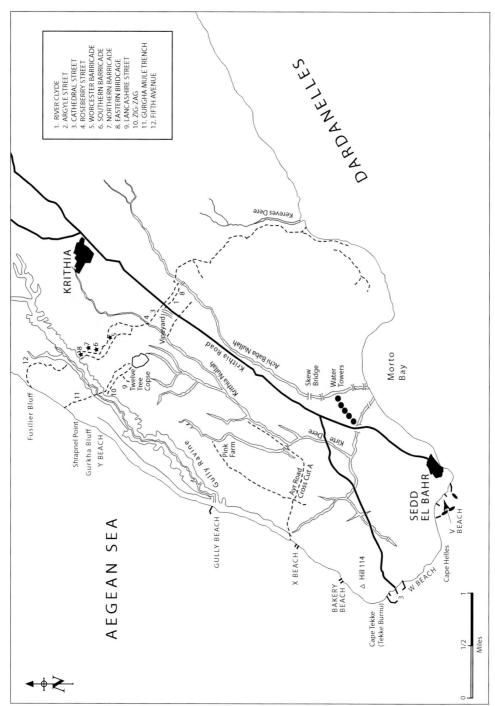

Lines of evacuation at Helles. (Terence Powell after War Diary, WO 95/4307 December 1915)

Evacuation: Tents Left Standing and Flags Flying 299

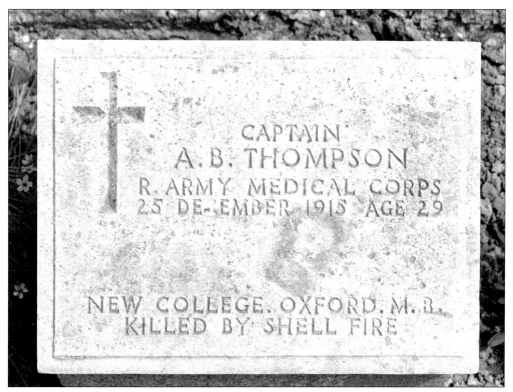

A routine death. Captain Arnold Bosanquet Thompson, aged 29, 1/3rd ELFA, acting RMO for the 1/5th Lancashire Fusiliers, was killed on a day that the war diary of his unit simply records, 'Routine'. (Author)

This meant that all MOs had to have a very thorough knowledge of the proposed lines of evacuation. Alterations to the general plan of evacuation on 6 January reduced the originally planned two-night departure to just one night, and the medical teams involved with the withdrawal were adapted to ensure any change to the evacuation routes were adequately covered.

On 31 December, the following medical units were at Helles:

- 42nd Division: 1/1st and 1/3rd ELFAs
- 52nd Division: 1/1st, 1/2nd and 1/3rd Lowland Field Ambulances
- RND: 1st, 2nd and 3rd Field Ambulances
- 11th CCS
- No. 17 Stationary Hospital.

It should be noted, however, that, although by this time the 42nd Division had been replaced by the 13th Division, the medical units of the 42nd Division remained. The 13th Division was not accompanied by its field ambulances, and the division was served by the units of the 42nd Division that it replaced. Also, the 29th Division had landed at Helles by 21 December, but its 'Field Ambulances scattered all over the place, 89th and 87th at Mudros – 88th in pieces

– part on the *Southland*, part on Imbros.'[33] It was arranged that the 29th Division would have the support of the 1/1st Lowland Field Ambulance of the 52nd Division and the 1/1st South Eastern Mounted Brigade Field Ambulance (SEMBFA) of the 42nd Division.[34] The ADMS of the 29th Division remained on Helles, overseeing these arrangements for his division until final evacuation.

The 42nd Division's field ambulances were posted to the left flank in and about Gully Ravine, the 52nd Division's field ambulances in the centre sector in and around the Pink Farm area, and the RND on the right flank, where it had taken over the section of trenches that had been held by the French colonial troops earlier in the month. The 11th CCS and No. 17 Stationary Hospital remained at W Beach.

The preliminary orders for evacuation were made known on 31 December. A meeting of all ADsMS was held, followed by a meeting of all COs of field ambulances. It was planned that there was to be a gradual withdrawal of men, baggage, vehicles and animals on a nightly basis until the final two nights. On the penultimate night, 11 officers and 220 men were to form the RAMC establishment to cope with casualties. Surgical and medical equipment sufficient to cover up to a seven-day period was to be retained, and all surplus material was evacuated.

The 1/1st SEMBFA and the 1/2nd ELFA embarked from V Beach for Mudros on 30 December. All wounded, sick, weakly and unreliable men were to be evacuated with the proviso that the strength of field ambulances was not reduced by more than 10 percent. All surplus stores and officer kits were collected and sent to ordnance for embarkation. Wagons no longer required had their wheels destroyed and were lined up on the beach ready to be destroyed by naval gunfire after evacuation of the beaches. To maintain an air of normality, tents were left standing, dugouts remained in normal condition, and Red Cross flags were kept flying. Men were encouraged to go about their normal duties, washing was to be hung out, ambulance wagons were to continue making regular visits whether needed or not, incinerators were to be kept burning, Thresh Disinfectors were to continue working, any packing of baggage was to be done indoors, and such ploys as empty boxes were stacked particularly at open-to-view storage areas. Throughout all this preparation, it should be mentioned that, during the entire evacuation process, the enemy continued artillery bombardment. During the following two days, the last of the French troops and their medical and support units (about 7,600 in total) left the peninsula.

The plan drawn up on 6 January to evacuate the wounded was that one bearer was attached to each group of 50 men to assist as necessary. Help was sought from troops to carry all wounded down to the divisional rendezvous. Each remaining division had its own rendezvous close to the beaches. At each of these positions, two officers and 45 bearers equipped with 56 stretchers, aided by three horse-drawn wagons and nine personnel, were available to transfer the wounded to the beach and then embark with the wounded men. This was meant to allow rapid embarkation of small groups, thus keeping the embarkation process moving at a controlled pace. The attendant beach officer and naval transport officer were to oversee the process. RMOs and stretcher-bearers were evacuated under regimental control. Inland evacuation routes were chosen that gave the best protection from enemy shellfire, and, where possible, they were

---

33   TNA: WO 95/4307: War Diary, 29th Division ADMS, 21 December.
34   TNA: WO 95/4307: War Diary, 29th Division ADMS, 31 December.

widened to make the journey easier for the wounded and bearers. Naval stretchers and blanket stretchers were made available to the RMOs.

The Turks began a severe bombardment on 7 January. This was followed by the detonation of four mines and a Turkish attack. The attack was not aggressive and was easily repulsed by the 7th North Staffordshire Regiment but not without loss – the medical units eventually treated and evacuated 114 wounded men. On the final day (8 January), the morning was dedicated to the removal of all remaining equipment. Any other materials and buildings no longer required were destroyed as far as possible. Notably, there was no time to destroy some motor ambulance wagons. A number of horses and mules were shot. At dusk, some tents were cut into ribbons and rendered useless.

At 9:00 p.m. on the final day, there was a report that the wind and sea were rising, which raised doubts that the evacuation process could be completed. The last party of 390 men of the 13th Division on the left flank was to be evacuated at Gully Beach using the last K2 boats. Of this number, 260 men were successfully taken away on the first boat, but the second ran aground because of the wind and rough sea. The remainder, including six MOs and 24 men of the RAMC, made a hasty march to W Beach, where they were finally evacuated. The remains of the K lighter that ran aground can still be seen at Gully Beach.

Captain W. W. Greer, ADMS 52nd Lowland Division, recorded the medical arrangements for the evacuation of the 52nd Division from the centre sector on 6 January 1916. The line of evacuation was along the Achi Baba Nullah route. Eight control posts were set up along the route, the common meeting point being the divisional rendezvous at the lower end of the route. At 6:00 a.m., the men at the existing relay posts found their way to Nos 1–7 Control Posts. At 4:00 p.m., the two remaining dressing stations were evacuated, and, again, the men found their way to the nearest control post.[35] MOs in charge did not allow any departure from the posts until entirely satisfied that there were no wounded parties left to arrive. Only then was the post closed to allow the party to make its way to the divisional rendezvous. At 9:30 p.m., the last party left No. 8 Control Post and reported at the divisional rendezvous. The remaining RAMC men, with three ambulance wagons, assembled at the divisional rendezvous. The men were added to the parties arriving from the front lines. As no casualties had occurred, there was an attempt to save the spare stretchers. They were taken down to the pier, but the rough seas made the quick transfer to the awaiting boats too difficult with stretchers, so they were abandoned.

Two men who had been carrying machine guns from the firing line reached the divisional rendezvous but were so exhausted they had to be sent to the beach in a wagon. This was the only occasion in which a wagon was used, and, as such, these two exhausted men could be classed as the only casualties in this area for the evacuation. At 1:20 a.m. on 9 January, the final party, consisting of Captains Greer, Black, Walker and Linklater accompanied by the remaining 47 RAMC men, left the divisional rendezvous. The divisional police were immediately behind them and were the last of the division to be evacuated.[36]

The RND followed very much the same procedures as the other divisions. The field ambulances were reduced to 10 officers and 200 other ranks and reduced further to just 60 medical personnel to leave with the final party. Excess baggage, equipment, vehicles and horses were

---

35   TNA: WO 95/4318: War Diary, 52nd Division ADMS, 6 January.
36   TNA: WO 95/4318: War Diary, 52nd Division ADMS, 9 January.

evacuated. No fewer than 600 men said to be of 'indifferent health or not considered fit for really hard work' were immediately sent off the peninsula.[37] Such a high number reflects the high level of incapacitated men to be found on the peninsula as the campaign came to an end. Field ambulances were closed on 6 January, and orders were issued for all cases to be sent direct to the 11th CCS. A small dressing station was established on V Beach. On 7 January, all field ambulance personnel for the final period proceeded to their positions in the trenches. At 8:00 p.m. on the final night (8 January), the initial party of troops began to make their way down to V Beach and embarked at 11:00 p.m., accompanied by a medical party consisting of six MOs and 144 men with two motor ambulances and two horse-drawn ambulance wagons. At 11:45 p.m., the final party made its way down to V Beach in the company of the two surgeons (Walker and Mayne), 42 other ranks, two ambulance wagons, four drivers and two wagon orderlies. There, they were joined by the ADMS, DADMS and Staff Sergeant Wilson, coming from the rendezvous point. The RND party embarked at V Beach at 2:00 a.m. on 9 January, arriving at Lemnos on the next day and proceeding to South Camp, Mudros West. Surgeon Rivers and six men remained at the dressing station on V Beach until the demolition party and beach guard had embarked. At 2:00 a.m. on 9 January, the last party embarked from the Gallipoli Peninsula, effectively bringing the campaign to an end.[38]

37   TNA: WO 95/429: War Diary, Royal Naval Division ADMS, 31 December.
38   TNA: WO 95/429: War Diary, Royal Naval Division ADMS, 8 January.

18

Not Equal to the Task

Following the failure of the Gallipoli Campaign and the MEF withdrawal from the peninsula, pressure was brought on the government in London to disclose the reasoning and processes that had brought about the disaster. The government was, at first, reluctant to make any such move, but eventually Prime Minister Herbert Asquith agreed to set up a Royal Commission under the Special Commissions (Dardanelles and Mesopotamia) Act 1916, which received Royal Assent on 17 August 1916. The remit of the 10 appointed commissioners was defined to be:

> … for the purpose of inquiring into the origin, inception, and conduct of operations of war in the Dardanelles and Gallipoli, including the supply of drafts, reinforcements, ammunition and equipment to the troops and Fleet, the provision for the sick and wounded, and the responsibility of those departments of Government whose duty it has been to minister to the wants of the forces employed in that theatre of war.[1]

Most of the work of the commission is outside the scope of this work, but 'the provision for the sick and wounded' is of direct relevance to that which has been described throughout and will be reviewed briefly in this chapter.

The 10 commissioners met for the first time on 23 August 1916 and, throughout the rest of the year, took evidence from 35 witnesses. Notably, among these was Winston Churchill, who occupied five days of the commissioners' time during October 1916 in bringing his case for the campaign to the front. The work of the first months of the commission brought about the publication of the *First Report* in February 1917, by which time the commission had already commenced taking evidence from more witnesses. It was during the second part of the commission's work that the medical services came under considerable scrutiny, and serving officers were called to give evidence of the manner in which the medical services had been conducted throughout the campaign. The *Final Report* of 1919 outlines the evidence collected from the witnesses, and significant emphasis is placed upon the organisation that had been put in place for the evacuation of the wounded in both April and August. From the evidence, general conclusions were drawn, which include a number with direct bearing upon the medical services:

---

1   Dardanelles Commission, *First Report* (London: HMSO, 1917), p.1, para.1.

> The provision for the evacuation of the wounded, especially in the matter of hospital ships, proved insufficient to meet the emergencies which actually arose. We think that, if the operations to be undertaken in landing on the peninsula had been considered before the expedition started and a general plan prepared, further provision of hospital ships might, and probably would have, been made.[2]

The provision for the evacuation of wounded was, at least to Hamilton and his staff, almost an afterthought. This is clear by the fact that Surgeon General Birrell's appointment occurred after the departure of Hamilton for the Dardanelles. This attitude is, at least, partly due to the attitudes in the army at this time, partly due to the fact that the medical services were seen as subordinate and had no presence on the Army Council and partly due to the time scales placed upon the campaign by the politicians, notably Churchill. The *Final Report* gives some recognition of the latter in subsequent paragraphs. There is also recognition of the subordination of the medical services: 'We think that the separation of the Administrative Staff including … Director of Medical Services, from the rest of Headquarters Staff during the time preceding the landing was a mistake and it would have been better if the Director of Medical Services had been kept more fully informed of the operations which were proposed'.[3] This refers directly to the weeks before the landing when Birrell was left in Egypt whilst the General Staff was at Lemnos, aboard the *Arcadian* and making plans in vacuo for the assault on the peninsula without direct reference to the support arms that would be needed in the event of a landing. Birrell's time in Egypt was not entirely wasted since he became involved in organising large-scale hospital accommodation in that country for the casualties that he, at least, anticipated. However, he had no input on the overall planning for the assault until it was almost too late.

The *Final Report* allows that the arrangements '… would probably have worked satisfactorily if the anticipation of a rapid advance after the landing had been fulfilled'.[4] This is recognition of the fact that, although a landing had been made, it had not been a success and the ground won, and held, particularly at Anzac, would not allow for the landing of medical services such as CCSs and the tent subdivisions of field ambulances. This led the commission to conclude, correctly, that there was little room on the beaches to sort out the wounded, which in turn led subsequently to issues of transport and the confusion that ensued as a result. Initially, the problem of space and lack of sorting meant that slightly wounded men reached the hospital ships first while the seriously wounded often found their way onto the transport – the so-called 'black ships'. This seems to have been more of an issue at Anzac than at Helles. This transport issue led the commission to conclude that '… a greater part of the suffering of the wounded in the first days after the landing seems to us to have been inevitable, but there appears to have been some want of organisation in the control of the boats and barges carrying wounded to the hospital ships and transports, which occasioned delay in their embarkation'.[5]

It is interesting to note that, while the commission readily pointed out the obvious, there is no indication as to where the responsibility for such organisation rested. There is acceptance that the military failure was not the fault of the DMS and that he could not be held responsible for

---

2   Dardanelles Commission, *Final Report* (London: HMSO, 1919), p.89, para.23.
3   Dardanelles Commission, *Final Report*, p.90, para.25.
4   Dardanelles Commission, *Final Report*, p.90, para.26.
5   Dardanelles Commission, *Final Report*, p.90, para.26.

that, but there is an implied criticism that the DMS should have been aware that there was a potential for failure.[6] However, the *Final Report* points out that, in the effectively rigid hierarchical structure then operating in the army, to have been able to plan for such a contingency was likely to be impossible. This rather contradictory approach seems to seek to blame everybody for the apparent failure of the medical services.

Noticeably, a large part of the criticism levelled at the medical services originated from officers serving at Anzac, where there appears to have been an inordinate level of confusion at the time of the landing. At Helles, where the troops were operating under similar conditions, with similar losses, there seems to have been considerably less problem. The experienced, thoroughly trained soldiers of the 29th Division appear to have coped better with their immersion in battle. Whilst the courage and fortitude of the ANZACs cannot be denied, it must be said that they were little more than untrained and inexperienced men being led by officers who were, generally, ill prepared for the difficulties that would face them in battle. Whilst some, like Lieutenant Colonel N. R. Howse VC, ADMS of the 1st Australian Division, had experience of warfare, they had little organisational experience to carry them through the confusion of the initial landing, although they learned very quickly.

In this context, Colonel A. E. C. Keble was critical of Howse for not stepping up to take the more senior role of DDMS ANZAC when asked. Keble pointed out that Howse was a small-town doctor and not really a soldier, with little experience of the matters required in warfare.[7] These comments before the commission have been identified as a slight on Howse by an Imperial officer.[8] In fact, Keble had stated the case simply. Howse may have had particular medical skill but, apart from exemplary service in South Africa, had little experience of the military or the administration of medical matters in the military context. It is unlikely that Howse would have held anything like the same seniority in anything but the emerging AAMC of this time. This does not detract from Howse or his later service, but the statement Keble made before the commission was factually correct when the Gallipoli Campaign was underway. To his credit, Howse did step up, and, with the experience gained during the Gallipoli Campaign and later, he reached the rank of surgeon general in the AAMC. It has to be accepted that the Gallipoli Campaign was a learning process for all the forces involved and in particular for the most recently raised forces of Australia and New Zealand. There seems to be scant recognition of this in the commission reports, where all elements of the landing forces are treated in the same manner.

During the campaign, improvements were made in the general approach to evacuation in time for the August Offensive, and this was recognised by the commission: '… the supply of hospital ships was much larger that at the first landing. On the whole, this scheme worked well, though again there were cases in which the transports were not satisfactory and the organisation for transporting the wounded to the ships was imperfect'.[9] Once again, this conclusion raises the issue of the adequacy of the shore-to-ship transfer. This was the Royal Navy's problem, in so far as it was their job to provide the boats to ferry the wounded that were also their responsibility for the length of the journey to the hospital ship. Whilst the Royal Navy needed to have, at the

---

6   Dardanelles Commission, *Final Report*, p.90, para.27.
7   TNA: CAB 19/29: Lieutenant Colonel A. E. C. Keble, Statement to the Dardanelles Commission.
8   Moncrieff, *Expertise, Authority and Control*, p.40.
9   Dardanelles Commission, *Final Report*, p.90, para.29.

306   The Fight for Life

very least, some idea of the requirements of the land forces, there often seemed to have been a breakdown in communications between the two arms, with the result that small boats and barges sometimes were not where they were needed most. There is no recognition of any failings on the part of the Royal Navy in the *Final Report* of the commission. In fact, as far as the medical services are concerned, there is little mention of the need for close cooperation with the navy. In the commission's eyes, the navy always did what was asked of it. Perusal of war diaries of various medical units would suggest that this was not always the case.

The penultimate conclusion of the *Final Report* states, in part, 'The Director of Medical Services, Surgeon General Birrell, did his best; we are of the opinion that he was not equal to the task of grappling with the exceptional conditions which arose.'[10] On the basis of the evidence presented in the report, it is difficult to understand this conclusion. The commission recognised the difficulties Surgeon General Birrell faced in the hasty preparation for the landing. In fact, it was down to Birrell and Lieutenant Colonel Keble that there was any sort of plan at all for the medical services at the time of the landing. The breakdown of the plan was also recognised as not being Birrell's responsibility but rather the result of the overall military failure. Surgeon General Birrell and Lieutenant Colonel Keble were critical of the fact that the ADMS of the 1st Australian Division, Lieutenant Colonel Howse, did not remain at divisional HQ to oversee the work of his medical units during the landing. They cited the fact that similar problems had not generally occurred at Helles. Furthermore, Lieutenant Colonel Fenwick, DADMS of the New Zealand and Australian Division, supported this view as correct from his experience with the conditions in his division. However, this argument was dismissed by the commission based upon contrary evidence from Howse. This would seem to be the commission demonstrating a bias towards the SMO of the ANZACs at that time.[11] Nevertheless, Howse was critical of Birrell and '… considered he was ill, when I saw him, and I did not think he was physically fit to grapple with such a big situation as existed, which required a good deal of initiative'.[12] Initiative seems to have been something that Howse did not take at the early stage of the campaign, preferring to complain of inadequacies rather than attempt to solve the enormous problems that faced him as ADMS of a division.

Surgeon General Babtie VC made a statement to the commission that was appended to the *Final Report*. In the course of this, he stated:

> I had gathered that there had been some difficulties as to Surgeon General Birrell's proposals for the evacuation of the wounded, and I feared from what I had heard he was not working well with the Principal Staff Officers of the Force. I consulted the IGC, the CGS, AG and QMG as to this and as all agreed that he was not a success, the AG and I saw the Commander-in-Chief on the subject. I said that although I had little fault to find with his work it was an impossible position if he had not the full confidence of the Staff, and that I thought he had better go home.[13]

---

10   Dardanelles Commission, *Final Report*, p.91, para.34.
11   Dardanelles Commission, *Final Report*, p.74, para.166.
12   Tyquin, *Australian Medical Perspective*, p.247.
13   Dardanelles Commission, *Final Report*, p.169, para.21.

This does not necessarily suggest that 'he was not equal to the task'; rather, he had fallen victim to the remoteness of Hamilton and his staff. This is, to some extent, borne out by the fact that Birrell was not allowed to be part of the GHQ, aboard the *Queen Elizabeth* when the landing took place, hence divesting him of any control or authority from day one over the medical services during the crucial landing phase of the operations and as the military failure proceeded.

There is much criticism of the use of transports for the evacuation of wounded in the *Final Report*. Indeed, one section is devoted to the conditions on the black ships. There can be little doubt that conditions on the black ships were far from ideal, and, in a number of cases, they were appalling. The report remarks upon the number of witnesses who gave details of the conditions but, at the same time, warns, 'It is a subject on which hearsay information should be received with caution, as a natural sympathy with the sufferings of the wounded may lead to some exaggeration.'[14] Whilst this was a sensible caution from the commissioners, it appears that more weight was given to those cases where conditions were little short of horrific than those that were acceptable. Lieutenant Colonel Keble was at pains to point out to the commission that transports sent to Helles at the time of the landing were supplied with at least four MOs. That this did not occur for those ships serving Anzac was not the cause of oversight or lack of planning so much as the misfortunes of war. The black ships intended for use at Anzac were to be staffed by the medical staff of No. 2 ASH, who were sent to Lemnos from Alexandria for that purpose, so that all four ships concerned would have a share of the medical staff of the stationary hospital. However, their transport, the *Hindoo*, arrived at Mudros late, and the allocated staff could not be transferred before the transports left for the start of the landings. The *Hindoo* was then effectively lost to the campaign for four days through lack of communication with the main body, although it spent those days within sight of the peninsula.[15] By this time, the transports were filling up with desperately wounded men, and, in the absence of medical care, conditions deteriorated rapidly. This confusion cannot be levelled at the lack of organisation of the medical services in general or Surgeon General Birrell in particular. It was more a problem of the inability to communicate and control the ships that were in use at this time – not a medical issue. Much of the problem of the use of black ships was caused by the military failure on the beaches and not a failure of the organisation of the medical services. The commission, writing of the overall scheme for medical services, concluded, 'The failure of the scheme was mainly due to the fact that no substantial advance was effected, and that no hospitals could therefore be established on land. This necessitated the immediate evacuation by sea of all casualties without any possibility of separating the serious cases from those of a slighter nature.'[16] The use of black ships, particularly those used immediate upon landing of the force, was inevitable, at least partly because of the number of casualties. The *Final Report* recognises the problem: 'It may be that it was not the number of casualties alone which was important, but that the number combined with the necessity of transporting them by sea, and the impossibility of sorting them into slight and serious cases, caused and unexpected confusion and crowding of the hospital ships and transports.'[17]

---

14   Dardanelles Commission, *Final Report*, p.76, para.172.
15   AWM: AWM4/26/71/1: War Diary, No. 2 Australian Stationary Hospital, April 1915.
16   Dardanelles Commission, *Final Report*, p.90, para.26.
17   Dardanelles Commission, *Final Report*, p.74, para.166.

308   The Fight for Life

Whilst the use of transports had, to some extent, been allowed for, the ships were never intended to carry seriously wounded, and it is here that the main criticism of conditions should lie. At Anzac, because of the poor military position at the close of the first day, all field ambulances and the CCS were ordered to evacuate their wounded men as soon as possible in case of a more general evacuation of the landed force. In this event, the use of transports could not have been avoided. Furthermore, the lack of space, which limited sorting of casualties, also limited space for treatment, which indicated rapid evacuation. Evacuation was preferable to men lying in exposed positions open to shell fire and small-arms fire. Whilst Colonel Ryan reported that the use of black ships had not caused '… much loss of life', there was no consideration given to the lives that may have been saved simply by getting wounded off the beaches, where further injury was likely.[18] Whilst, undoubtedly, the use of black ships could have been avoided if more hospital ships had been available, the simple fact is that they were not, and the evacuation of men proceeded by the only method available. Perhaps Colonel Ryan gave the best summation of the use of black ships when he commented to the commission, '… that if all these transports had been fitted up as hospital ships more lives, but not a great many, would have been saved'.[19]

The commission, in summarizing its findings on black ships, stated:

> In our opinion, most of the suffering was due to the causes mentioned, but we also think that there was, in some instances a lack of organisation. Evidence of this was given by … Surgeon General Howse. The last named witness described the conditions as 'extremely difficult' and exceptional and said – 'We were in the unfortunate position of having no history to guide us of a previous landing on such a large scale in modern times, so that we could get no idea of what medical arrangements should have been made.' We think many of the difficulties might have been avoided if a general plan of the operations had been carefully marked out before the expedition was undertaken.[20]

This conclusion is nothing more than hindsight, and it is unlikely that any of the senior officers involved would not have changed the planning process if they had been aware of the events subsequent to the start of the campaign. However, Howse, who seems to have had an opinion on every aspect of the medical services, made a fair assessment that no one had any '… idea of the medical arrangements that should have been made'. This should have been enough for the commission.

The *Final Report* of the commission, as far as it applies to the medical services, appears to be selective, in that it appears to deal largely with those criticisms raised by the problems of the military condition at Anzac. It seems to rely heavily upon the statements by Howse to the detriment of those received from other, more senior and, indeed, more experienced officers of the medical services. There can be little doubt that, given the conditions, things could have been better and, if the military solution had been achieved, they would have been. Unfortunately for Surgeon General Birrell, he seems to have become a scapegoat for the overall failings of the campaign in which he was but a bit player.

18   Dardanelles Commission, *Final Report*, p.77, para.172.
19   Dardanelles Commission, *Final Report*, p.77, para.172.
20   Dardanelles Commission, *Final Report*, p.80, para.174.

Conclusions

The medical services of the British Army were, at the start of the war, reasonably well developed and well organised. However, as a result of the internal reorganisation of the British Army as a whole in the early years of the century, the medical services were subordinate to the operational sections of the army. This meant that the medical services were relegated to a support role and had little or no executive control and only a subsidiary role within the War Council. This position meant that, when the time came to plan for a campaign such as the Gallipoli Campaign, the service was not the first to be consulted, with operational concerns naturally taking precedence.

By the time the Gallipoli Campaign started, the medical services of Australia, New Zealand and Canada were organised along the lines of the RAMC for the most part. However, they were inexperienced, and many of the MOs, often former general practitioners, had little knowledge of surgery or military medicine. This undoubtedly impacted upon the treatment of battle casualties, particularly at Anzac during the opening exchanges of the campaign. This general lack of experience should be remembered when considering the care of wounded during the campaign.

The IMS differed somewhat in detail from the other Empire forces present at the campaign but was certainly better experienced than other colonial medical units of the Empire and operated well within the difficulties of the campaign. In a general sense, the IMS was not dissimilar to the RAMC. Indeed, its officers were all commissioned into the RAMC. The differences in the organisation of the IMS were largely a function of the cultural and, in some instances, racial differences between the Indian Army and the other Empire forces at that time.

The French *Service de Santé des Armées* differed substantially to its allies and was not as well developed overall. The regimental structure in the French Army differed to that of the Allies, and the allocation of MOs was dependent on this structure. MOs were assigned to regiments, comprising three battalions. The SMO of the regiment was akin, but not identical, to the ADMS of a British division, in that he controlled the needs of the three battalions and the MOs whom he assigned to those battalions. He was, however, more closely involved with the treatment of wounded and such things as the organisation of the dressing stations. In general, the evacuation along their lines of communication was similar but, perhaps, not as well defined as in the British Army. The French Medical Service performed well at Helles and was subject to the same difficulties as its British ally.

It is clear that, at the time of the landing on the peninsula, the medical services were rather unprepared for the large numbers of casualties that they were expected to handle following the heavy fighting at the landing. This would appear to be a direct result of the subsidiary role played by the medical services during the planning phase and the hasty and limited preparations for the military campaign as a whole. The short time allowed for the planning for the campaign as a whole left little time to ensure that all was in place for the medical services when the landings on the peninsula took place.

The ability of the medical services to carry out their work efficiently immediately after the landing was impacted by the lack of success of the landings at Helles and particularly at Anzac. Whilst the organisation and planning of the medical services may have been better, there is seldom any emphasis on how poorly the military side of the campaign performed when criticism is levelled at the medical services. The medical services required that the military operation was a success if they were to perform their duty efficiently.

Under the adverse circumstances of the landing, the medical services performed extraordinarily well, but the lack of transport for evacuation tends to colour any consideration of the work they were able to carry out. This does not indicate a failure of the medical services; rather, it is a failure in understanding of the overall situation on the peninsula and elsewhere. Their work was only part of a much more complex story. A more holistic approach is necessary when considering the efficacy of the medical services during the Gallipoli Campaign.

Whilst it is true that there were insufficient hospital ships provided at the beginning of the campaign and that the provision of alternatives was often unsatisfactory, there is seldom recognition that lives were probably saved by getting casualties off fire-exposed beaches even where the transports were unsuitable. The whole story of the medical services has been predicated upon this one oft repeated and generally imprecise aspect of the campaign. Though much of the work was reactive, the ability of the medical services to adapt only adds credit to the work carried out at this critical phase.

Whilst it is true that there had been some consideration for the provision of MOs for black ships, this was probably inadequate, in so far as there was a lack of success in the military operation. Many of the casualties needing treatment on black ships would have received their initial treatment on shore had it been possible to establish suitable hospitals when the attacking force moved away from the beachhead. This meant that there was an increased need for transportation and for MOs on that transportation. Once again, the problem was not one created by the medical services; rather, it was one created by an underestimate of the effects of the hard fighting that was to be the result of a landing on an enemy shore.

The planning for hospitals in places such as Egypt and Malta had started before the campaign. Preparations for the care of wounded were considerably advanced by the start of the campaign. Nevertheless, during the opening weeks of the fighting, these hospitals were almost overwhelmed by casualties as they adapted and grew to meet the difficulties. The result of this growth was that, by the end of the campaign, there were 36,000 beds in Egypt. This gives a clear indication of how the medical services had changed as a direct result of the needs forced upon them by the ultimate failure of the campaign on the peninsula. Whilst it can be said that better planning of the medical services may have alleviated some of the problems that were forced upon them in Egypt, this is generally with the benefit of hindsight. The medical services needed to evolve as quickly as the military situation was failing on the peninsula. It may have been better prepared for success had there been such, but, in the light of the events that followed the landings, this probably would have made little difference.

The development of Lemnos as a forward base had not been thought necessary at the planning stage of the campaign. It became inevitable when the landings failed to produce the immediate success against the Turks upon which much of the planning had been based. The development of hospitals on Lemnos was necessary, although it was not an ideal location for the care of wounded for a number of reasons, not least the shortage of a good water supply. The hospitals were closer to the fighting, and transport over the shorter distance was less of an issue, as wounded men were transferred more quickly into hospital care. The medical services did much to overcome the difficulties at Lemnos, but it remained a difficult place to serve and care for wounded. Great credit should be afforded to all medical personnel who served on Lemnos for the work that was carried out on the dry, windswept island.

Disease became a major issue during the summer months, and the impact on the medical services was as severe as at any time of fighting. The outbreaks of dysentery, enteric and jaundice in epidemic proportions stretched a service that was struggling to meets its commitments to battle casualties. There had been little planning or preparation for handling infectious diseases on the scale experienced during the Gallipoli Campaign. Nevertheless, there is evidence to suggest that the medical services adapted as best they could under the stress produced by significant sickness across the peninsula and under the adverse conditions of such places as Lemnos.

The shortages of all kinds of stores, equipment and food played its part in the difficulties faced by the medical services, and perhaps this feature troubled MOs more than many other issues, as they fought to get everything from bed pans to drugs for their patients. This reflects badly on the planning of the campaign as a whole and on the home government in particular, as shortages were faced in all aspects of the campaign. These shortages affected the work of the medical services significantly. It is perhaps easy to understand the frustration that can be seen in contemporary records when diseases such as scurvy should have been easily avoided by a regular supply of fresh food.

The procrastination of both political and military leaders as winter approached prevented suitable planning for winter on the peninsula. The devastating effects of the blizzard in November could have been avoided if there had been early action in providing warm clothes and some shelter for the men in the field. Once again, the medical services were in the forefront and bore the brunt of dealing with the difficult situations, such as frostbite and exposure, that could have been avoided. Once again, they excelled.

On the basis of the evidence gathered during the course of this work, it appears that the medical services performed well during the entire campaign. There were places where things could, or even should, have been better, but, overall, the duty performed by the entire service was good. The medical services were heavily criticised by the Dardanelles Commission, and this would seem to be unjustified and biased towards the conditions described at Anzac. It should be reflected upon that most of the problems raised about the medical services were raised by the AAMC and its commanders on the peninsula. There is little criticism from those serving at Helles or Suvla. This must indicate upon not only the lack of planning by the Imperial Government but also the lack of readiness of the inexperienced Australian forces. Interestingly, there seems to be less criticism arising from the New Zealand contingent. It was perhaps unfortunate that the Australians were thrown into this difficult campaign as their first experience of warfare, for their presence had little or no impact on the final outcome. Not all of the problems of handling casualties can be laid at the door of British SMOs, for there are other aspects to be considered. The Dardanelles Commission was clearly a political attempt to address questions raised about problems that politicians, notably Winston Churchill, had caused in the first place, and, in the case of the medical services, it appears to have failed to address the issues even-handedly.

Appendix I

A Note on the Turkish Medical Services during the Çanakkale Wars

Ahmet Senol Ozbeck

The First World War is seen today as the last struggle of a failing Ottoman Empire after 200 years of decline and unrest within its borders. Day by day, the Empire was losing its power, and the chaos in all aspects of life within its borders was destroying the organised state. It was in an effort to bring about change that one idealistic, young man, Enver Pasha, drew close to the Kaiser's Germany. Enver Pasha was a staff officer who was unhappy with the state of affairs in his country during the reign of Abdulhamid II and, with great courage, sought to change how the country was being governed. He lacked experience on the international stage and, somewhat naïvely, trusted the Germans to help produce the stability that the Ottoman's were lacking in the early years of the twentieth century. This drew the nations inexorably closer together, but the only positive results of this approach were a rejuvenation of the Turkish Army and some logistical support from Germany. The latter was never enough for the Empire.

When the Ottoman Empire entered the war, it came as a surprise to many. There were no mobilisation plans in place for such an event, and there was no mobilisation budget or funds for the furtherance of the war. All the plans were based on wishes and dreams and not on the materiel of war that was available to the Empire at that time. Likewise, all the logistic planning was imaginary.

At the beginning of the Çanakkale Wars, all the supply services of *Çanakkale Müstahkem Mevki Komutanlığı*, the command HQ in Çanakkale for the protection of the strait (the Narrows), were provided by the Ministry of Defence. Later, on 25 March 1915, the 5th Army was established to defend the area and took on the supply responsibility after 5 April.

The geography around this area could be expected to be very convenient for the roads, railroads and shipping. Although there were some possibilities for the ships, the seaway was soon blockaded. The railroads were insufficient, and there were great difficulties in transportation by roads due to the deficiencies in both the infrastructure and road vehicles. The İstanbul–Edirne line was the only railroad connecting the battlefields to İstanbul. There were macadam roads from Uzunköprü station to Keşan (about 70km) and Bolayır–Gelibolu (about 110–120km or a six- or seven-day marching distance for a soldier). That railroad was repaired just before the war and maintained for use as much as possible later to be sufficient for use in emergency. However, it was not possible to run this line smoothly due to its construction style with its steep inclines and sharp bends. In spite of the inadequacy of this line for the needs of such a large army, it was used increasingly for the transportation of the soldiers, particularly after the Allies started to use their submarines in the Sea of Marmara.

There was no uninterrupted land route going from one end of the peninsula to the other at the time of the war. There were mostly paths suitable for pedestrians and beasts of burden. The situation was such that there was no road suitable for motorised vehicles. It was impossible to drive even between Gelibolu and Mydos, which were the two main points of the battle zone. This was not as much of a problem as the shortage of motor vehicles. The total number of motor vehicles in the country in 1914 was only 187. More than half of them were in İstanbul, and the rest were in the other big cities. This meant that, at the time of entry into the war, the most efficient and fastest vehicle of the time was the double-horse carriage.

At the start of the conflict, there were a number of different categories of hospitals such as clearing hospitals, field hospitals, Red Crescent hospitals and central hospitals. These hospitals had accommodation starting from 180 beds up to 2,000 beds in central hospitals. The clearing hospitals of the 8th, 9th and 12th Divisions were active around Gelibolu and Çanakkale shortly after the opening of the Çanakkale front. In addition, a number of ferries of the company *Şirket-i Hayriye* were assigned for use as hospital boats for transportation within the Sea of Marmara. Both wounded soldiers and refugees were transported on these boats, and supplies such as tea, cereal, milk, ayran and cigarettes were distributed to the sick and injured in the region via these boats in an effort to keep morale high. The company sent a letter to the presidency of the Turkish Red Crescent Society on 12 May 1915 stating that it was honoured to provide humanitarian aid in this manner.

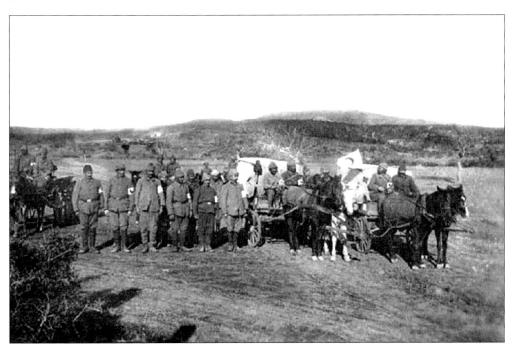

Turkish field medical unit during the Çanakkale Wars (Gallipoli Campaign). Note the use of the two-horse ambulance wagons. (Ahmet Senol Ozbeck)

314   The Fight for Life

The Red Crescent hospitals also served in the Çanakkale Wars. When war intensified, the Red Crescent Association increased its aid activities both at the front and directly behind it and fought against diseases such as malaria, cholera, typhoid fever, dysentery and smallpox.

Until March 1915, the hospitals in the area – Çanakkale Central Hospital with a 350-bed capacity, Erenköy Hospital with 50-bed capacity, Ezine Hospital with 200-bed capacity, Umurbey Hospital with 200-bed capacity, Kilitbahir Hospital with 50-bed capacity and Eceabat Hospital with 200-bed capacity – were used only for public health services. However, most of the needs of these hospitals, such as medical personnel and relevant equipment, were supplied locally, and the people of the region were mobilised to meet these needs. It is a fact that, when the Ottoman Empire was fighting on many fronts, the population of Anatolia decreased dramatically, not only because of epidemic diseases but also because so many volunteers from İstanbul and nearby provinces went to the Çanakkale front. In İstanbul, the students of the Faculty of Medicine, which had been closed for a year and had become a military hospital, were recruited into army medical service and sent to the fronts and the training camps. These students were not able to do internships and complete their studies. As a result, after a one-year obligatory closure, the Faculty of Medicine, which could not graduate any students in 1915, resumed its teaching on 4 March 1916.

The troops of the 9th Division, which were assigned with the defence of the peninsula before 18 March, were deployed in a wide area on both sides of the Dardanelles, and two clearing hospitals were put into operation in order to provide the necessary medical intervention as quickly as possible. For this purpose, clearing hospitals were opened with 100-bed capacity in Eceabat and Kilitbahir and 500-bed capacity in Erenköy. In addition, the clearing hospital of the 19th Division in Kilitbahir and the clearing hospital of the 9th Division in Sarıacaali were ready to accept casualties.

When the fighting of May was at its peak, the accommodation for casualties on the Çanakkale front reached 5,050 beds: 1,450 in Tekirdağ, 400 in Şarköy, 150 in Gelibolu, 300 in Lapseki, 500 in Ezine, 450 in Dümrek, 1,300 in Biga and 500 in Dimetoka Village. By July 1915, this capacity was increased to 14,280 beds.

On the other hand, due to the growing ferocity of the land battles, large dressing stations were opened behind the front line at locations such as Tengerderesi, Soğanlıdere, Havuzlarderesi, Kocadere and Matikdere, and the medical squadrons served the wounded soldiers in these positions.

Upon the declaration of mobilisation, following the secret agreement signed with Germany on 2 August 1914, a letter was sent to the General Directorate of the Range Inspector from the Ministry of War Sanitary Department on 5 August. In that letter, it was ordered that 7,000 of the hospital beds, out of a total of 10,000, in İstanbul would be administered by the army and that the remaining 3,000 beds would be administered by the Red Crescent Society. It was decided that the shipping piers for wounded would be Ayastefanos, Tekirdağ, Gelibolu and Çanakkale. Accordingly, the wounded would be brought to Gülhane Military Hospital in İstanbul, and, from there, they would be transferred to other hospitals by cars rented by the Red Crescent Society. In addition, two ferries would be given to the Red Crescent Society for the dispatch of the wounded from the front. Furthermore, the GHQ of the Field Medical Inspectorate of the General Staff notified the Red Crescent HQ that the new hospitals were needed to be opened in İstanbul for the wounded coming from Çanakkale. The Red Crescent Society made extraordinary efforts, and the wounded from the front were placed in *Galatasaray*

Appendix I 315

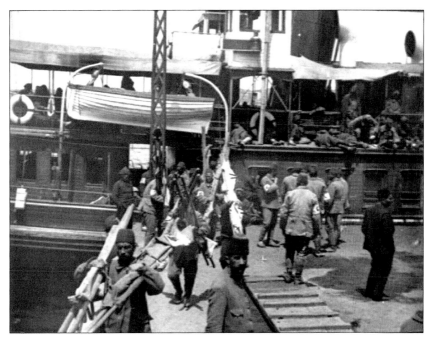

Embarking wounded on a hospital ship for transfer to Istanbul. The ship is not carrying the internationally recognised livery for a hospital ship and is essentially a black ship. (Ahmet Senol Ozbeck)

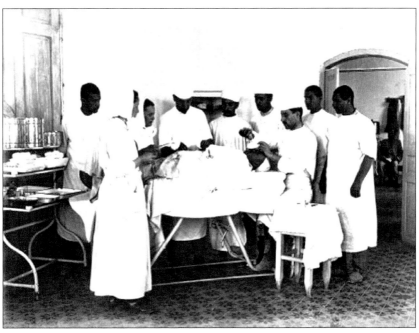

An operating theatre in one of the larger, more permanent hospitals during the Çanakkale Wars (Gallipoli Campaign). Two nurses are assisting. (Ahmet Senol Ozbeck)

316   The Fight for Life

Mekteb-i Sultani (Galatasaray High School in Beyoğlu today) and *Darüşşafaka* (High School), and their treatment and care began.

It soon became clear that there was a need to open a hospital near Çanakkale for the seriously wounded soldiers who could not be immediately transferred to İstanbul. It was decided to evacuate the French girls' school and use it as a hospital. For this hospital, which was thought to have accommodation for 200 beds, the necessary furnishings were completed, and it was opened on 19 April 1915 as 'Gelibolu Red Crescent Hospital'. Since this hospital was reserved for the seriously injured soldiers, those who were brought here were injured generally by shrapnel, howitzer shells or bombs. The casualties were transferred to İstanbul after the necessary medical intervention, and the beds were again occupied by the seriously injured ones in a very short time. The hospital, which tried to provide service despite much difficulty, was moved to Şarköy by the Plevne ferry on 8 May 1915 since it could not carry out further activities due to the heavy bombardment of the town of Gelibolu by the Allies. Therefore, Gelibolu Red Crescent Hospital was able to serve for about three weeks before the exigencies of war required its removal from its first site. This hospital continued its activities in Şarköy. Although Şarköy Red Crescent Hospital treated the soldiers coming from the front with considerable devotion to duty and under great difficulties, it was decided to move the hospital from Şarköy to Tekirdağ. This move was forced upon the hospital as a result of an increase in the number of wounded and sick, as well as the problems experienced in transportation and security. The hospital in Tekirdağ continued its activities until the end of December. Therefore, the services of this hospital in Gelibolu, Şarköy and Tekirdağ lasted for eight months.

A significant proportion of injuries among the soldiers were caused by bombs, shrapnel or the infantry bullet. The wound of a soldier at the front was first bandaged by using the 'war pack' (first field dressing) in his bag, and then he was transported to the 'wounded nests' (RAPs) created behind the trenches by the field soldiers or medics. The wounded who were brought to the 'aid station' (ADS) from here were examined by the battalion doctors. According to their injury, they were either transferred to the 'assembly places' (collection posts) or, if their injuries were serious, carried to the 'bigger aid stations' (field ambulances) via medical vehicle stops. The increasing number of wounded soldiers on the front line increased the importance of transport services. The vehicles working among the 50-bed medical stations established every 20km were assigned to transfer sick and injured soldiers to the main transportation centres. Some of the wounded who needed to be transferred to the hinterland after their initial treatment were brought to the Eceabat or Akbaş piers, and then they were sent to İstanbul by the ferry, boat, barge or sailboat returning from there. From 25 April to the end of November, 150,868 soldiers (99,275 wounded, 33,794 sick and 17,799 sick-leave) were transferred from Akbaş and Ağaderesi Post Hospitals.

From time to time, some hospitals were bombed by the Allied forces. Thus, hospitals with limited opportunities could not always provide the desired services uninterruptedly. This also caused disruption of the medical services behind the front. The Ottoman State vigorously protested this situation. For example, it was reported in the letter sent by the Red Crescent Çanakkale Centre to the presidency of the Red Crescent on 30 April that, on 29 April, a heavy bombardment was carried out from Saros Gulf to Maydos and, as a result of the bombing of the military hospital carrying the Red Crescent flag, a number of wounded, estimated to be hundreds, died. Acting Commander-in-Chief Enver Paşa stated in a telegram he sent to the Ministry of Foreign Affairs on 10 May, conveyed to the British Government through the American Embassy, that, if the British bombed the hospital ships or hospitals again, the Ottoman State would respond violently by using the British civilian or military prisoners. In another document dated to 25 May, it was stated that Allied planes bombed the Akbaş Tekkesi Hospital tent with the Red Crescent signs on it. In a series of telegrams sent by Enver Paşa to United States Ambassador Henry Morgenthau, it was requested that necessary precautions were taken to prevent this situation from recurring.

Although great effort and devotion was expended on the transport of the wounded to the hospitals, it was not without problems. The medics tried to move the wounded to the safe areas quickly by entering the firing line in order to carry in the wounded. The transport of the wounded in these areas could not be carried out quickly as the medics would have liked because the hospitals and the aid stations near the front were exposed to bombardment and fire from time to time. Thus, the commander of the 33rd Regiment, Lieutenant Colonel Şevki Bey, was killed when he entered Karayörük Stream to rescue a wounded soldier. As a result of these issues, the wounded soldiers had to wait in open areas where their wounds gradually worsened, sometimes causing gangrene. Sometimes, soldiers who were wounded and should have been treated within six hours could not reach a hospital until six or seven days later, by which time the wounds were often infested with maggots. This was seen frequently among the wounded soldiers brought to Gelibolu Hospital throughout the war.

In the first intervention to the wounded soldiers, morphine was used primarily to relieve and alleviate the pain of the patient. Boric acid, ointment or Vaseline, which has softening properties, was used to clean the wound and remove clothes that were mixed into the skin or tissues and fused to the wound. Since tetanus, which is transmitted to humans through dirty and open wounds, posed a significant risk in such wounds, anti-tetanus serum was used in the preventative treatment of the disease.

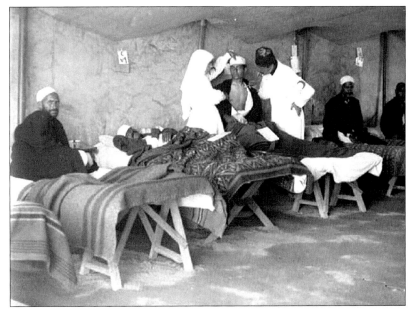

A temporary hospital nearer the front. The wounded soldier is receiving treatment from a doctor assisted by a nurse. (Ahmet Senol Ozbeck)

318   The Fight for Life

The Red Crescent Society played an important role in the supply of this kind of medical supplies and made an effort to procure a large number of syringes, operating-room linoleum and bandages. However, the medical measures that were taken were insufficient due to the increase in the number of wounded from the front and when most of the medical supplies sent from Germany were either unusable or unsuitable for their needs. The shortages and desperation were covered to some extent by the devotion of the medical services personnel.

In the medical services, treatment continued through such supply shortages, and sometimes it was necessary for practical solutions to be found instead of relying upon the products that could not be supplied. For example, the use of chewing gum instead of mastisol, which is a liquid adhesive used for surgical purposes, was a very common practical solution in the hospitals short of supplies.

The aid provided by the Red Crescent Society to the hospitals was not limited to medical supplies: socks, underwear, beds and quilts needed by the sick and wounded were also sent to the hospitals and the military units. The society increased its aid activities both at the front and in the rear area after the war intensified, where it also fought against diseases such as malaria, cholera, typhoid fever, dysentery and smallpox.

Malaria, diarrhoea, lice and scurvy were common diseases seen on the Çanakkale front. Malaria, especially, was one of the most common diseases among the local people and soldiers due to the swamps and the stagnant water in and around Kumkale and the surrounding areas. Since it was not possible to dry these swamps located on the Anatolian side of the war zone, it was attempted to prevent the spread of malaria by measures such as protecting the places where the soldiers were billeted with mosquito nets as much as possible, preventing mosquito bites by keeping the body covered by various means and removing the disease-carrying individuals. These were detected by taking the blood of the infected patients and sending them to the Asian Group Laboratory. In order to prevent the spread of malaria, which was frequently seen in the 15th Corps units on the Anatolian side, six mobile bacteriology units and a laboratory that could perform all kinds of analysis were put into operation at the Kalvert Farm. However, despite these efforts, the epidemic of malaria could not be completely prevented. As a matter of fact, the lack of sufficient quinine used in the treatment of the disease caused 6,661 deaths out of 116,985 malaria cases recorded across the front.

Another disease seen in the Çanakkale front was diarrhoea. The damp and wet nature of the trenches, which were dug deep for protection from bombardment, caused the spread of diarrhoea among the soldiers. Sometimes, soldiers had to be removed from the trenches. For example, complaints of vomiting, bloody diarrhoea, headache and stomach-ache arose in approximately 500 soldiers at the front on 26–28 August 1915. Dysentery and cholera, which started because the water used in the front was not clean, was treated by feeding those who fell sick with these diseases with clay soil since there was not enough medicine. This was another practical solution forced upon the medical services by supply shortages. An attempt to halt the spread of the diseases was made by vaccinations given to soldiers newly arrived in the area. As a result of these measures, the number of deaths from typhoid fever was significantly reduced.

One of the issues that worried the military authorities on the Çanakkale front was a possible lice epidemic. Typhus, popularly known as 'spotted fever', was spread by lice and could pose a serious threat to the soldiers at the front. As a matter of fact, it was seen that 36 of 149 soldiers who fell ill with typhus during the period lost their lives. In this case and in an effort to prevent further spread of typhus, one or two wells were drilled by the drilling team of the engineering

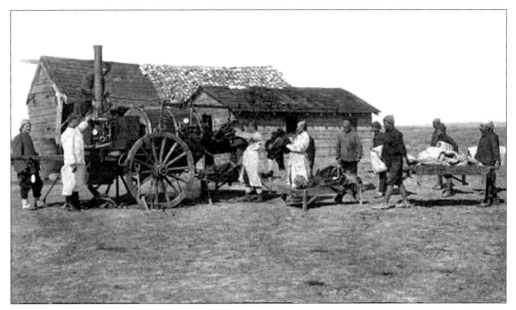
Field disinfector or steriliser. (Ahmet Senol Ozbeck)

battalions near the baths and kitchens of each division to provide a clean water supply in order to avoid a serious epidemic. In addition, three mobile sterilisation ovens and a range of cleaning stations were opened in Keşan on the Uzunköprü–Keşan–Gelibolu road. The newly recruited soldiers began to be cleaned systematically to eradicate lice. Mobile sterilisation ovens were given to the troops, but, because of the insufficiency, it was preferred to pass the clothes, or equipment, through the field sterilisation ovens. As a result of these measures, it was possible to prevent typhus from becoming an epidemic during the combat.

Scurvy, caused by vitamin C deficiency, was another disease seen at the front. This disease, which usually manifests itself in the form of swelling and bleeding in the gums, emerged especially as a result of the nutritional deficiencies caused by the winter season. In the winter months, precautions were taken by ensuring the consumption of the sorrel plant, which was known by the soldiers, could be found in the foothills of the mountains and contained vitamin C. The spread of the disease was prevented by providing vegetables and fresh food as much as possible during the summer months.

To summarise, the Ottoman medical services were largely unprepared for the scale of fighting that took place on the Gallipoli Peninsula and found themselves often short of all sorts of supplies and medical equipment. Their transportation of wounded relied on the very poor infrastructure of the peninsula, which caused delay in treatment for many of the wounded. Fortunately, the use of ferries as hospital ships assisted in the rapid transportation of wounded to Istanbul. The structure of the medical services close to the front would have been familiar to most of the forces engaged in the fighting but with some differences as necessity dictated. Field hospitals and clearing hospitals were used to give immediate care before transferring wounded to central hospitals. This staged process of evacuation and treatment was essentially similar to that found amongst the Allies.

Appendix II

List of Hospital Ships Serving during the Gallipoli Campaign

The following vessels have been identified as carrying patients in the Mediterranean theatre during the campaign. Most made at least one voyage to the peninsula, but some were used to carry wounded from Alexandria to Great Britain and never direct to or from the peninsula. The list is based on *History of the Great War Based on Official Documents: Medical Services* volume 1 by Major General Sir W. G. MacPherson and is supported by war diaries of the various units identified:

HMHS *Aberdonian* (TNA: WO 95/4142/1; see war diary of 13th CCS, December 1915)
HMHS *Aquitania* (TNA: WO 95/4142/1)
HMHS *Assaye* (see war diaries of 13th CCS and Pocock)
HMHS *Braemar Castle* (TNA: WO 95/4142/5)
HMHS *Brighton*
HMHS *Britannic*
HMHS *Caledonia* (TNA: WO 95/4143/1)
HMHS *Carisbrook Castle* (see war diary of No. 16 BSH)
HMHS *Clan MacGillivray* (see war diary of 1st ALHFA, July 1915; painted as 'HS', 24.7.15)
HMHS *Delta* (see war diary of 13th CCS)
HMHS *Devanha* (see war diary of 13th CCS)
HMHS *Dongola* (see war diary of 13th CCS)
HMHS *Dover Castle* (identified in war diaries of 54th CCS and No. 1 CSH)
HMHS *Dunluce Castle*
HMHS *Ebani* (see war diary of No. 16 BSH, October 1915)
HMHS *Egypt*
HMHS *Essequibo*
HMHS *Euryalia* (see war dairy for the *Seang Choon*)
HMHS *Formosa* (see war diary of 13th CCS)
HMHS *Galeka* (see war diary of 13th CCS)
HMHS *Gascon* (TNA: WO 95/4145/1)
HMHS *Glenart Castle* (TNA: WO 95/4145/2)
HMHS *Gloucester Castle*
HMHS *Goorkha* (TNA: WO 95/4145/5)

HMHS *Grantully Castle*
HMHS *Guildford Castle* (TNA: WO 95/4145/7; see war diary of 13th CCS)
HMHS *Kanowna*
HMHS *Karapara* (identified in war diary of 13th CCS)
HMHS *Karoola*
HMHS *Kildonan Castle* (identified in war diary of No. 16 BSH, 1.11.15)
HMHS *Kyarra*
HMHS *Lanfranc* (TNA: WO 95/4146/5)
HMHS *Letitia*
HMHS *Loyalty* (TNA: WO 95/4146/8)
HMHS *Maheno* (see war diary of 13th CCS)
HMHS *Mauretania* (TNA: WO 95/4146)
HMHS *Morea* (see war diary of 16th CCS, January 1916)
HMHS *Neuralia* (diary from 1.1.17)
HMHS *Nevasa* (diary from 1.7.16)
HMHS *Oxfordshire* (identified in war diary of the 13th CCS)
HMHS *Panama* (to Malta to collect Dardanelles casualties – see *3rd London General Hospital Gazette*)
HMHS *Rewa* (see war diary of 13th CCS)
HMHS *Salta*
HMHS *Seang Choon* (identified in war diary of 110th IFA; TNA: WO 95/4148/2; temporary hospital ship in 1915 only)
HMHS *Sicilia* (TNA: WO 95/4148/3)
HMHS *Somali* (see war diary of 13th CCS)
HMHS *Soudan* (see war diary of 13th CCS)
HMHS *Syria* (see war diary of 13th CCS, November 1915)
HMHS *Tagus* (see war diary of No. 16 BSH)
HMHS *Takada*
HMHS *Valdivia* (see war diary of 13th CCS)

Temporary Hospital Ships (Ambulance Carriers or Black Ships), Ferries and Transports

The following vessels have been identified in war diaries of various medical units as accepting wounded or sick from the peninsula:

HMT *Aeneas* (see war diary of No. 16 BSH)
HMT *Alania* (see war diary of No. 16 BSH)
HMT *Alaunia* (see war diary of No. 16 BSH)
SS *Ansconia* (see war diary of No. 18 BSH)
HMT *Ascanius* (see war diary of No. 16 BSH)
HMT *Ausonian* (see war diary of 52nd CCS, July)
SS *Beachy* (see war diary of No. 16 BSH, December)
HMT *Boliviana* (see war diary of No. 16 BSH)

322   The Fight for Life

SS *Borda* (see war diary of No. 16 BSH; described as 'HS' in war diary of No. 18 BSH)
HMT *Canada* (see war diary of No. 16 BSH)
HMAT *Clan MacEwen* (see war diary of No. 16 BSH)
HMT *Demosthenes* (see war diary of No. 16 BSH)
RMS *Empress of Britain* (see war diary of No. 16 BSH)
SS *Ermine* (see war diary of No. 16 BSH; ferry used between Suvla and Mudros)
SS *Folkestone* (see war diary of No. 16 BSH)
AC *Grampian* (see war diary of No. 16 BSH)
SS *Huntsgreen* (see war diary of No. 16 BSH)
SS *Itonus* (see war diary of No. 18 BSH)
HMT *Ivernia* (see war diary of No. 16 BSH)
SS *Kalyan* (see war diary of No. 16 BSH)
SS *Kingstonian* (see war diary of No. 16 BSH)
SS *Malta* (see war diary of No. 16 BSH)
SS *Marathon* (see war diary of No. 18 BSH)
SS *Mashobra* (see war diary of 2nd AFA, April 1915)
SS *Minneapolis* (see war diary of No. 16 BSH)
SS *Northland* (see war diary of No. 16 BSH)
SS *Orsova* (see war diary of No. 18 BSH)
SS *Osmanieh* (see war diary of No. 16 BSH)
SS *Prince Abbas* (see war diary of 1st ALHFA, July 1915)
SS (HMS?) *Redbreast* (see war diary of No. 16 BSH)
SS *Royal George* (see war diary of No. 16 BSH)
SS *Saturnia* (see war diary of No. 18 BSH)
HMT *Scotian* (see war diary of No. 16 BSH)
SS *Seang Bee* (see war dairy of 1st ACCS, May 1915)
HMT *Simla* (see war diary of No. 16 BSH)
HMT *Southland* (see war diary of No. 16 BSH)
RMS *Transylvania* (see war diary of No. 16 BSH)
SS *Willow Branch* (see war diary of No. 16 BSH)

Bibliography

Primary Sources

Personal Accounts

Australian War Memorial (AWM)
1DRL/0499, RCDIG0000181: Typescript Extracts from Diary of Sir Reginald Jeffery Millard
1DRL/0560, AWM2020.22.104: Wallet 1 of 1 – Interview with Surgeon-General Charles Snodgrass Ryan Regarding the Australian Army Medical Corps, 1919
2DRL/0778, RCDIG0000252: Diary of Frederick Trouton Small, 1915
2DRL/0786, RCDIG0001478: [Transcript] Diaries of Thomas James Richards, Vol. 2
AWM41: Official History, 1914-18 War: Records of A.G. Butler, Historian of Australian Army Medical Services
AWM41/937: [Nurses Narratives] Margaret Aitken
AWM41/975: [Nurses Narratives] Principal Matron Ellen Julia Gould
AWM41/988: [Nurses Narratives] Matron A Kellett
AWM41/998: [Nurses Narratives] Sister I G Lovell
AWM41/1013: [Nurses Narratives] Head Sister N C Morrice
AWM41/1045: [Nurses Narratives] N F S Smith
AWM41/1053: [Nurses Narratives] Sister E J Tucker
AWM41/1065: [Nurses Narratives] Sister Louise E Young
AWM41/1072: [Official History, 1914-18 War: Records of Arthur G Butler:] Interviews Containing Accounts of Nursing Experiences in the AANS [Australian Army Nursing Service]. These Nurses Were Interviewed by Matron Kellett [Index to Interviews of Members of AANS Included in File]
AWM224/407: Narrative of Colonel J. A. Dick
AWM2018.666.1, AWM2018.785.52: Diary of Oberlin Herbert Gray, August 1915 to March 1916
PR85/374: Samsing, Hilda Theresa Redderwold (Sister, b.1871–d.1957), 'Diary of Samsing (1914-1918)'
PR02082, RCDIG0000976: Transcript of Diaries of Alice Ross-King, 1915-1919
PR04297, RCDIG0000269: Diary for Roy Rowe, 1915-1916
PR04710, RCDIG0001342: Transcript of Diary of Laurie John Smee, 1915-1917
PR05050, RCDIG0001389: Transcript of Diary of Mary Ann 'Bessie' Pocock, 1914-1918 (Vol. 1)

324   The Fight for Life

PR05050, RCDIG0001390: Transcript of Diary of Mary Ann 'Bessie' Pocock, 1914-1918 (Vol. 2)
PR05050, RCDIG0001394: Diary of Mary Anne 'Bessie' Pocock, May–December 1915

Museum of Military Medicine (MMM)
PE/1/715/Corb.: Diary of Staff Sergeant Corbridge, 87th Field Ambulance

The National Archives (TNA)
CAB 19/29: Lieutenant Colonel A. E. C. Keble, Statement to the Dardanelles Commission

Australian War Memorial War Diaries
1st Australian Casualty Clearing Station: AWM4/26/62
DDMS ANZAC Corps: AWM4/26/14
DMS MEF: AWM4/26/3
General Staff, Headquarters New Zealand and Australian Division: AWM4/1/53
No. 1 Australian Stationary Hospital: AWM4/26/70
No. 2 Australian Stationary Hospital: AWM4/26/71
PDMS: AWM4/26/2

1st Australian Division
1st Australian Field Ambulance: AWM4/26/44
1st Australian Light Horse Field Ambulance: AWM4/26/39
2nd Australian Field Ambulance: AWM4/26/45
2nd Australian Light Horse Field Ambulance: AWM4/26/40
3rd Australian Field Ambulance: AWM4/26/46
3rd Australian Light Horse Field Ambulance: AWM4/26/41
3rd Infantry Brigade: AWM4/23/3
4th Australian Field Ambulance: AWM4/26/47
ADMS: AWM4/26/18

2nd Australian Division
5th Australian Field Ambulance: AWM4/26/48
6th Australian Field Ambulance: AWM4/26/49
7th Australian Field Ambulance: AWM4/26/50
ADMS: AWM4/26/19
New Zealand Field Ambulance: AWM4/35/27
New Zealand Mounted Field Ambulance: AWM4/35/26

The National Archives (Kew) War Diaries

2nd Mounted Division
1/1st Highland Mounted Brigade Field Ambulance: WO 95/4292
1/4th London Mounted Brigade Field Ambulance: WO 95/4292
ADMS: WO 95/4292

VIII Corps
ADMS: WO 95/4275

10th Division
30th Field Ambulance: WO 95/4295
31st Field Ambulance: WO 95/4295
32nd Field Ambulance: WO 95/4295
ADMS: WO 95/4294

11th Division
6th Lincolnshire Regiment: WO 95/4299
7th South Staffordshire Regiment: WO 95/4299
22nd Sanitary Section: WO 95/4298
35th Field Ambulance: WO 95/4298
ADMS: WO 95/4298

13th Division
1/2nd South Western Mounted Brigade FA: WO 95/4303
39th Field Ambulance: WO 95/4301
40th Field Ambulance: WO 95/4301
41st Field Ambulance: WO 95/4301
ADMS: WO 95/4300

29th Division
29th Divisional Field Ambulance and Workshop Unit: WO 95/4309
87th Field Ambulance: WO 95/4309
89th Field Ambulance: WO 95/4309
ADMS: WO 95/4307

42nd Division
1/1st East Lancashire Field Ambulance: WO 95/4314
1/1st South Eastern Mounted Brigade Field Ambulance: WO 95/4316
1/2nd East Lancashire Field Ambulance: WO 95/4314
1/3rd East Lancashire Field Ambulance: WO 95/4314
ADMS: WO 95/4313

52nd Division
1/1st Lowland Field Ambulance: WO 95/4319
1/1st Lowland Mounted Brigade Field Ambulance: WO 95/4321
1/2nd Lowland Field Ambulance: WO 95/4319
1/3rd Lowland Field Ambulance: WO 95/4319
ADMS: WO 95/4318
Sanitary Section: WO 95/4319

326   The Fight for Life

53rd Division
1/1st Welsh Field Ambulance: WO 95/4322
1/2nd Welsh Field Ambulance: WO 95/4322
1/3rd Welsh Field Ambulance: WO 95/4322
ADMS: WO 95/4322
Sanitary Section: WO 95/4322

54th Division
1/1st Eastern Mounted Brigade Field Ambulance: WO 95/4325
1/3rd East Anglia Field Ambulance: WO 95/4324
2/1st East Anglia Field Ambulance: WO 95/4324
ADMS: WO 95/4324
Sanitary Section: WO 95/4324

MEF General Headquarters
108th Indian Field Ambulance: WO 95/4272
ADMS: WO 95/4267
DDMS: WO 95/4267
DMS: WO 95/4267

Lines of Communication
11th Casualty Clearing Station: WO 95/4356
13th Casualty Clearing Station: WO 95/4356
14th Casualty Clearing Station: WO 95/4356
16th Casualty Clearing Station: WO 95/4356
16th Sanitary Section: WO 95/4356
24th Casualty Clearing Station: WO 95/4356
26th Casualty Clearing Station: WO 95/4356
52nd Casualty Clearing Station (Lowland): WO 95/4356
53rd Casualty Clearing Station (Welsh): WO 95/4356
54th Casualty Clearing Station: WO 95/4356
110th Indian Field Ambulance: WO 95/4356
137th Indian Field Ambulance: WO 95/4279
ADMS (Mudros – Two Diaries): WO 95/4355
HMHS *Aberdonian*: WO 95/4142/1
HMHS *Aquitania*: WO 95/4142/1
HMHS *Braemar Castle*: WO 95/4142/5
HMHS *Caledonia*: WO 95/4143/1
HMHS *Gascon*: WO 95/4145/1
HMHS *Glenart Castle*: WO 95/4145/2
HMHS *Goorkha*: WO 95/4145/5
HMHS *Guildford Castle*: WO 95/4145/7
HMHS *Lanfranc*: WO 95/4146/5
HMHS *Loyalty*: WO 95/4146/8
HMHS *Mauretania*: WO 95/4146

HMHS *Seang Choon*: WO 95/4148/2
HMHS *Sicilia*: WO 95/4148/3
No. 4 Advanced Depot Medical Stores: WO 95/4357
No. 4 Base Depot Medical Stores: WO 95/4357
No. 5 Advanced Depot Medical Stores: WO 95/4357
No. 5 Base Depot Medical Stores: WO 95/4357
No. 8 Advanced Depot Medical Stores: WO 95/4357
No. 16 Stationary Hospital: WO 95/4357
No. 17 Stationary Hospital: WO 95/4357
No. 18 Stationary Hospital: WO 95/4357

Royal Naval Division
2nd Field Ambulance: WO 95/4290
ADMS: WO 95/429

Published Sources

Adami, John G., *War Story of the Canadian Army Medical Corps: The First Contingent, to the Autumn of 1915* (London: The Rolls House Publishing Co., 1918), vol. 1

Annabell, Norman, *History of the New Zealand Engineers, 1914–1919* (Wanganui: Evans, Cobb & Sharpe, 1927)

Anon. [a sergeant major], *With the RAMC in Egypt* (London: Cassell & Company, 1918)

Anon. [Joseph Vassal], *Uncensored Letters from the Dardanelles* (London: William Heinemann, 1916)

Ashwood, Rodney, *Duty Nobly Done: The South Wales Borderers at Gallipoli 1915* (Solihull: Helion & Company, 2017)

Aspinall-Oglander, Brigadier General C. F., *Official History of the Great War, Military Operations: Gallipoli* (London: William Heinemann, 1932), vols 1–2 and appendices

Atkinson, C. T., *The History of the South Wales Borderers, 1914–1918* (London: Medici Society, 1931)

Badsey, Phylomena, 'Care-Giving and Naval Nurses at Gallipoli', in R. Crawley and M. LoCicero (eds), *Gallipoli: New Perspectives on the Mediterranean Expeditionary Force, 1915–16* (Warwick: Helion & Company, 2018), pp. 568–84

Baker, Anthony, *Battle Honours of the British and Commonwealth Armies* (London: Ian Allen, 1986)

Baly, Lindsay, *Horseman, Pass By: The Australian Light Horse in World War 1* (Staplehurst: Spellmount, 2004)

Banks, Arthur, *A Military Atlas of the First World War* (Barnsley: Leo Cooper, 1975)

Barrett, James W., and Deane, P. E., *The Australian Army Medical Corps in Egypt During the First World War* (London: H. K. Lewis and Son, 1918)

Bassett, Jan, *Guns and Brooches: Australian Army Nursing from the Boer War to the Gulf War* (Melbourne: Oxford University Press, 1992)

Bean, Charles E. W., *Anzac to Amiens* (Canberra: Australian War Memorial, 1968)

Bean, Charles E. W., *Official History of Australia in the War of 1914-18: The Story of ANZAC* (Sydney: Angus and Robertson, 1940), vols 1–2

Becke, Major A. F., *History of the Great War Based on Official Documents: Order of Battle of Divisions* (London: HMSO, 1945), parts 1–5

Beecroft, Arthur, *Gallipoli: A Soldier's Story* (London: Robert Hale, 2015)

Beeston, Joseph L., *Five Months at Anzac: A Narrative of Personal Experiences of the Officer Commanding the 4th Field Ambulance, Australian Imperial Force* (Angus & Robertson, 1916, Kindle e-book)

Benson, Sir Irving, *The Man with the Donkey: John Simpson Kirkpatrick, The Good Samaritan of Gallipoli* (London: Hodder & Stoughton, 1965)

Birdwood, General Sir William R., *Khaki and Gown. An Autobiography* (London: Ward, Lock, & Co., 1941)

Bou, Jean, *Light Horse: A History of Australia's Mounted Arm* (Melbourne: Cambridge University Press, 2010)

Bourne, J. M., *Britain and the Great War, 1914-1918* (London: Edward Arnold, 1989)

Broadbent, Harvey, *Defending Gallipoli: The Turkish Story* (Melbourne: Melbourne University Press, 2015)

Broadbent, Harvey, *Gallipoli: The Fatal Shore* (Camberwell: Penguin, 2009)

Brooks, Jane, and Hallett, Christine E. (eds), *One Hundred Years of Wartime Nursing Practices, 1854–1953* (Manchester: Manchester University Press, 2015)

Brown, Malcolm, *The Imperial War Museum Book of the First World War: A Great Conflict Recalled in Previously Unpublished Letters, Diaries, Documents, and Memoirs* (London: Guild Publishing, 1991)

Burness, Peter, *The Nek: A Gallipoli Tragedy* (Barnsley: Pen and Sword, 2013)

Butler, A. G., *The Official History of the Australian Army Medical Services in the War of 1914–1918: Volume I: Gallipoli, Palestine and New Guinea* (Facsimile edition of 1938 edition, Uckfield: Naval & Military Press, 2019)

Cameron, David W., *The August Offensive: At Anzac, 1915* (Canberra: Army History Unit, 2011)

Carberry, A. D., *The New Zealand Medical Service in the Great War 1914–1918* (Facsimile edition, Uckfield: Naval & Military Press, n.d.)

Carlyon, Les A., *Gallipoli* (London: Doubleday, 2001)

Carver, Field Marshal Lord, *The National Army Museum Book of the Turkish Front, 1914–1918* (London: Pan Macmillan, 2003)

Cassar, George H., *Reluctant Partner: The Complete Story of the French Participation in the Dardanelles Expedition of 1915* (Warwick: Helion & Company, 2019)

Chambers, Stephen, *Anzac: Sari Bair* (Barnsley: Pen and Sword, 2014)

Chambers, Stephen, *Anzac: The Landing* (Barnsley: Pen and Sword, 2008)

Chambers, Stephen, *Gully Ravine: Gallipoli* (Barnsley: Pen and Sword, 2003)

Chambers, Stephen. *Suvla: August Offensive* (Barnsley: Pen and Sword, 2011)

Chataway, Lieutenant T. P., *History of the 15th Battalion AIF, 1914-1918* (Facsimile edition, Uckfield: Naval & Military Press, n.d.)

Chasseaud, Peter, and Doyle, Peter, *Grasping Gallipoli: Terrain, Maps and Failure at the Dardanelles, 1915* (Staplehurst: Spellmount, 2005)

Churchill, Alexandra, 'The Decision to Evacuate the Gallipoli Peninsula', in R. Crawley and M. LoCicero (eds), *Gallipoli: New Perspectives on the Mediterranean Expeditionary Force, 1915–16* (Warwick: Helion & Company, 2018), pp.157–89

Churchill, Winston S., *The World Crisis: 1915* (London: Thomas Butterworth, 1923), vol. 2

Clint, Mabel B., *Our Bit: Memories of War Service by a Canadian Nursing-Sister* (Montreal: Barwick, 1934)

Corbett, Sir Julian S., *Naval Operations* (London: Longmans, Green and Co., 1920), vols 1–3

Crawford, Lieutenant Colonel D. G., *A History of the Indian Medical Service, 1600–1913* (London: W. Thacker & Co., 1914), vol. 2

Crawley, Rhys, and LoCicero, Michael (eds), *Gallipoli: New Perspectives on the Mediterranean Expeditionary Force, 1915-16* (Warwick: Helion & Company, 2018)

Curran, Tom, *Across the Bar: The Story of 'Simpson', The Man with the Donkey: Australia and Tyneside's Great Military Hero* (Brisbane: Ogmios Publications, 1994)

Curran, Tom, *The Grand Deception: Churchill and the Dardanelles* (Newport: Big Sky Publications, 2015)

Dardanelles Commission, *First Report* (London: HMSO, 1917)

Dardanelles Commission, *Final Report* (London: HMSO, 1919)

Davidson, George, *The Incomparable 29th and the 'River Clyde'* (James Gordon Bisset, 1919, Kindle e-book)

Denning, Roy and Lorna, *Anzac Digger: An Engineer in Gallipoli and France* (Loftus: Australian Military History Publications, 2004)

Dixon, John, *A Clash of Empires: The South Wales Borderers at Tsingtao, 1914* (Wrexham: Bridge Books, 2008)

Dixon, John, *A Vital Endeavour*: *Military Engineering in the Gallipoli Campaign* (Warwick: Helion & Company, 2019)

Dixon, John, *Army Nurse: The Matron Who Went to War* (Llangan: Cwm Press, 2019)

Dixon, John, *Magnificent but Not War: The Second Battle of Ypres 1915* (Barnsley: Pen and Sword, 2003)

Doyle Peter, *Battle Story: Gallipoli 1915* (Staplehurst: Spellmount, 2012)

East, Sir Ronald (ed.), *The Gallipoli Diary of Sergeant Lawrence of the Australian Engineers – 1st A.I.F. 1915* (Melbourne: Melbourne University Press, 1981)

Erickson, Edward J., *Gallipoli: The Ottoman Campaign* (Barnsley: Pen and Sword, 2010)

Ewing, John, *The Royal Scots 1914-1919* (Edinburgh: Oliver and Boyd, 1925), vol. 1

Fell, A. S., 'The Mobilization and Experience of Nurses in the First World War', in P. Liddle (ed.), *Britain Goes to War: How the First World War Began to Reshape the Nation* (Barnsley: Pen and Sword, 2015), pp.259–72

Fell, Alison S., and Hallett, Christine E. (eds), *First World War Nursing: New Perspectives* (Abingdon: Routledge, 2013)

Fewster, Kevin, Başarın, Vecihi, and Başarın, Hatice H., *Gallipoli: The Turkish Story* (Crows Nest: Allen and Unwin, 2003)

Forbes, Major General A., *A History of the Army Ordnance Services* (Facsimile edition of 1929 edition, Uckfield: Naval & Military Press, 2010)

Ford, Roger, *Eden to Armageddon: World War 1 in the Middle East* (London: Phoenix, 2010)

Gallishaw, John, *Trenching at Gallipoli: The Personal Narrative of a Newfoundlander with the Ill-Fated Dardanelles Expedition* (Location unknown: Alpha Editions, 2020)

Gardam, John, *Seventy Years After 1914–1984* (Sittsville: Canada's Wings, 1983)

Gillon, Captain Stair, *The K.O.S.B. in the Great War* (London: Thomas Nelson and Sons, 1930)

Gillon, Captain Stair, *The Story of the 29th Division: A Record of Gallant Deeds* (London: Thomas Nelson and Sons, 1925)

Glen, Alec, *In the Front Line: A Doctor's Life in War and Peace* (Edinburgh: Birlinn, 2013)

Gough, Barry, *Churchill and Fisher: The Titans at the Admiralty Who Fought the First World War* (Barnsley: Seaforth Publishing, 2017)

Grimwade, F. C., *The War History of the 4th Battalion, The London Regiment (Royal Fusiliers) 1914–1919* (London: HQ of the 4th London Regiment, 1922)

Hallett, Christine E., *Containing Trauma: Nursing Work in the First World War* (Manchester: Manchester University Press, 2009)

Hallett, Christine E., *Veiled Warriors: Allied Nurses of the First World War* (Oxford: Oxford University Press, 2014)

Halpern, Paul G., *A Naval History of World War I* (London: UCL Press, 1995)

Hamilton, General Sir Ian, *Gallipoli Diary* (Woking: Unwin Brothers, 1920), vols 1–2

Hamilton, John, *Goodbye Cobber, God Bless You* (Sydney: Pan MacMillan, 2005)

Hammerton, Sir J. A., *A Popular History of the Great War: Extension of the Struggle* (London: The Fleetway House, n.d.), vol. 2

Hargrave, John, *The Suvla Bay Landing* (London: MacDonald & Co., 1964)

Harris, Kirsty, *More Than Bombs and Bandages: Australian Army Nurses at Work in World War I* (Newport: Big Sky Publications, 2011)

Harrison, Mark, *The Medical War: British Military Medicine in the First World War* (Oxford: Oxford University Press, 2010)

Hart, Peter, *The Gallipoli Evacuation* (Manly: Living History, 2020)

Hay, Ian, *One Hundred Years of Army Nursing* (London: Cassell & Company, 1953)

Heffer, Simon, *Staring at God: Britain in the Great War* (London: Random House Books, 2019)

Herbert, A. P., *The Secret Battle* (Oxford: Oxford University Press, 1982)

Holt, Tonie, and Valmai, *Major & Mrs Holt's Battlefield Guide to Gallipoli* (Barnsley: Leo Cooper, 2000)

James, Brigadier E. A., *British Regiments, 1914–18* (London: Samson Books, 1978)

James, Robert R., *Gallipoli* (London: Pan Books, 1984)

Jerrold, Douglas, *The Royal Naval Division* (Facsimile edition of 1923 edition, Uckfiled: Naval & Military Press, n.d.)

Jordan, Humfrey, *Mauretania: Landfalls and Departures of Twenty-five Years* (Wellingborough: Patrick Stephens, 1988)

Keegan, John, *The First World War* (London: Hutchinson, 1998)

Kinross, Patrick, *Ataturk: The Rebirth of a Nation* (Istanbul: Remzi Kitabevi, 2001)

Klein, Maury, *Days of Defiance: Sumter, Secession, and the Coming of the Civil War* (New York: Vintage Books, 1999)

Kyle, Roy, *An Anzac's Story* (Camberwell: Viking, 2003)

Lee, John, *A Soldier's Life: General Sir Ian Hamilton 1853-1947* (London: MacMillan, 2000)

Liddle, Peter, *Gallipoli 1915: Pens, Pencils and Cameras at War* (London: Brassey's Defence Publishers, 1985)

Liddle, Peter, *The Gallipoli Experience Reconsidered* (Barnsley: Pen and Sword Military, 2015)

Lloyd George, David, *War Memoirs* (London: Odhams Press, 1938), vol. 1

MacKenzie, Compton, *Gallipoli Memories* (London: Cassel & Company, 1929)

MacKinnon, Rev. Albert G., *Malta: The Nurse of the Mediterranean* (London: Hodder & Stoughton, 1916)

MacPherson, Major General Sir W. G., *History of the Great War Based on Official Documents: Medical Services* (Facsimile edition, Uckfield: Naval & Military Press, n.d.), vols 1–5

MacPherson, Major General Sir W. G., *History of the Great War Based on Official Documents: Medical Services, Diseases of the War* (London: HMSO, 1922), vol. 1

Masefield, John, *Gallipoli* (London: William Heinmann, 1916)

Massie, Robert K., *Castles of Steel: Britain, Germany, and the Winning of the Great War at Sea* (London: Jonathan Cape, 2004)

McEwen, Yvonne, *In the Company of Nurses: The History of the British Army Nursing Service in the Great War* (Edinburgh: Edinburgh University Press, 2014)

Merewether, Lieutenant Colonel J. W. B., and Smith, Lieutenant Colonel Sir Frederick, *The Indian Corps in France* (London: John Murray, 1918)

Meyer, Jessica, *An Equal Burden: The Men of the Royal Army Medical Corps in the First World War* (Oxford: Oxford University Press, 2019)

Mitchell, T. J., and Smith, G. M., *Official History of the Great War: Medical Services: Casualties and Medical Statistics* (Facsimile edition of 1931 edition, Uckfeld: Naval & Military Press, n.d.), vol. 5

Moncrieff, Alexia, *Expertise, Authority and Control: The Australian Army Medical Corps in the First World War* (Cambridge: Cambridge University Press 2020)

Moorehead, Alan, *Gallipoli* (London: Andre Deutsch, 1989)

Morton-Jack, George, *The Indian Empire at War* (London: Abacus 2020)

Murdoch, Keith, *The Gallipoli Letter* (Crows Nest: Allen and Unwin, 2010)

Mure, A. H., *This Bloody Place: With the Incomparable 29th* (Barnsley: Pen and Sword Military, 2015)

Murray, Joseph, *Gallipoli 1915* (Bristol: Cerberus, 2004)

Newton, L. M., *The Story of the Twelfth: A Record of the 12th Battalion AIF during the Great War 1914–18* (Facsimile edition of 1925 edition, Uckfield: Naval & Military Press and IWM, n.d.)

Olden, Lieutenant Colonel A. C. N., *Westralian Cavalry in the War: The Story of the Tenth Light Horse Regiment, A.I.F., in the Great War, 1914–1918* (Facsimile edition of 1921 publication, Uckfield: Naval & Military Press, n.d.)

O'Neill, H. C., *The Royal Fusiliers in the Great War* (Facsimile edition, Uckfield: Naval & Military Press, 2002)

Owen, Bryn, *Owen Roscomyl and the Welsh Horse* (Caernarfon: Palace Books, 1990)

Parsons, W. D., *Pilgrimage: A Guide to the Royal Newfoundland Regiment in World War One* (St John's: Creative Publishers, 1994)

Penn, Geoffrey, *Fisher, Churchill and the Dardanelles* (Barnsley: Leo Cooper, 1999)

Perry, F. W., *History of the Great War Based on Official Documents: Order of Battle of Divisions: Part 5a. The Divisions of Australia, Canada and New Zealand and Those in East Africa* (Newport: Ray Westlake – Military Books, 1992)

Prior, Robin, *Gallipoli: The End of the Myth* (London: Yale University Press, 2009)

Pugsley, Christopher, *Anzac: The New Zealanders at Gallipoli* (New Zealand: Reed Children's Books, 2000)

Pugsley, Christopher, *Gallipoli: The New Zealand Story* (Auckland: Hodder & Stoughton, 1984)

Purdom, C. B. (ed.), 'Account of Lieutenant Colonel F. W. D. Bendall', in *Everyman at War* (London: Dent & Sons, 1930), pp.290–97

Rae, Ruth, *Scarlet Poppies: The Army Experience of Australian Nurses during the First World War* (Ruth Rae Consultancies, 2015, Kindle e-book)

Rae, Ruth, *Veiled Lives: Threading Australian Nursing History into the Fabric of the First World War* (2nd edition, Australian College of Nursing, 2012, Kindle e-book)

Rees, Peter, *The Other Anzacs: Nurses at War, 1914–1918* (Crows Nest: Allen and Unwin, 2008)

Regimental History Committee [C. T. Atkinson], *History of the Dorsetshire Regiment 1914-1919. Part III: The Service Battalions* (Dorchester: Henry Ling, 1932)

Richardson, Pat, and Skinner, Anne (eds), *Queenie: Letters from an Australian Army Nurse, 1915–1917* (New South Wales: Gumleaf Press, 2012)

Rignault, Daniel P., *The History of the French Military Medical Corps* (Paris: Ministère de la défense, Service de Santé des Armées, 2004)

Roberts, Chris, *The Landing at Anzac: 1915* (Sydney: Big Sky Publishing, 2013)

Rodge, Huw and Jill, *Helles Landing: Gallipoli* (Barnsley: Pen and Sword, 2003)

Roynon, Gavin (ed.), *A Prayer for Gallipoli: The Great War Diaries of Chaplain Kenneth Best* (London: Simon & Schuster, 2011)

Sandes, Lieutenant Colonel E. W. C., *The Military Engineer in India* (Chatham: Institution of Royal Engineers, 1935), vols 1–2

Schembri, Gioconda S., *Three Anzacs from Malta: A True Story of Friendship, Love, and Loss* (Australia: Gioconda S. Schembri, 2016)

Smith, E. D., *Valour: A History of the Gurkhas* (Staplehurst: Spellmount, 1997)

Stacey, A. J., *Memoirs of a Blue Puttee: The Newfoundland Regiment in World War One* (St John's: DRC Publishers, 2002)

Stanley, Peter, *Quinn's Post: Anzac, Gallipoli* (Crow's Nest: Allen and Unwin, 2005)

Steel, Nigel, *Gallipoli* (Barnsley: Leo Cooper, 1999)

Steel, Nigel, and Hart, Peter, *Defeat at Gallipoli* (London: MacMillan, 1994)

Strachan, Hew, *The First World War: Volume I: To Arms* (Oxford: Oxford University Press, 2001)

Taylor, Eric, *Wartime Nurse: One Hundred Years from the Crimea to Korea 1854-1954* (London: Robert Hale, 2001)

Taylor, Phil, and Cupper, Pam, *Gallipoli: A Battlefield Guide* (Kenthurst: Kangaroo Press, 1989)

Teichman, Captain O., *Diary of a Yeomanry M.O.: Egypt, Gallipoli, Palestine and Italy* (London: T. Fisher Unwin, 1921)

Toman, Cynthia, *Sister Soldiers of the Great War: The Nurses of the Canadian Army Medical Corps* (Vancouver: UBC Press, 2016)

Tyquin, Michael B., *Gallipoli: An Australian Medical Perspective* (Newport: Big Sky Publishing, 2012)

Tyquin, Michael B., *Gallipoli: The Medical War. The Australian Army Medical Services in the Dardanelles Campaign of 1915* (Kensington: New South Wales University Press, 1993)

Wahlert, Lieutenant Colonel Glenn, *Exploring Gallipoli: An Australian Army Battlefield Guide* (Canberra: Army History Unit, 2008)

Waite, Fred, *The New Zealanders at Gallipoli* (Auckland: Whitcombe and Tombs, 1921)

Walker, Rob W., *To What End Did They Die? Officers Died at Gallipoli* (Worcester: R. W. Walker Publishing, 1985)

Ward, C. H. D., *Regimental Records of the Royal Welch Fusiliers* (Wrexham: Royal Welch Fusiliers, 1995), vol. 4

Weeks, Alan, *Tea, Rum & Fags: Sustaining Tommy, 1914-18* (Stroud: The History Press, 2009)

Westlake, Ray, *British Regiments at Gallipoli* (Barnsley: Leo Cooper, 1996)
Westlake, Ray, *The Territorial Force, 1914* (Newport: Ray Westlake, Military Books, 1988)
Wolf, Klaus, *Victory at Gallipoli 1915: The German–Ottoman Alliance in the First World War* (Barnsley: Pen and Sword Military, 2020)
Young, Margaret O. (ed.), *We Are Here, Too: The Diaries and Letters of Sister Olive L. C. Haynes, November 1914 to February 1918* (3rd edition, South Australia: Margaret O. Young, 2014)

Journals & Periodicals

Anon., 'The French Medical Services during the War of 1914-1918', *BMJ Military Health*, 52 (1929), pp.38–46
Cleverly, Jeff, 'More Than a Sideshow? An Analysis of GHQ Decision Making during the Planning for the Landings at Suvla Bay, Gallipoli, August 1915', *War in History*, 24:1 (2017), pp.44–63
Collingwood, Fleet Surgeon T., 'Notes on the Work of the RN Hospital Ship *Soudan* at the Dardanelles', *Journal of the Royal Naval Medical Service*, 1 (1916), pp.315–21
Collingwood, Fleet Surgeon T., 'Notes on the Work of the RN Hospital Ship *Soudan* at the Dardanelles', *Journal of the Royal Naval Medical Service*, 2 (1916), pp.200–07
Dalton, Fleet Surgeon F. J. A., 'Notes on the Work of the RN Hospital Ship *Rewa* at the Dardanelles', *Journal of the Royal Naval Medical Service*, 2 (1916), pp.1–29
James, Robert R., 'A Visit to Gallipoli, 1962', *Stand-To*, 9:2 (1964), p.5
Lambert, Temporary Surgeon J., 'Two Months' Work in the Royal Navy Hospital Ship *Rewa* at the Gallipoli Beaches: By the Staff of the *Rewa*', *Journal of the Royal Naval Medical Service*, 2 (1916), pp.1–29
MacDonald, Donald, 'The Indian Medical Service. A Short Account of Its Achievements 1600–1947', *Proceedings of the Royal Society of Medicine*, 49:1 (1955), pp.13–17
Macleod, Jenny, 'General Sir Ian Hamilton and the Dardanelles Commission', *War in History*, 8:4 (2001), pp.418–41
Mirsky, Samuel, 'Epidemic Jaundice (Viral Hepatitis)', *Canadian Medical Association Journal (CMAJ)*, 70:3 (1954), pp.308–11
Moritz, S., 'Epidemic Jaundice in War Time', *BMJ*, 2:2860 (1915), p.602
Phipson, Colonel E. S., 'With the Gurkhas on Sari Bair', *Gallipolian*, 147 (Autumn 2018), pp.37–39
Smith, Lucian A., 'Shiga Dysentery', *Journal of the American Medical Association (JAMA)*, 130:1 (1946), pp.18–22
Symmers, Douglas, 'Epidemic Jaundice', *Journal of the American Medical Association (JAMA)*, 123:16 (1943), p.1066

Electronic Sources

Bruce, Captain G. R., 'Military Hospitals in Malta during the War: A Short Account of Their Inception and Development', *ScarletFinders* <http://www.scarletfinders.co.uk/190.html>
Canadian Great War Project <https://canadiangreatwarproject.com/>

'Diary of Service with No. 15 Stationary Hospital on Lemnos during the Dardanelles Campaign, June 1915-Jan 1916, and in East Africa, May 1916-Jan 1917', *Welcome Collection* <https://wellcomecollection.org/works/yfvzvc4a>

'Go-Gr', *Australian Nurses in World War 1* <http://ausww1nurses.weebly.com/go-gr.html>

'Image Number 42871_635001_11844_00099', *Ancestry* <https://www.ancestry.com/>

McCarthy, Perditta M., 'Ellen Julia (Nellie) Gould (1860–1941)', *Australian Dictionary of Biography* (2006) <https://adb.anu.edu.au/biography/gould-ellen-julia-nellie-6437/text11013>

'New Zealand History', *NZHistory* <nzhistory.govt.nz>

'New Zealand Military Nursing', *NZANS* <nzans.org>

Savona-Ventura, C., 'Military Hospitals in Malta', *Vassallo History* <https://vassallohistory.wordpress.com/military-hospitals-in-malta/>

Index

People

Asquith, Prime Minister H.H., 282, 303

Battye, Major W.R., 115–18, 126–28, 131, 234–35, 238, 242–43, 267–68, 288–89
Bedford. Surgeon General W.G.A., 221, 236
Begg, Lieutenant Colonel C.M., 150
Birdwood, Lieutenant General Sir W., 92, 284, 328
Birrell, Surgeon General W.G., 43, 55, 57–58, 60–65, 108, 112–13, 179–82, 196–98, 304, 306–8
Braithwaite, Major General Sir W.P., 58, 92
Brown, Sister M., 196

Casson, Lieutenant Colonel H.G., 72
Chibnall, Sister H.F., 248, 249
Churchill, Winston, 295, 297, 304, 328-31
Clint, Sister M., 270-72, 279
Corbridge, Staff Sergeant, 82, 121–22, 211, 215

Dalton, Fleet Surgeon F.J.A., 245, 247, 248-49
Davidson, Lieutenant G., 74-6, 214, 254

Fawcett, Matron K.F., 50, 153
Ford, Surgeon General R., 51

Gallishaw, Corporal J. 250-1, 329
Giblin, Lieutenant Colonel W.W., 193
Gould, Matron N., 34-6, 52, 104
Gray, Private O.H., 185-86
Grierson, Sister M.E.M, 52

Hamilton, General Sir I.S.M., 50–51, 56–58, 108, 132, 177, 180–82, 215–16, 281–83, 304, 307

Howse, Colonel N.H., 52, 61–62, 64, 94-95
Hunter-Weston, Lieutenant-General Sir A., 88
Husband, Captain G.S., 116-17, 126, 131, 133-34

Jaggard, Matron J.B., 174, 272
Johnston, Sister J.B., 104

Keble, Lieutenant Colonel A.E.C., 61–62, 306–7
Kellet Sister A.M., 53, 54, 105, 164, 172, 197
Kitchener, Field Marshal Lord H.H., 281–84

Maxwell, General Sir J., 51
McNaught Lieutenant Colonel J.G., 193-5
Medical Officer (MO), 27–29, 34–36, 39–44, 46–47, 55–57, 111–14, 122–24, 129–31, 138–39, 150–52, 158–63, 189–92, 217–20, 222–26, 232–35, 242–43, 259–72, 276–79, 309–10
Miles Walker, Matron J., 164-5
Millard, Sir R.J.M., 102–4, 107, 227
Monro, General Sir C.C., 283-84
Morrice, Sister N.C., 104, 274–75
Munro, Sister M.F., 174, 272.

Phipson, Captain E.S., 191, 333
Pocock, Sister M.A. (Bessie), 93, 182, 226, 251, 273
Principal Medical Officer (MO), 28, 32, 34–36

Regimental Medical Officer (RMO), 29, 36, 39, 150, 152, 156, 158, 160, 189, 191–92, 231–32, 286–87, 289, 291, 299–301

336   The Fight for Life

Richards, Private T.J., 93, 95, 100-1, 182-83, 188

Ryan, Colonel C.S., 112, 308

Samsing, Sister H.S.R., 49, 105

Simpson, Private J., 144–47, 161, 329

Stopford, Lieutenant General Sir F., 200, 203, 205

Tucker, Sister E., 84, 96, 97, 103, 193, 195, 197, 225

Vassal, Major J., 44, 86–88, 116, 121–23, 129–30, 132

Wilson, Principal Matron G., 170, 172, 270

Woodward, Brigadier General E.M. 63-5

Woodward, Brigadier General E.M., 60, 109

Wooler, Matron S., 225

Yarr, Colonel M.T., 61–62, 81–82, 118, 120–21, 123–24, 219, 221

Zwar, Major B.T., 98, 162-63

Places

Achi Baba, 81, 88, 137, 140

Achi Baba Nullah, 85, 135–37, 211, 298, 301

Aegean Sea, 73, 85–86, 91, 201, 298

Aghyl Dere, 187–89, 201, 227, 289

Alexandria, 44–45, 48, 51–52, 54, 58, 63–64, 84, 88–89, 97–98, 103–6, 140, 142–43, 162–63, 167–69, 171–72, 196–97, 199–200, 202, 225–26, 251

Anzac Cove, 73, 91, 144, 149, 155, 178, 189, 201, 236, 267

Ari Burnu, 73, 91–92

Asiatic Coast, 84, 86, 88

Asmak Dere Bridge, 296

Bombay Presidency General Hospital (BPGH), 42, 54

Brighton Beach, 142–43, 184, 190, 228

Brown's Dip, 183–85, 188–89, 228

Cairo, 48, 51–52, 54, 93, 104–5, 144, 164, 197, 199, 251

Cape Helles, 70–73, 75–89, 98, 109–11, 139–41, 157, 178–80, 182, 203–4, 210, 216–18, 220–23, 247, 249, 260–61, 264–65, 282–83, 285, 297–300, 304–7, 309–11

Chailak Dere, 91, 181, 186–90, 235, 240, 267, 289

Chocolate Hill, 201, 208, 253, 295–96

Chunuk Bair, 90, 178, 186–87, 190, 201, 290

Dressing Stations, Main, 122–23, 129, 132, 135–36, 140, 204–5, 262

Egypt, 38, 42–44, 48–58, 60–62, 66–68, 70, 84, 107–8, 110, 139–40, 153, 163–64

Fisherman's Hut, 90–92

Gaba Tepe, 73, 86, 92, 95–96, 98, 102, 143, 161, 166, 168

Gibraltar, 50, 57, 112, 237, 258

Gully Beach, 85, 117, 126–27, 130–34, 180, 214–15, 298, 301

Gully Ravine, 85, 117, 125–28, 130–33, 135, 211, 214, 218, 300, 328

Gurkha Beach, 131–35

Imbros, 46, 177, 179–80, 182, 193, 195, 197–98, 204, 296–97, 300

Krithia, 73, 77–78, 81, 85, 88, 116, 118, 121, 127, 129–30, 298

Kum Kale, 74, 78, 84, 86, 88–89, 116

Lala Baba, 201, 203, 295–96

Lemnos, 47–48, 58–59, 62–63, 66, 69–70, 112, 139–41, 155–56, 162, 166–72, 174, 177–79, 195–99, 224–28, 231, 249, 271–76, 278–80, 291–92, 310–11

Lone Pine, 91, 178, 183–85, 189, 192

Luna Park, 52–53, 105–6

Mal Tepe Dere, 127, 135–36, 211

Malta, 45–46, 48, 55–57, 66, 70, 153, 155, 169, 171, 195, 197, 225–26, 229–30, 332–34

Mena House, 52, 104–5, 164–65

Mudros, 42–43, 45–46, 50, 52, 59, 62, 64, 96–97, 118, 137–40, 166–71, 174, 176-177, 179–80, 196, 199, 202, 227–29, 273, 275–78, 280, 291–92, 299–300, 302

Narrows, 50, 71, 73, 312
Newfoundland, 38, 144, 250
New South Wales, 32, 34, 36, 197, 237, 332
New Zealand, 36–38, 54, 64, 96, 187, 224, 305, 311, 331
North Beach, 90, 235

Pink Farm, 85, 117, 127, 132, 135, 211–12, 214, 298

Quinn's Post, 159–60, 186, 332

Regimental Aid Post (RAP), 45–47, 82, 128, 131, 134–36, 159, 188, 214–15, 291, 316

S Beach, 72, 80
Salonika, 38, 177, 241, 249–50, 281, 284
Salt Lake, 201, 203, 205–6, 253, 260, 293, 295–96

South Africa, 29, 32–33, 35–37, 305
South Pier, 294–96
Suvla Bay, 73, 169, 171, 178, 180-82, 200–3, 205–9, 217, 244–47, 249–51, 253, 255–57, 260–63, 279–80, 282–83, 285, 291–93, 297

V Beach, 72, 74, 76, 78, 88, 115-116, 140-141, 254, 300, 302
Victoria Gully, 142, 183–84, 189

W Beach, 72, 76-78, 80, 115, 117, 122-123, 127, 133, 135-136, 212, 214, 221, 254, 300-1
West Beach, 251, 263, 292, 294–95
Western Front, 31, 47–48, 109, 124, 170, 283
West Krithia Road, 117, 127, 132, 135–36

X Beach, 71-72, 77, 135-136

Y Beach, 71-72, 77, 127-128, 131, 134, 221

Formations & Units

Armies
Mediterranean Expeditionary Force (MEF), 50, 54, 56, 57, 61, 62, 64, 108, 124, 156, 166, 219, 232, 239, 303

Army Corps
VIII Corp, 219, 220, 221, 283, 325
IX Corps, 38, 39, 40, 44, 71, 86, 174, 178, 180, 200, 203, 219, 220, 221, 231, 232, 239, 283, 293
Australian and New Zealand Army Corps (ANZAC), 61-64, 147, 229, 238, 288, 234
Corps Expéditionnaire D'Orient, 86

Divisions
1st Australian Division, 33, 52, 61, 64, 94, 110, 149, 181, 183, 188, 190, 227, 228, 229, 233, 305, 306
2nd Australian Division 287
10th (Irish) Division 200, 202, 203, 204, 249, 253, 253
11th (Northern) Division, 200, 203, 204, 205, 217, 245, 253, 254, 260, 293, 294, 295, 296
13th Division, 140, 183, 188, 193, 194, 253, 246, 293, 294, 295, 299, 301, 325
29th Division, 38, 51, 61, 62, 63, 64, 65, 66, 71, 72, 78, 81, 82, 88, 110, 115, 118, 120, 121,

123, 124, 125, 126, 128, 129, 130, 132, 134, 135, 157, 159, 168, 203, 206, 210, 211, 212, 214, 215, 219, 249, 250, 254, 256, 260, 262, 292, 294, 295, 299, 300, 305, 329.
42nd (East Lancashire) Division, 51, 52, 54, 104, 117, 118, 122, 123, 124, 135, 136, 138, 210, 212, 214, 215, 216, 218, 219, 221, 222, 223, 299, 300
52nd (Lowland) Division, 135, 136, 137, 138, 139, 140, 141, 211, 215, 217, 218, 219, 264, 299, 301
53rd (Welsh) Division 203, 206, 249, 262, 326
54th (East Anglian) Division 231, 232, 236, 243, 267, 288
2nd Mounted Division 206, 207, 293, 294
New Zealand & Australian Division, 37, 52, 61, 186, 187, 227, 287, 306
Royal Naval Division (RND), 61, 66, 71, 72, 76, 110, 113, 117, 117, 123, 124, 129, 135, 136, 140, 157, 200, 204, 215, 220, 245, 299, 300, 301, 302

French
1st Division, 86, 137

Brigades
1st Australian Brigade, 90, 92, 99

2nd Australian Brigade, 90, 92
3rd Australian Brigade, 50, 90, 92, 99, 166, 167
4th Australian Brigade, 149, 183
5th Australian Brigade, 291
6th Australian Brigade, 227, 291
5th Cavalry Brigade 30
29th Brigade, 249
32nd Brigade, 203, 295
33rd Brigade, 203, 204
34th Brigade, 203
38th Brigade, 295
39th Brigade, 189, 296
86th Brigade, 80, 141, 212, 262
87th Brigade, 81, 128
88th Brigade, 210, 212, 215, 250
125th Brigade, 210
126th Brigade, 223
127th Brigade. 210
7th Indian Mountain Artillery Brigade, 42, 144, 232, 233, 235
29th Indian Brigade, 42, 115, 116, 126, 128, 132, 134, 181, 183, 190, 232, 234, 288, 291
New Zealand Brigade, 92, 183, 291
New Zealand Mounted Rifle Brigade, 183, 291

Regiments/Battalions
10th Australian Light Horse 265
2nd Battalion AIF, 100
4th Battalion AIF, 100, 158
9th Battalion AIF 90, 92, 165
10th Battalion AIF 90, 92
11th Battalion AIF 90, 92, 182
12th Battalion AIF 90, 92
14th Battalion AIF, 196
15th Battalion AIF, 265
20th Battalion AIF, 229
1st Border Regiment, 71, 82
5th Dorsetshire Regiment, 261, 262
1st Essex Regiment, 211
1/5th Gurkhas, 128, 134, 242, 243
1/6th Gurkhas, 127, 128, 191, 238
1/10th Gurkhas, 128
2/10th Gurkhas 233, 267, 268
2nd Hampshire Regiment, 72, 211
1st King's Own Scottish Borderers (KOSB), 71, 82, 125
1/4th KOSB, 264

1st Lancashire Fusiliers, 72, 76, 128, 254
1/5th Lancashire Fusiliers 299
6th Lincolnshire Regiment, 260
1/5th Manchester Regiment, 210
4th London Regiment, 260
69th Punjabis, 116.
97th Punjabis, 242
1st Royal Dublin Fusiliers, 72, 74, 76
2nd Royal Fusiliers, 71, 260
1st Royal Inniskilling Fusiliers, 71, 83
1st Royal Munster Fusiliers, 72, 74, 133
1/5th Royal Scots, 72, 249, 250, 261
14th Sikhs, 128, 133, 134, 242
6th South Lancashire Regiment, 189
7th South Staffordshire Regiment, 260, 301
2nd South Wales Borderers (SWB), 71, 72, 77, 122, 130, 258
4th SWB, 183, 191
1/5th Welsh Regiment, 170, 171
5th Wiltshire Regiment, 183
4th Worcestershire Regiment, 72, 211
13th Worcestershire Regiment, 133
6th Yorkshire Regiment, 203

Anson Battalion, 71, 72, 76
Auckland Battalion, 186
Auckland Mounted Rifles 186
Canterbury Battalion, 160
Canterbury Mounted Rifles 186
Hawke Battalion, 157
Herefordshire Regiment, 262
London Regiment, 55
Malta Militia, 55
Newfoundland Regiment, 38, 249, 250, 254
Otago Mounted Rifles, 186
Plymouth Battalion, 71
Royal Marine Light Infantry (RMLI), 79, 101
Wellington Battalion, 159, 160, 187
Wellington Mounted Rifles, 186, 188, 190
Worcestershire Yeomanry, 206, 281

French
4th Colonial Regiment, 117
6th Mixed Colonial Regiment, 44, 86, 88, 122
Miscellaneous Units
Army Bearer Corps, 41, 42, 140
Army Hospital Corps, 41, 42
Army Medical Corps of the Militia, 39
Army Ordnance Corps, 177

Index 339

Army Service Corps, 71, 122, 272
Australian Army Medical Corps. 32, 33, 34, 36, 51, 52, 61, 108, 112, 226, 239, 273, 274, 305, 311
Australian Engineers, 153, 261, 329
Australian Medical Service, 32, 44, 55, 60, 61, 62, 68, 70, 96, 108, 113, 156, 157, 158, 159, 162, 169, 171, 176, 187, 287
Canadian Army Medical Corps, 38, 40, 174
Indian Medical Service, 40, 41
Indian Mule Cart Corps, 236
New South Wales Army Medical Corps, 35
New Zealand Engineers, 327
New Zealand Medical Corps, 36, 37, 61, 63, 95, 157, 158, 159, 160, 328
Permanent Active Medical Corps, 39
Royal Army Medical Corps (RAMC), 27, 29–31, 32, 33, 34, 35, 37, 39, 40, 41, 42, 43, 45, 46, 47, 49, 51, 52, 54, 55, 56, 57, 71, 72, 74, 79, 84, 96, 98, 103, 128, 133, 163, 171, 180, 189, 206, 231, 240, 244, 251, 253, 255, 262, 276, 300, 301, 309
Royal Engineers, 27, 62, 71, 74, 109, 115, 117, 129, 130, 139, 166, 219, 260
West Riding Field Company RE, 74

French
Service de Santé des Armée, 42, 44, 45, 80, 89, 122, 166, 309

Advanced Depot Medical Stores
4th Advanced Depot Medical Stores, 288, 327
5th Advanced Depot Medical Stores, 62, 123, 168, 219
Base Depot Medical Stores
4th Base Depot Medical Stores, 168

Field Ambulances
1st Australian Field Ambulance, 52, 70, 93, 94, 99, 100, 102, 103, 142, 158, 181, 182, 183, 184, 185, 188, 189, 190, 226, 227, 228, 239
1st Australian Light Horse Field Ambulance, 186, 188
1st London Field Ambulance, 55
1st Royal Navy Field Ambulance, 113, 136, 245, 299
1/1st East Lancashire Field Ambulance, 52, 104, 264
1/1st Eastern Mounted Brigade FA, 267, 326

1/1st Highland Mounted Brigade FA, 256, 297, 324
1/1st Lowland Field Ambulance, 135, 136, 212, 219, 264, 300, 325
1/1st South Eastern Mounted Brigade Field Ambulance, 300
1/1st Welsh Field Ambulance, 206, 209, 244, 253, 262
1/2nd Lowland Field Ambulance, 135, 219
1/2nd Welsh Field Ambulance, 254
1/2nd South Western Mounted Brigade FA, 294
1/3rd East Lancashire Field Ambulance, 129
1/3rd Lowland Field Ambulance, 135, 136, 218, 299
1/3rd Welsh Field Ambulance, 202, 206, 254
1/4th London Mounted Brigade FA, 208
2nd Australian Field Ambulance, 93, 143, 184, 227, 322
2nd Australian Light Horse Field Ambulance, 185, 187
2nd Royal Navy Field Ambulance, 117, 200, 204, 299
2/1st East Anglia Field Ambulance, 326
3rd Australian Field Ambulance, 93, 94, 97, 99, 101, 143, 144, 146, 157, 184, 185, 187, 188, 189, 227
3rd Australian Light Horse Field Ambulance, 187
3rd Royal Navy Field Ambulance, 136, 299
4th Australian Field Ambulance, 102, 149, 161, 184, 187, 194, 228, 266
5th Australian Field Ambulance, 181, 226, 227, 234, 287, 291
6th Australian Field Ambulance, 228, 287, 240, 324
7th Australian Field Ambulance, 228, 287, 324
30th Field Ambulance, 202, 204
31st Field Ambulance, 202, 204, 205, 253
32nd Field Ambulance, 204, 205
33rd Field Ambulance, 205
34th Field Ambulance, 200
35th Field Ambulance, 204, 255, 294
39th Field Ambulance, 188, 189, 253, 254, 294, 295, 296
40th Field Ambulance, 188, 189, 193, 257, 293, 294, 296
41st Field Ambulance, 85, 140, 188, 294, 296

87th Field Ambulance, 72, 77, 78, 79, 82, 83, 84, 117, 118, 121, 122, 124, 125, 126, 127, 128, 129, 130, 132, 133, 134, 211, 212, 215, 249, 292

88th Field Ambulance, 72, 80, 117, 127, 130, 132, 292, 294

89th Field Ambulance, 72, 74, 75, 76, 77, 80, 81, 83, 115, 117, 121, 123, 124, 125, 127, 130, 132, 133, 134, 135, 140, 141, 214, 254, 262, 292, 294

108th Indian Field Ambulance, 42, 115, 116, 117, 118, 125, 126, 127, 128, 130, 131, 132, 133, 135, 139, 140, 181, 190, 191, 192, 217, 225, 233, 234, 235, 238, 239, 240, 241, 242, 243, 260, 267, 268, 276, 288, 289, 291

110th Indian Field Ambulance, 42, 140, 168, 276, 277, 279, 280, 321

137th Indian Field Ambulance, 264, 326, 224, 288

NZFA, 93, 103, 150, 151, 152, 156

New Zealand Mounted Field Ambulance, 153, 155, 157, 158, 266, 291

Casualty Clearing Stations

1st Australian Casualty Clearing Station (ACCS), 34, 53, 93, 94, 95, 99, 100, 101, 111, 113, 142, 149, 152, 155, 161, 162, 176, 181, 182, 187, 188, 192, 193, 199, 224, 225, 235, 261, 266, 267, 288, 291

11th Casualty Clearing Station (BCCS), 11, 62, 69, 72, 77, 78, 81, 115, 118, 119, 121, 123, 124, 127, 128, 129, 133, 134, 136, 137, 139, 212, 215, 265, 299, 300

13th Casualty Clearing Station, 91, 194, 202, 224, 240, 241, 288

14th Casualty Clearing Station, 200, 201, 204, 256, 263, 294, 295, 296

16th Casualty Clearing Station, 91, 201, 240, 241, 288, 321

24th Casualty Clearing Station, 326

26th Casualty Clearing Station, 200, 201, 202, 205, 293, 294

52nd Casualty Clearing Station, 176, 177, 321, 326

53rd Casualty Clearing Station, 200, 201, 205, 244, 256, 294

54th Casualty Clearing Station, 262, 263

Indian Clearing Hospital, 44

Hospitals
Stationary
1st Australian Stationary Hospital, 34, 58, 97, 167, 168, 201, 288, 291

1st Canadian Stationary Hospital, 40, 174, 175, 176, 177, 270. 271, 278, 279, 32

2nd Australian Stationary Hospital, 34, 97, 98, 102, 168, 170, 176, 270, 271, 272, 273, 274, 275, 307

3rd Canadian Stationary Hospital, 40, 174, 176, 177, 270, 271, 272, 273, 278, 280

5th Canadian Stationary Hospital, 40

10th Canadian Field Hospital, 39

15th Stationary Hospital, 62, 156, 167, 168, 268, 279, 280

16th Stationary Hospital, 98, 168, 278, 279, 280

18th Stationary Hospital, 174, 177, 270, 278, 279

19th Stationary Hospital, 177

No 1 New Zealand Stationary Hospital, 38

No 2 New Zealand Stationary Hospital, 54

General
Indian Bombay Presidency General Hospital, 42

No. 1 Australian General Hospital, 34, 48, 52, 53, 54, 105, 197, 239

No. 2 Australian General Hospital, 34, 52, 54, 93, 104, 105, 163, 164, 165, 197, 198, 239

No. 3 Australian General Hospital, 48, 170, 171, 172, 173, 174, 176, 270, 271, 274, 278

No. 4 Canadian General Hospital, 241

No. 5 Indian General Hospital, 42, 54

No. 8 Indian General Hospital, 42, 54

No. 15 General Hospital, 54, 197

No. 17 General Hospital, 54

No. 21 General Hospital, 21, 251

No. 27 General Hospital, 176, 177, 279, 280

Auxiliary
No 1 Australian Auxiliary Hospital, 48, 53

Malta Hospitals
Cottonera Military Hospital, 55, 56, 57

Imtarfa Military Hospital, 55

Forrest Hospital, 56, 57

Valletta (Old) Military Hospital, 55, 57

Fort Chambray Convalescent Hospital, 55

Nursing Corps
New South Wales Army Nursing Service, 35
South Australian Transvaal Nurses, 35
Australian Army Nursing Corps (AANS), 33, 34,36, 53, 69, 80, 84, 85, 93, 96, 106, 153, 195, 225, 252, 27, 273, 274, 275
Canadian Army Nursing Sisters, 40, 176, 228, 270, 272
French Flag Nursing Corps, 45
New Zealand Army Nursing Service, 37
New Zealand Medical Corps Nursing Service, 37, 38
Princess Christian's Army Nursing Service (PCANS), 31
Princess Christian's Army Nursing Service Reserve (PCANSR), 34, 35, 37
Queen Alexandra's Imperial Military Nursing Service (QAIMNS), 31, 36, 37, 51, 52, 55, 56, 80, 153, 195, 197, 225, 252
Queen Alexandra's Imperial Military Nursing Service Reserve (QAIMNSR), 31, 31, 36, 252
Queens Alexandra's Royal Navy Nursing Service (QARNNS), 31, 245
Queens Alexandra's Royal Navy Nursing Service (QARNNSR), 31, 248
Territorial Force Nursing Service (TFNS), 31
Territorial Force Nursing Service Reserve (TFNSR), 31

Sanitary Sections
18th Sanitary Section, 249
21st Sanitary Section, 288
24th Sanitary Section, 288
Royal Navy
Royal Navy, 31, 50, 56, 60, 62, 66, 74, 113, 118, 127, 174, 245, 248, 275, 305, 306

Warships
HMS *Agamemnon*, 275
HMS *Clacton*, 70, 152
HMS *Cornwallis*, 174, 275
HMS *Endymion*, 204
HMS *Euryalus*, 76
HMS *Hythe*, 70
HMS *Implacable*, 76, 83
HMS *Majestic*, 155
HMS *Newmarket*, 70
HMS *Redbreast* 182, 193, 292

HMS *Ribble* 93
HMS *Talbot*, 127
HMA *Queen Elizabeth*, 64, 88
Bretagne (French Battleship) 137

Fleet Sweepers, 46, 47, 70, 74, 78, 118, 120, 130, 139, 152, 155, 179, 180, 182, 193, 224, 245

Transports
HMT *Ajax*, 116, 118
HMT *Arcadian*, 64
HMT *Aragon*, 63
HMT *Caledonia.* 63
HMT *City of Benares*, 102
HMT *Clan MacGillivray*, 98
HMT *Derflinger*, 63, 170
HMT *Dongola*, 167
HMT *Franconia*, 163
HMT *Hindoo*, 64, 66, 98, 168, 307
HMT *Huntsgreen*, 170, 206
HMT *Ionian* 98
HMT *Ivernian*, 142
HMT *Lutzow*, 63 98
HMT *Marquette*, 38, 72, 80, 176
HMT *Mooltan*, 170
HMT *Rowan*, 296
HMT *Royal Edward*, 122
HMT *Seang Bee*, 63
HMT *Seang Choon*, 98
HMT *Simla*, 170
HMT *Southland*, 63, 117 226, 227
HMT *Themistocles*, 170

SS *Abassiah (Abbassiyeh)*, 140, 289
SS *Alvania*, 202
SS *Ausonia*, 169
SS *Carron*, 202
SS *Ceylan*, 86
SS *Euripides*, 202
SS *Georgian*, 202
SS *Hunsgate*, 202
SS *Japanese Prince*, 116
SS *Karroo*, 169
SS *La Savoie* (French), 86
SS *Minnetonka*, 177
SS *Melville*, 202
SS *Stetonian*, 202
SS *Wiltshire* 202, 206

342   The Fight for Life

SS *Transylvania*, 202
SS *Umsinga*, 177
SS *Vinh Long* (French), 86
Black Ships, 69, 70, 84, 100, 102, 106, 107, 114, 144, 155, 162, 168, 199, 226, 304, 307, 308, 310

Hospital Ships
HS *Aquitania*, 251, 278
HS *Ascania,* 136
HS *Asturias*, 174
HS *Assaye*, 182, 226, 251, 252, 273
HS *Carisbrooke Castle*, 241
HS *Charles Roux*, (French) 89
HS *Devanha,* 98, 102, 195, 196
HS *Dongola*, 139, 291
HS *Duguay-Trouin*, (French) 89
HS *Dunluce Castle*, 112, 116, 171

HS *Formosa, 169*
HS *Galeka*, 216
HS *Gascon*, 60, 63, 65, 69, 96, 95, 96, 97, 100, 102, 103, 105, 111, 143, 152, 165, 182, 193, 195, 197, 225, 226
HS *Gloucester Castle*, 102, 163
HS *Guildford Castle*, 69, 97, 120
HS *Grantully Castle*, 80, 154
HS *Letitia,* 57
HS *Maheno*, 224
HS *Mauretania*, 200, 269, 278
HS *Neuralia*, 140, 227
HS *Rewa* 66, 245, 247, 248, 249, 251, 254
HS *Seang Choon*, 98, 140, 181, 192, 193, 276
HS *Sicilia*, 60, 63, 69, 75, 78, 79, 80, 84, 152, 153, 154, 181, 192, 213
HS *Somali*, 237
HS *Soudan*, 66, 84, 182, 245